W0050580

Current Topics in Pathology
90

Managing Editors

C.L. Berry   E. Grundmann

Editorial Board

W. Böcker, H. Cottier, P.J. Dawson, H. Denk
C.M. Fenoglio-Preiser, P.U. Heitz, O.H. Iversen
U. Löhrs, F. Nogales, U. Pfeifer, N. Sasano
G. Seifert, J.C.E. Underwood, Y. Watanabe

Springer

Berlin
Heidelberg
New York
Barcelona
Budapest
Hong Kong
London
Milan
Paris
Santa Clara
Singapore
Tokyo

Gerhard Seifert (Ed.)

Oral Pathology

Actual Diagnostic and Prognostic Aspects

Contributors
A. Burkhardt, J.K. Field, N.W. Johnson
R.C.K. Jordan, P.A. Reichart, A.G.M. Scholes
C. Scully, P.J. Slootweg, P.M. Speight
K.A.A.S. Warnakulasuriya, D.M. Williams

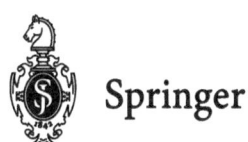 Springer

GERHARD SEIFERT, Prof. Dr. med.
Institute of Pathology
University of Hamburg
Martinistr. 52 UKE
20246 Hamburg, Germany

With 44 Figures, Some in Colour, and 16 Tables

ISBN-13:978-3-642-80171-6   e-ISBN-13:978-3-642-80169-3
DOI: 10.1007/978-3-642-80169-3

Library of Congress Cataloging-In-Publication Data. Oral pathology: actual diagnostic and prognostic aspects/Gerhard Seifert, ed.; contributors, A. Burkhardt ... [et al.].   p.   cm. – (Current topics in pathology;v.90)Includes bibliographical references and index.ISBN-13:978-3-642-80171-6(ha rdcover)1. Mouth – Pathophysiology. I. Seifert. Gerhard, 1921–**. II. Burkhardt, Anne. III. Series. [DNLM: 1. Mouth Diseases – diagnosis. 2. Mouth – pathology. 3. Mouth – virology. 4. Head and Neck Neoplasms – genetics. 5. Oral Manifestations. W1 CU821H v. 90 1996/WU 140 0628 1996] RB1. E6 vol. 90 [RC815] 616.07 s – dc20 [616.3'107] DNLM/DLC for Library of Congress 96-18025

This work is subject to copyright. All rights are reserved, whether the whole or part of the material is concerned, specifically the rights of translation, reprinting, reuse of illustrations, recitation, broadcasting, reproduction on microfilm or in any other way, and storage in data banks. Duplication of this publication or parts thereof is permitted only under the provisions of the German Copyright Law of September 9, 1965, in its current version, and permission for use must always be obtained from Springer-Verlag. Violations are liable for prosecution under the German Copyright Law.

© Springer-Verlag Berlin Heidelberg 1996
Softcover reprint of the hardcover 1st edition 1996

The use of general descriptive names, registered names, trademarks, etc. in this publication does not imply, even in the absence of a specific statement, that such names are exempt from the relevant protective laws and regulations and therefore free for general use.

Product liability: The publishers cannot guarantee the accuracy of any information about dosage and application contained in this book. In every individual case the user must check such information by consulting the relevant literature.

Cover design: Design & Production, Heidelberg

Typesetting: Best-set Typesetter Ltd., Hong Kong

SPIN: 10523903   25/3134/SPS – 5 4 3 2 1 0 – Printed on acid-free paper

List of Contributors

BURKHARDT, A., Prof. Dr. Pathologisches Institut
Kreiskrankenhaus Reutlingen
Steinenbergstr. 31
72764 Reutlingen, Germany

FIELD, J.K., MA PhD, Molecular Genetics and Oncology Group
BDS, MRCPath Department of Clinical Dental Sciences
School of Dentistry
The University of Liverpool
Liverpool L69 3BX, England

JOHNSON, N.W., Prof. Dr. Royal College of Surgeons
Department of Dental Sciences/
Department of Oral Medicine and
Pathology
King's College
School of Medicine and Dentistry
Caldecot Road
London SE5 9RW, England

JORDAN, R.C.K., Department of Dentistry
DDS, Diplo O Path, MSc, Sunnybrook Health Sciences Centre
PhD, FRCD(C) University of Toronto
2075 Bayview Avenue
Toronto, Ontario M4N 3M5, Canada

REICHART, P.A., Prof. Dr. Abteilung für Oralchirurgie
und Zahnärztliche Röntgenologie
Universitätsklinikum Charité
Medizinische Fakultät der
Humboldt-Universität zu Berlin
Zentrum für Zahnmedizin,
Föhrerstr. 15
13353 Berlin, Germany

SCHOLES, A.G.M., Dr.   Molecular Genetics and Oncology Group
                               Department of Clinical Dental Sciences
                               School of Dentistry
                               The University of Liverpool
                               Liverpool L69 3BX, England

SCULLY, C.,   Eastman Dental Institute for
Prof. Dr., MD, PhD, MDS,   Oral HealthCare Sciences
FDSRCPS, FFDRCSI,   University of London
FDSRCS, FRCPath   256 Gray's Inn Road
                               London WC1X 8LD, England

SLOOTWEG, P.J., Prof. Dr.   Department of Pathology, H 04.312
                               University Hospital
                               3508 GA Utrecht, The Netherlands

SPEIGHT, P.M.,   Department of Oral Pathology
BDS, PhD, FDSRCPS,   Eastman Dental Institute for Oral
MRCPath   Health Care Sciences
                               256 Gray's Inn Road
                               London WC1X 8LD, England

WARNAKULASURIYA,   Royal College of Surgeons
K.A.A.S.,   Department of Dental Sciences/
BDS, PhD, FDSRCS   Department of Oral Medicine and
                               Pathology
                               King's College
                               School of Medicine and Dentistry
                               Caldecot Road
                               London SE5 9RW, England

WILLIAMS, D.M.,   Department of Oral Pathology
BDS, MSc, PhD, FRCPath,   Faculty of Clinical Dentistry
FDSRCS   St. Bartholomew's and
                               The Royal London
                               School of Medicine
                               and Dentistry
                               Turner Street
                               London E1 2AD, England

Preface

Oral pathology is a field of pathology which is well established in the United States, in Japan and, within Europe, in the United Kingdom and Scandinavia. In these countries, oral pathology is practised in institutes and departments of oral pathology which are mostly integrated in a special faculty of dentistry, a dental school or a dental institute. In many other countries, oral pathology is integrated as a special field in institutes of general pathology and as part of a faculty of medicine. These different patterns have led to the different development of science and practice in this area. The scientific expansion of oral pathology is documented by the foundation of new scientific societies of oral pathology, such as the International Association of Oral Pathologists (IAOP), and new journals, such as the *Journal of Oral Pathology and Medicine*, *Oral Oncology* (as Part B of the *European Journal of Cancer*) and *Oral Diseases*. Recently, oral pathology has also been recognised as a part of head and neck pathology, an interdisciplinary field of science. Many new methods have been integrated into the scientific work and diagnostic repertoire of oral pathology.

In this volume, a comprehensive review of the importance of new methods in the diagnosis and prognosis of non-malignant disease and malignant tumours in this area is provided. Eight reputed specialists of oral pathology give a concise survey concerning new aspects of diseases of the oral mucosa. The oral mucosa is not only the point of attack in local injuries, but also reflects many systemic diseases of the organism. It is therefore a valuable indicator of diagnosis and prognosis of various pathological processes.

The chapter by D.M. WILLIAMS deals with mucocutaneous conditions affecting the mouth. Most of these diseases are either auto-immune or immunologically mediated. This chapter will review the advances in the understanding of their aetiology and suggests an approach to systematic diagnosis.

The chapter by C. SCULLY gives a survey of the great number and the diversity of oral viral diseases. The past decade has seen intense and increasing interest in the oral health care consequences of viral infection, particularly the possible relationships between viruses and oral diseases, such as malignant neoplasms, the possible infectivity of saliva and oral secretions and, more recently, the oral consequences of infection with the human immunodeficiency viruses (HIV).

The third chapter is a supplement to the previous one and reviews the numerous connections between oral mucosa, acquired immunodeficiency syndrome (AIDS) and oro-facial Kaposi's sarcoma. The diagnostic criteria for both the clinical and histopathological aspects are considered to be of particular importance.

The fourth chapter concerns the new concept of extranodal non-Hodgkin's lymphomas (NHL) of the oral cavity. The head and neck area is the second most common site of extranodal NHL after the gastro-intestinal tract. The importance of identifying the subtle histological features of each, coupled with immunological and molecular biological studies of biopsy tissues, has been discussed.

The fifth chapter focuses on the importance of proliferation markers in oral pathology as indicators of the clinical aggressiveness of human neoplasms. The value of the different methods and their clinical application in the diagnosis and prognosis of oral lesions are compared.

The sixth chapter analyses the special role of the suppressor protein p53 and its occurrence in oral tumours. This contribution focuses on the occurrence of p53 alterations in oral tumours and their significance as well as on the various means currently available for analysis of the p53 gene.

The seventh chapter gives new insights into genomic instability in head and neck cancer. In this chaper, potentially important chromosome regions identified by cytogenetic and loss of heterozygosity analysis in squamous cell carcinomas of the head and neck are reviewed.

The eighth chapter rounds off the volume with a contribution about oncogenes and growth factor receptors as diagnostic and prognostic markers in precancers and cancers of the oral mucosa.

In all the chapters, the most recent methods of immunocytochemistry, in situ hybridisation techniques and molecular pathology are integrated in the classification of the different types of precancerous lesions and cancers, and their value in diagnosis and prognosis is discussed. This volume is an important source of information about new scientific results in the field of oral medicine and pathology. Illustrations, tables and references to the most important literature make this volume a valuable publication for all readers interested in the field of oral medicine.

The editor would like to thank all the authors for their excellent cooperation in completing their manuscripts accurately and carefully; thanks are also due to Mrs. STEPHANIE BENKO of Springer-Verlag, Heidelberg, for her continued support during the planning, preparation and completion of this volume in the present version and to Mrs. MONIKA SCHACHT for her excellent work in the extensive correspondence with the authors and the publisher.

Hamburg, May 1996   GERHARD SEIFERT

Contents

Mucocutaneous Conditions Affecting the Mouth

D.M. WILLIAMS

1 Introduction

Diseases affecting the oral mucosa are divisible into neoplasms and conditions which are either auto-immune or immunologically mediated. This chapter is prin-

Current Topics in Pathology
Volume 90, G. Seifert (Ed.)
© Springer-Verlag Berlin Heidelberg 1996

cipally concerned with those which have an immunological basis, including pemphigus vulgaris, mucous membrane pemphigoid (MMP), linear immunoglobulin A (IgA) bullous dermatosis (LABD), dermatitis herpetiformis, epidermolysis bullosa (EB), erythema multiforme and lichen planus. These may all appear as vesicles, bullae, ulcers and erosions which, in addition to affecting the mouth, may also involve the skin, eyes and other mucosal sites. Accurate diagnosis is often not possible from oral presentation alone, and even systematic clinical evaluation may fail to yield a definitive diagnosis. However, recent advances in understanding the aetiology of a number of these diseases has now made specific, accurate diagnosis possible. Major advances have been made in understanding pemphigus, pemphigoid and the diseases which make up the EB group. This chapter will review the advances in understanding their aetiology and suggest an approach to systematic diagnosis.

2 Pemphigus Vulgaris

Pemphigus presents in two main forms: pemphigus vulgaris, which is characterised by low-level intra-epithelial bulla formation, and pemphigus foliaceus, in which epithelial separation occurs at a higher level. Pemphigus vulgaris is far more common in the mouth than pemphigus foliaceus.

2.1 Epidemiology

Incidence rates for all forms of pemphigus range between 0.5 and 3.2 per 100000 per annum, affecting both sexes with equal frequency (KORMAN 1988). It occurs principally in the fifth and sixth decades, although cases have been recorded in children (AHMED et al. 1980) and adolescents (AHMED 1983). There is a strong genetic predisposition, and the highest frequency is seen in Ashkenazi Jews (PISANTI et al. 1974).

2.2 Oral Manifestations

Pemphigus affects the mouth in up to 70% of cases (KORMAN 1988), and it is the only site to be affected in over 50% of patients (AHMED and SALM 1983). Vesicles in the mouth (Fig. 1) rupture extremely early (CORRELL and SCHOTT 1985), and patients usually present with one or two painful areas of ulceration. Lesions do not heal, leading to extensive oral ulceration (AHMED et al. 1980). The sites most commonly affected are palate, buccal mucosa and gingivae (ZEGARELLI and ZEGARELLI 1977), and lesions may extend directly to the oesophagus (RAQUE et al. 1970), pharynx (ZEGARELLI and ZEGARELLI 1977) and larynx (AHMED et al. 1980).

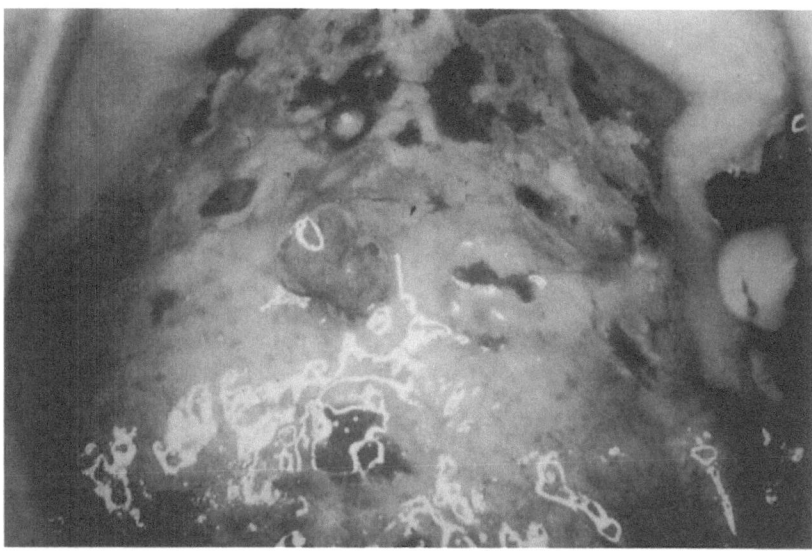

Fig. 1. Oral lesions in pemphigus vulgaris. An intact blister on the palate can be seen in the centre, surrounded by areas of ulceration which show no tendency to heal

2.3 Skin Lesions

The typical skin lesions in pemphigus vulgaris are fluid-filled blisters which rupture, resulting in areas of denudation. In severe disease, patients may develop electrolyte loss due to the extent of the lesions, together with wound infections, causing management problems. Ocular lesions in pemphigus are usually of minor significance, consisting of a mild, transient conjunctivitis which heals without scarring.

2.4 Histopathological Features

Histological examination with immunofluorescence (IF) (BEUTNER and JORDAN 1964; BEUTNER et al. 1965) is crucial in the diagnosis of pemphigus vulgaris. Acantholysis, with separation low in the stratum spinosum, is the diagnostic characteristic of the disease, and this is usually preceded by intercellular oedema and loss of intercellular contacts in the immediately suprabasal cell layers. As separation progresses, bulla formation occurs (Fig. 2a,b), and groups of rounded acantholytic cells, with uniformly hyperchromatic nuclei and homogeneous eosinophilic cytoplasm, are seen floating within the blister fluid. The basal cells remain attached to the basement membrane until the blister ruptures, but secondary inflammation then obscures the diagnostic features. Auto-antibodies directed against an antigen on the surface of stratified squamous epithelial cells are found

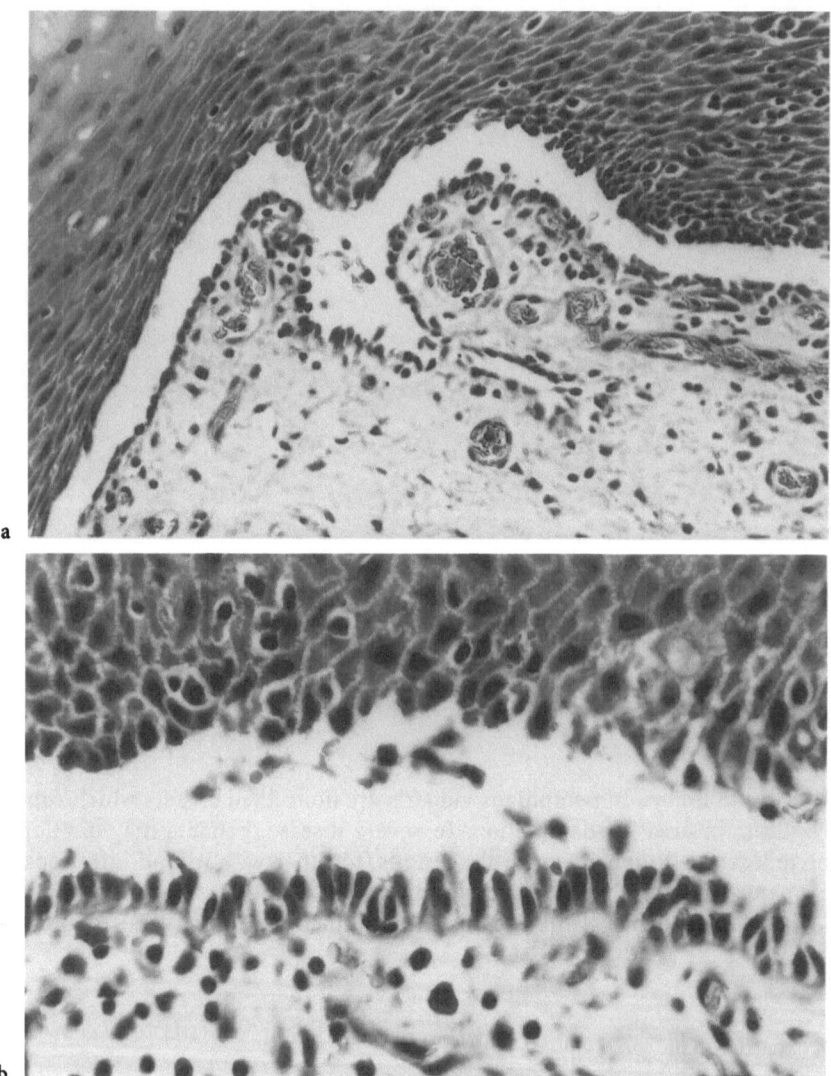

a

b

Fig. 2. a Medium-power photomicrograph showing the classical features of pemphigus vulgaris. Extensive suprabasal separation has occurred within the epithelium, leaving an intact basal cell layer in the floor of the bulla. There is a striking absence of inflammation in the underlying connective tissue. **b** High-power view of the separation zone in pemphigus vulgaris. The basal cell layer is intact, with separation in the immediate suprabasal layer. Darkly staining acantholytic cells are present, free within the bulla in the centre of the field. The cells in the roof of the bulla also show early features of acantholysis. Their cytoplasm is somewhat shrunken, and there is evidence of intercellular oedema

in pemphigus (Fig. 3), and their presence is the most reliable diagnostic test for the disease. Patients with active disease generally have circulating auto-antibodies, and titres tend to reflect the severity of the disease (Fitzpatrick and Newcomer 1980; Cresswell et al. 1981).

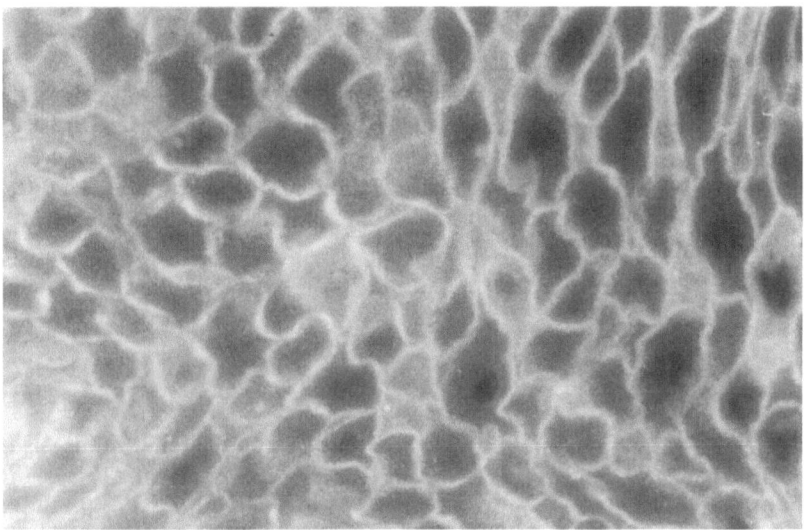

Fig. 3. Direct immunofluorescence in pemphigus vulgaris. Binding of autoantibodies to the antigen located in the cell membrane of keratinocytes has produced the fishnet appearance which is diagnostic of pemphigus

2.5 Pathogenesis

Recent studies have focused on the molecular basis of normal cell–cell interaction in epithelium and on understanding how interference with this leads to intra-epithelial blister formation. Pemphigus foliaceus is associated with the presence of circulating auto-antibodies to desmoglein-1 (HASHIMOTO et al. 1990; CALVANICO et al. 1991), a transmembrane E cadherin present in all desmosomes. The cadherins are crucial in mediating cell–cell contact, which takes place through their calcium-dependent homophilic interaction (TAKEICHI 1991). The pemphigus vulgaris antigen (PVA) now appears to be the E cadherin desmoglein-3 (AMAGAI et al. 1994), which shows significant homology with desmoglein-1 (AMAGAI et al. 1991). The latter is probably a constant core component of all desmosomes (KOCH et al. 1992), whereas PVA seems to be a site-specific desmoglein (AMAGAI et al. 1991). The different localisation of the site of intra-epithelial blistering and the minor antigenic differences in these two closely related variants of pemphigus reflect heterogeneity in desmosomal structure (KOCH et al. 1992) in relation to both site (IOANNIDES et al. 1991) and stage of differentiation. The production of antibodies against epithelial cadherins interferes with their function as attachment proteins, and the specificity of the auto-antibody then determines the site at which blister formation begins. Once blistering has been initiated, complement- and protease-dependent mechanisms may lead to propagation of the blisters (WILLIAMS 1989).

2.6 Treatment

The first line of treatment in pemphigus vulgaris is oral prednisolone at a dose of 150 mg per day (LEVENE 1982), although this dose is increased in severe disease (EYRE and STANLEY 1987). Response to treatment is usually rapid and, once the development of new lesions has ceased, medication can be sharply reduced. In some cases, it may be possible to withdraw active treatment, but otherwise low-dose maintenance therapy is indicated.

3 Mucous Membrane Pemphigoid

The two principal forms of pemphigoid are bullous pemphigoid and MMP, also called cicatricial pemphigoid. Whilst bullous pemphigoid is essentially a skin disease, MMP mainly affects the oral and genital mucosa and the eyes, with only minor skin involvement. Discrimination between these two diseases on clinical grounds may be difficult, but it is now apparent that there are antigenic differences between them, and this should lead to precise diagnosis in the future.

3.1 Epidemiology and Oral Manifestations

The mean age of onset of pemphigoid is 60 years (BEAN 1974; SILVERMAN et al. 1986; VENNING et al. 1988), with symptoms having a mean duration of 3–5 years (VENNING et al. 1988; SILVERMAN et al. 1986). The gingivae are affected in almost all patients (AHMED and HOMBAL 1986; SILVERMAN et al. 1986), and the buccal mucosa and palate are involved in between one quarter and one third of patients, with several sites often affected at the same time. MMP typically presents with bullae (Fig. 4), which appear rapidly and then rupture, producing ulcers which heal slowly. Although MMP is often referred to as cicatricial pemphigoid, scarring is not usually a marked feature of oral involvement. MMP is one of the principal causes of desquamative gingivitis (Fig. 5), characterised by the presence of erythematous, shiny lesions confined to tooth-bearing areas (FINE and WEATHERS 1980). Desquamative gingivitis also occurs in lichen planus, pemphigus vulgaris and psoriasis (LASKARIS et al. 1981; PENG et al. 1986), so that further clinical or laboratory investigation is necessary to establish a definitive diagnosis.

3.2 Skin and Ocular Lesions

Skin lesions have been reported in up to a third of patients with MMP, and these affect the face, neck and scalp (PERSON and ROGERS 1977; AHMED and HOMBAL 1986). However, it is ocular involvement which gives rise to the major problems in

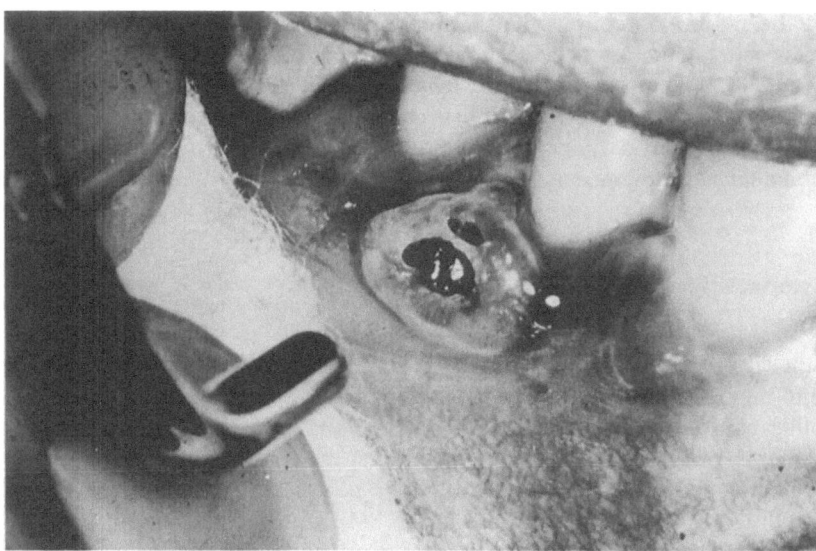

Fig. 4. A recently ruptured intra-oral blister in a patient with mucous membrane pemphigoid. A jet of air directed at the lesion has reinflated it

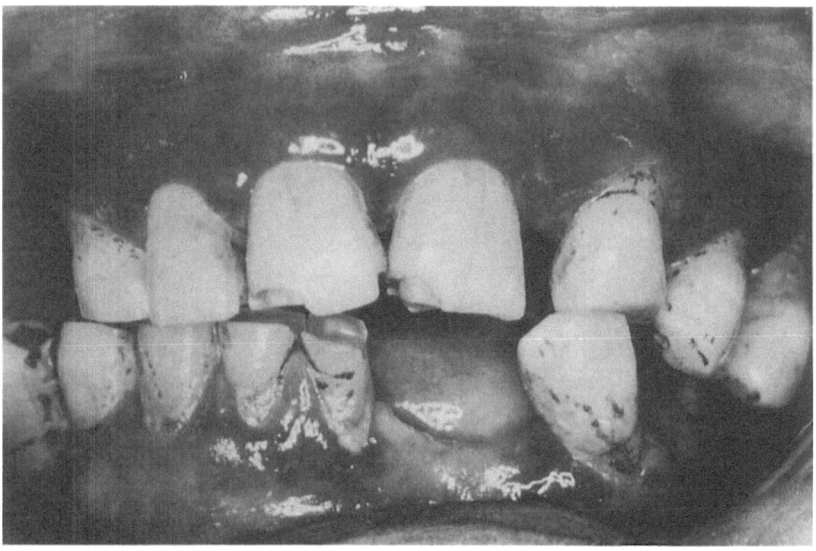

Fig. 5. Desquamative gingivitis in a patient with mucous membrane pemphigoid. Bright erythema of the gingivae is seen, confined to tooth-bearing areas. These features are particularly marked in the upper jaw, and the gingivae appear normal in the edentulous lower incisor region

MMP. Patients develop conjunctivitis which progresses to acute ulceration, and blindness occurs in the most severe cases (PERSON and ROGERS 1977; AHMED and HOMBAL 1986). Asymptomatic ocular signs have been detected in a high proportion of patients with oral MMP (WILLIAMS et al. 1984), and it is recommended that all patients diagnosed as having MMP should receive a thorough, competent, ophthalmological examination.

3.3 Histopathological Features

Subepithelial blister formation (Fig. 6) is characteristic of MMP, but it is not unique to the disease. Both bullous pemphigoid and MMP can be discriminated from other clinically similar conditions on the basis of direct IF, which reveals linear binding of Ig to the basement membrane zone (BMZ) at the site of the earliest pathological changes (Fig. 7). Bullous pemphigoid is characterised by linear binding of IgG, usually with C3, to the BMZ, and the majority of patients have circulating anti-BMZ IgG, although antibody titres do not reflect disease severity (IMBER et al. 1987).

In MMP, linear BMZ binding of Ig to the oral mucosa and conjunctiva is seen (PERSON and ROGERS 1977; AHMED and HOMBAL 1986), but recent studies have reported significant frequency of both IgM and IgA deposition in addition to IgG and C3 (WILLIAMS et al. 1984). Attempts to detect circulating auto-antibodies in patients with MMP are usually disappointing using indirect IF, but

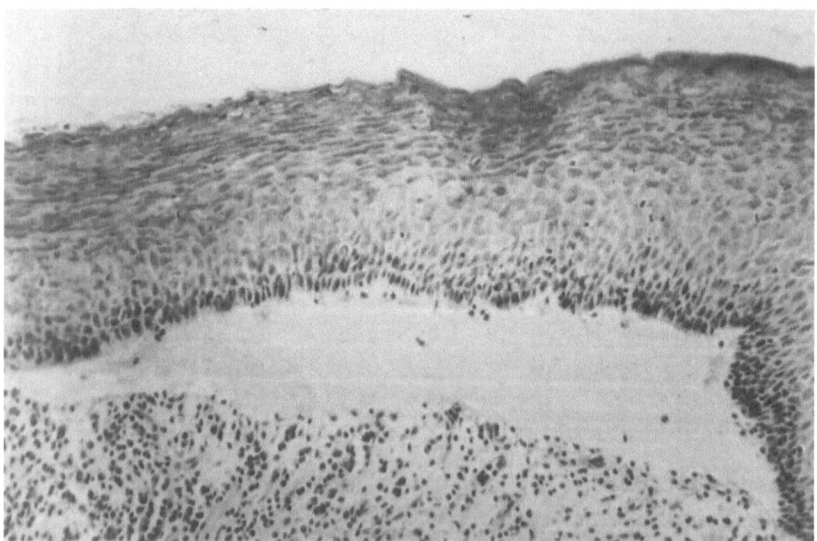

Fig. 6. Photomicrograph of an intact bulla in mucous membrane pemphigoid. The bulla is subepithelial in location, and the plane of separation in the basement membrane zone can be seen in the bottom right of the field

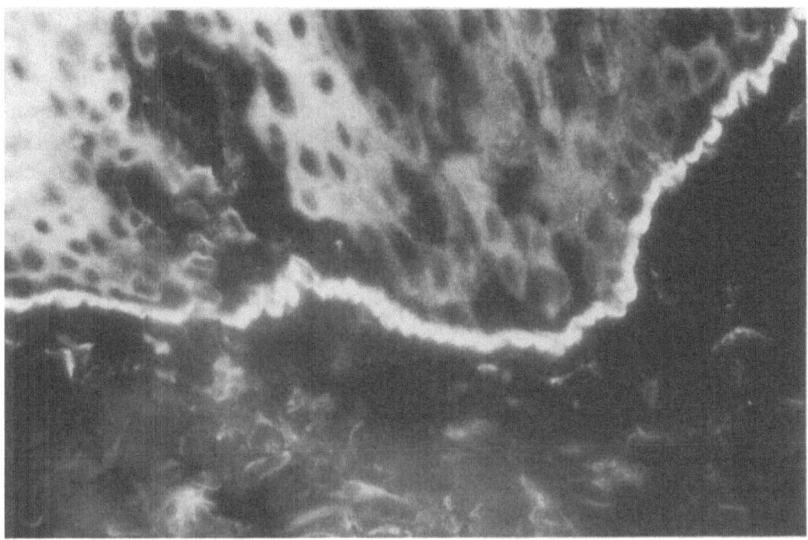

Fig. 7. Direct immunofluorescence in mucous membrane pemphigoid, showing bright, linear fluorescence in the basement membrane zone, indicating the site of autoantibody binding

immunoblotting and immunoprecipitation have been claimed to be more sensitive (BERNARD et al. 1990; MUTASIM et al. 1992).

Interestingly, direct IF performed on clinically normal skin from patients with MMP has revealed linear BMZ Ig deposition in up to 40% of patients (LEONARD et al. 1984). Whilst the pathological significance of these observations is uncertain, they may be a reflection of the overlap between MMP and other subepithelial bullous diseases. The presence of IgA in particular raises the possibility of overlap with linear IgA bullous dermatosis (WILLIAMS et al. 1984), and precise differentiation of these diseases will depend on identification of the antigen in each case.

3.4 Pathogenesis

Just as investigation of the pathogenesis of pemphigus has elucidated the mechanism of cell–cell contact in epithelium, so the study of pemphigoid has revealed the mechanism of epithelial attachment to the basement membrane. Two of the principal components of the basement membrane, which appears ultrastructurally as the lamina lucida and lamina densa, are laminin and type IV collagen (YURCHENCO et al. 1992). Attachment of this complex to the deeper connective tissue occurs by anchoring of the fibrils, which are mainly composed of type VII collagen that appears to be of epithelial origin (REGAUER et al. 1990). Anchorage of keratinocytes to the basal lamina is mediated via members of the integrin superfamily (RUOSLAHTI and PIERSCHBACHER 1987) which form stable anchoring complexes (SAC) and focal adhesions (FA). The former are composed of the $\alpha_6\beta_4$-heterodimer and are located at sites of hemidesmosome formation (CARTER et al. 1990a), where they are surrounded by a ring of FA, composed of $\alpha_3\beta_1$-integrin (CARTER et al. 1990b). The ligand for both of these integrins is thought to be an isoform of laminin, known as epiligrin (CARTER et al. 1991; DOMLOGE-HULTSCH et al. 1992), which appears ultrastructurally as the anchoring filaments which traverse the lamina lucida.

In bullous pemphigoid, patients have circulating antibodies against hemidesmosome-associated proteins of 230 and 180 kDa, known as bullous pemphigoid antigen-1 (BPAG1) and bullous pemphigoid antigen-2 (BPAG2), respectively (for a review, see WILLIAMS 1990). BPAG1 is located intracellularly and is involved in the linkage between the $\alpha_6\beta_4$-integrin and the intermediate filament system in hemidesmosomes (CARTER et al. 1990a). The antigen has been shown to have substantial sequence homology with desmoplakin (GIUDICE et al. 1992a), which is a component of desmosomes (KOCH et al. 1992). BPAG2, which has been sequenced and cloned (GIUDICE et al. 1992b; LI et al. 1992) and shown to be a 180-kDa hemidesmosome-associated protein (HOPKINSON et al. 1992), has a collagenous extracellular domain and is likely to be involved in cell–matrix interactions. As with antibody binding to desmoglein-3 in pemphigus vulgaris, it is probable that antibody binding with BPAG2 could lead to blister formation in bullous pemphigoid. Whether auto-antibody binding to BPAG1 also leads to blister formation is less clear.

Because patients with MMP generally lack circulating antibodies, precise identification of the antigen has been extremely difficult, although it has been recognised that it is different from the BP antigen (BERNARD et al. 1990, 1992). Indirect immunolectron microscopy has indicated that the MMP antigen is located extracellularly and is probably epiligrin, the key component of anchoring filaments (BEDANE et al. 1991; DOMLOGE-HULTSCH et al. 1992).

3.5 Treatment

Although there is no really effective management for MMP (AHMED and HOMBAL 1986), lesions appear to respond to topical steroids (LOZADA-NUR and SILVERMAN 1980). There are anecdotal reports of the use of sulphapyridine and dapsone is severe cases of MMP and in patients who are unresponsive to topical steroids (PERSON and ROGERS 1977; NISENGARD and ROGERS 1987), but there does not appear to have been a well-controlled study of the efficacy of this form of treatment.

4 Linear Immunoglobulin A Bullous Dermatosis

LABD is fundamentally a skin disease in which there is spontaneous formation of blisters associated with linear deposition of IgA in the BMZ (WILLIAMS et al. 1984).

Clinical features overlap substantially with those of MMP and dermatitis herpetiformis, with the result that definitive diagnosis depends on laboratory investigation.

Although histopathological examination reveals IgA deposition in the BMZ, this may also be found in MMP, and the antigen against which the antibodies are directed has not yet been identified. However, it appears to differ from that found in both MMP and EB acquisita (EBA) (WOJNAROWSKA et al. 1991), so diagnosis may be made by exclusion.

5 Dermatitis Herpetiformis

Although oral mucosal lesions have been described in up to 70% of patients with dermatitis herpetiformis (FRASER et al. 1973), these are not specific, and it is principally a skin disease, with an intensely itchy papulovesicular rash on a background of erythema.

Diagnosis depends on the demonstration of a gluten-sensitive enteropathy and granular deposition of IgA beneath the BMZ in clinically normal skin (FRY and SEAH 1974). The mechanism by which IgA becomes bound in the region of the BMZ and the antigen to which it binds are unknown. However, the disease has a strong genetic predisposition (KATZ and STROBER 1978).

Dermatitis herpetiformis is included here because it must be differentiated clinically from pemphigoid and related conditions and, on histological and IF grounds, from LABD and MMP.

6 Epidermolysis Bullosa

6.1 Clinical Features

EB is a disease complex comprising at least 20 hereditary and non-hereditary conditions (WRIGHT et al. 1993), all associated with epidermal and mucosal blistering of differing severity (see Table 1). The different forms of the disease are differentiated on the basis of the level at which blistering occurs. These develop within the epithelium in EB simplex, in the BMZ in junctional EB and below the BMZ in dystrophic EB and EBA. Skin and mucous membranes are the primary targets of this group of conditions, although other systems may be involved, and the skin is involved in all of them. The teeth are also affected in some forms of EB.

EB simplex is the most minor of the genetic forms of EB, and blisters generally heal without scarring. Dystrophic EB can occur in dominant and recessive forms and, although both are associated with scarring, this is most severe in the recessive form. Junctional EB may occur in mild and severe forms, and the latter is the most severe of all the forms of EB, due to the fact

Table 1. Classification of the hereditary types of epidermolysis bullosa (EB)

General EB type	Suptype	Mode of inheritance	Distribution of skin lesions	Scarring
Simplex	Localised (Weber-Cockayne)	AD	Palms/soles	Rare
Simplex	Generalised (Koebner)	AD	Principally extremities	Rare
Simplex	Herpetiformis (Dowling-Meara)	AD	Generalised	Variable
Simplex	Localised with hypodontia (Kallin)	AR	Hands and feet	Absent
Junctional	Generalised (Herlitz, Gravis)	AR	Generalised	Common
Junctional	Generalised (Mitis, non-Herlitz)	AR	Generalised	Common but focal
Junctional	Localised (minimus)	AR	Hands, feet, pretibial	Absent
Dystrophic	Generalised (Pasini, Cockayne-Touraine)	AD	Generalised	Common
Dystrophic	Localised (minimus)	AD	Acral	Absent
Dystrophic	Generalised (Gravis, Hallopeau-Siemens)	AR	Generalised	Common
Dystrophic	Generalised (mitis)	AR	Generalised	Present

After Wright et al. (1993).
AD, autosomal dominant; AR, autosomal recessive.

that the skin and mucosa become detached from the underlying connective tissue in response to the most minimal trauma. Patients seldom survive beyond the third year of life, with most dying shortly after birth because of overwhelming infections.

EBA is a very different condition from the other genetic diseases in this group. It is a pemphigoid-like disease associated with fragility and blistering of skin and mucosa. This presentation may give rise to confusion with both bullous pemphigoid and MMP on clinical grounds. Furthermore, the histological picture of BMZ separation and the IF appearance of linear IgG and C3 deposition in the BMZ also prevent clear differentiation from pemphigoid (Gammon et al. 1984).

6.2 Oral Involvement in Epidermolysis Bullosa

The extent of oral involvement in EB is variable, depending on the particular form of the disease (see Table 2). In the more minor forms of EB simplex, there may only be a few blisters or vesicles, which heal without scarring. Some degree of oral involvement seems to occur in all forms of junctional and dystrophic EB, but it is particularly associated with the more severe dystrophic forms of EB where it gives rise to major problems of management (Nowak 1988; Wright et al. 1993). The scarring which occurs on healing results in severe gingival retraction, shallowing

Table 2. Oral manifestations in inherited forms of epidermolysis bullosa (EB)

General EB type	Subtype	Erosions	Scarring	Ankylo-glossia	Micro-stomia	Dental defects
Simplex	Localised (Weber-Cockayne)	Occasional	Absent	Absent	Absent	Absent
Simplex	Generalised (Koebner)	Occasional	Absent	Absent	Absent	Absent
Simplex	Herpetiformis (Dowling-Meara)	Common	Absent	Absent	Absent	Absent
Simplex	Localised with hypodontia (Kallin)	Present?	Absent	Absent	Absent	Absent
Junctional	Generalised (Herlitz, Gravis)	Common	Mild/variable	Absent/mild	Moderate	Severe
Junctional	Generalised (mitis, non-Herlitz)	Common	Absent/mild	Absent/mild	Absent	Moderate
Junctional	Localised (minimus)	Common	Absent	Absent	Absent	Absent/mild
Dystrophic	Generalised (Cockayne-Touraine)	Mild/moderate	Absent	Absent	Absent	Absent
Dystrophic	Generalised (Gravis, Pasini, Hallopeau-Siemens)	Severe	Severe	Severe	Severe	Absent, except severe caries

After WRIGHT et al. (1993).

of the vestibule and partial or total tethering of the tongue to the floor of the mouth. Perioral scarring over a period of time causes microstomia, which is particularly severe in recessive dystrophic EB, although it may also occur in the Herlitz variant of junctional EB (WRIGHT et al. 1993).

Involvement of the teeth may be seen in EB, and hypoplastic enamel defects are seen in patients with all forms of junctional EB (WRIGHT et al. 1993), associated with a smooth amelo-dentinal junction. However, there is no consensus on the frequency and extent of dental involvement in all of the EB variants.

6.3 Pathogenesis

There have been major advances in understanding EB as a result of clarification of the molecular basis of cell–matrix interaction (UITTO and CHRISTIANO 1992). The Dowling-Meara variant of EB simplex results from structural abnormalities of the keratin filament system (ISHIDA-YAMAMOTO et al. 1991) associated with mutations in the keratin-5 (LANE et al. 1992) and keratin-14 (COULOMBE et al. 1991) genes. Severe recessive dystrophic EB is associated with failure to form normal type VII collagen, leading to abnormalities of the anchoring fibril system (LEIGH et al. 1988; BRUCKNER-TUDERMAN et al. 1989; IWASAKI et al. 1992). The aetiology of the lethal form of junctional EB has recently been clarified with the observation that epiligrin, which is associated with anchoring fibrils, is absent (DOMLOGE-

HULTSCH et al. 1992). It is important to recognise, as described in Sect. 3, that the antibodies in MMP are directed at the same protein as is absent in junctional EB.

Antibodies in EBA are directed against part of the type VII collagen molecule (WOODLEY et al. 1988), the same crucial matrix protein which is absent in hereditary dystrophic EB. Recent comparative IF studies using specific monoclonal antibodies and immunoblotting have shown that the antigen in EBA is probably one of the globular termini of type VII collagen (WOODLEY et al. 1988). Additionally, it has also been reported that expression of the hemidesmosome-associated $\alpha_6\beta_4$-integrin is normal in EBA, but is altered in bullous pemphigoid (MICHALAKI et al. 1992). The application of these results to modified diagnostic methods may lead to more reliable differentiation in the future.

7 Erythema Multiforme

Erythema multiforme is a mucocutaneous disease predominantly affecting young adults. The oral and skin manifestations vary both in severity and appearance. Attacks are usually of acute onset and may be isolated or recurrent. There are two principal forms of the disease, namely erythema multiforme minor, which is more common, and erythema multiforme major (BRICE et al. 1990). The latter is a bullous form of the disease, often termed Stevens-Johnson Syndrome, which is characterised by severe mucosal involvement. As its name implies, erythema multiforme minor is less severe, with relatively minor oral symptoms. It is becoming apparent that these two forms of the disease may be different conditions, with erythema multiforme minor being the more common.

7.1 Oral Manifestations

It has been reported that approximately 25% of patients with typical erythema multiforme minor have oral lesions (BRICE et al. 1990), although our own observations indicate that they are significantly more common (FARTHING et al. 1995). The tongue, buccal mucosa and lips are the most commonly affected oral sites (LOZADA-NUR et al. 1989), but gingival involvement is also seen. Patients typically present with lesions that are rather non-specific discrete erosions (Fig. 8) with an erythematous margin, although gingival lesions may be more extensive and confluent.

The mouth is usually involved in Stevens-Johnson syndrome, or erythema multiforme major, which is characterised by severe involvement of at least two mucosal sites (BRICE et al. 1990). In classical cases, large, fluid-filled blisters develop rapidly on the lips (Fig. 9), but these usually burst within a day (Fig. 10) to produce crusted lesions which can persist for up to 4 weeks. In the case of severe oral involvement, eating can prove extemely uncomfortable and difficult, and patients may require hospitalisation for supportive therapy.

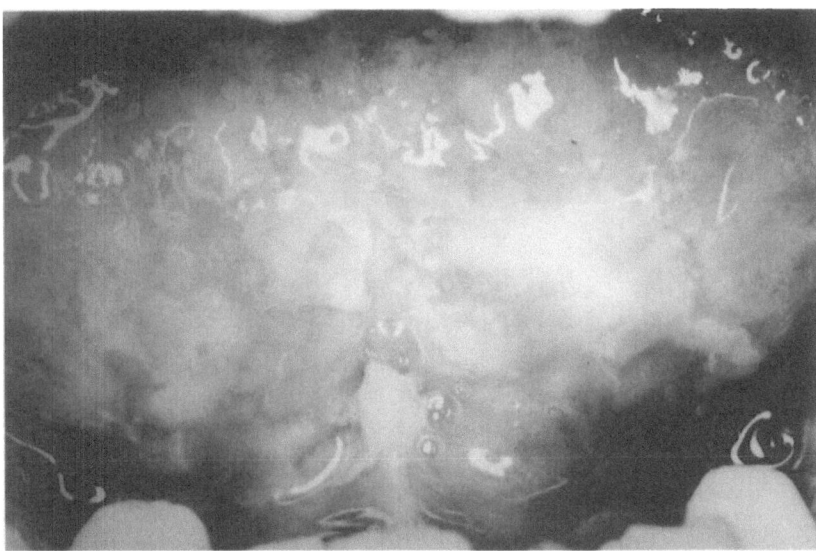

Fig. 8. Lesions of erythema multiforme on the ventral surface of the tongue. These comprise extensive, non-specific, sloughing erosions. The appearances seen here are not sufficiently characteristic to permit diagnosis without further clinical information

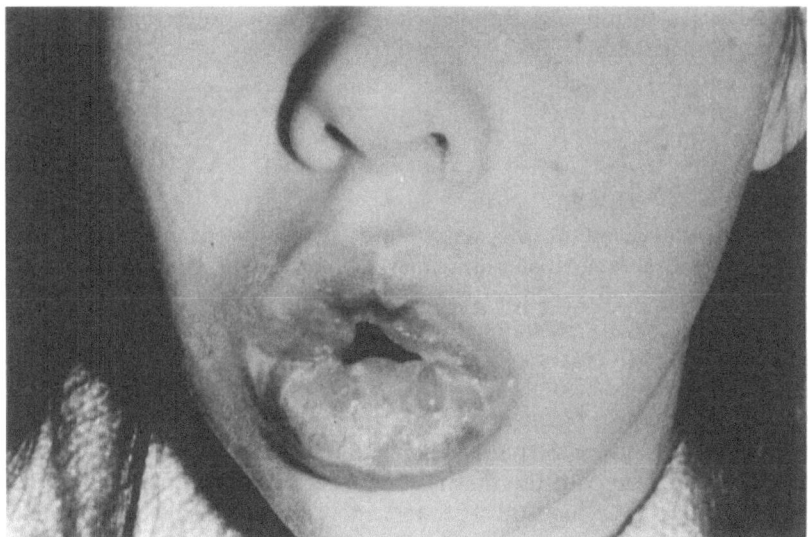

Fig. 9. Large fluid-filled blisters on the lips of a 10-year-old girl with Stevens-Johnson syndrome. The blisters do not extend beyond the vermilion border of the lips

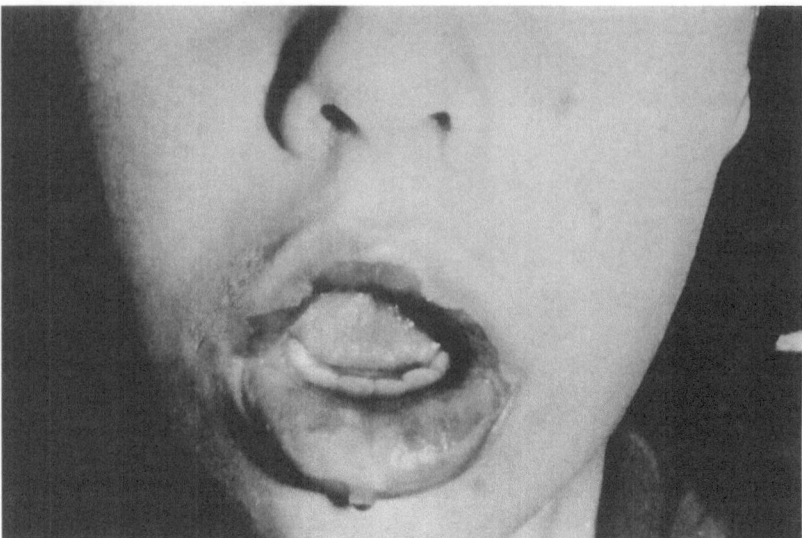

Fig. 10. The same patient as in Fig. 9, 24h later; the blisters have burst, leaving extensive areas of ulceration which subsequently became encrusted

Important insights into the aetiology of erythema multiforme have come from the observation that, although it can occur as a single attack, it is recurrent and has a strong association with herpes simplex virus (HSV) infections, episodes often being preceded by herpes labialis.

7.2 Skin Lesions

The onset of erythema multiforme may be preceded by prodromal symptoms, which tend to be more frequent and more marked in erythema multiforme major. Patients who experience frequent recurrences often report discomfort at the site where lesions subsequently develop approximately 24h before the appearance of physical signs (D.M. WILLIAMS and I.M. LEIGH, unpublished observation). The cutaneous characteristics of both erythema multiforme major and minor have been reviewed by BRICE et al. (1990). Erythematous macules which expand, giving rise to typical "iris" or "target" lesions, with a central dusky zone surrounded by an erythematous outer zone, are the first lesions to appear in both forms of the condition. In some sites, blood-filled blisters may develop in the central area. Individual lesions subsequently expand and merge to produce extensive, irregularly shaped areas. Lesions are often bilaterally symmetrical, affecting the hands, feet, arms and legs, but the basis of this pattern of distribution is unknown.

The lesions of erythema multiforme minor generally heal within 3 weeks, although some patients with continuously recurrent erythema multiforme develop new lesions before those from a previous episode have healed. Both the oral and cutaneous lesions of erythema multiforme major tend to be more extensive and long-lasting than in the minor form of the condition.

7.3 Histopathological Features

Virtually all studies on the histopathological features of erythema multiforme are based on biopsies of established clinical lesions, and the earliest stages in the process have gone largely unreported. However, if patients with recurrent erythema multiforme are biopsied in the prodromal phase, before there is clinical evidence of a lesion, distinctive histological changes can be seen (D.M. WILLIAMS, I.M. LEIGH and P.M. FARTHING, unpublished observations), which point to the conclusion that the keratinocyte is the initial target for cell-mediated immunological damage (MARGOLIS et al. 1983; ZAIM et al. 1987).

We have observed that Langerhans cells migrate from their customary suprabasal position in the epithelium to the upper cell layers, associated with a reduction in the length of dendritic processes. This is accompanied by intercellular oedema within the epithelium and the accumulation of helper/inducer and suppressor/cytotoxic T cells in the epithelium and adjacent connective tissue. With the progressive increase in the lymphocytic infiltrate, keratinocyte damage becomes apparent, followed by necrosis of the epithelium and sloughing. It is at this relatively advanced stage of lesion development in histological terms that the lesion is evident clinically.

An additional feature of the established lesion, as the influx of inflammatory cells in and around the epithelium progresses, is marked perivascular lymphocyte accumulation. Given that most earlier studies were of well-developed lesions, it is not suprising that attention focused on the importance of a vasculitic process in the aetiology of erythema multiforme (TONNESON et al. 1983). Circulating immune complexes can be detected in a significant proportion of patients with recurrent erythema multiforme (LEIGH et al. 1985), and direct immunofluorescence often reveals complement activation in the walls of blood vessels in early lesions (D.M. WILLIAMS, unpublished observation). However, the significance of complement activation is unclear, and the perivascular accumulation of lymphocytes is not specific to erythema multiforme.

With the progression of lesion development, keratinocyte damage becomes marked, with the influx of a mixed inflammatory infiltrate containing significant numbers of polymorphonuclear leukocytes (PMN). This is accompanied by bulla formation and sloughing of the epithelium. By this stage, the histological features are non-specific, and diagnosis is made on the basis of the clinical features.

7.4 Pathogenesis

A large number of agents have been implicated in the etiology of erythema multiforme (for a review, see BRICE et al. 1990):

1. Herpes simplex virus
   a) Especially in recurrent erythema multiforme minor
   b) HLA-related susceptibility
2. Ultraviolet (UV) light – associated with HSV activation
3. Drugs – especially in erythema multiforme major
4. Foodstuffs
5. Unknown

Drugs have been particularly associated with the triggering of Stevens-Johnson syndrome (GEBEL and HORNSTEIN 1984), leading to the view that allergic mechanisms might be implicated in the pathogenesis of lesions. This conclusion was supported by the finding of circulating immune complexes and complement deposition in intralesional blood vessels, as described above. More recently, attention has shifted to the keratinocyte as the principal target in erythema multiforme, with increasing evidence for the role of HSV infection in the pathogenesis of lesions (BRICE et al. 1989; HUFF and WESTON 1989; ASLANZADEH et al. 1992; MIURA et al. 1992). HSV DNA has been identified both in the active (BRICE et al. 1989; ASLANZADEH 1992) and healed (MIURA et al. 1992) lesions of erythema multiforme in patients who develop recurrent disease following episodes of herpes labialis. The role of HSV DNA in lesion development is further supported by the observation that prophylactic acyclovir therapy can suppress recurrent erythema multiforme (MOLIN 1987). Whilst there is accumulating evidence that keratinocyte infection by HSV triggers the cycle of lymphocyte-mediated damage, as described above, the mechanism by which HSV DNA becomes localised to keratinocytes, and why this should lead to erythema multiforme, remains to be established. Interestingly, an increased likelihood of developing erythema multiforme following HSV infection has been noted in patients with HLA DQw3 (KAMPGEN et al. 1988), which raises the possibility that the linkage of the two conditions is related to genetic factors. This matter merits further investigation.

The pathogenic mechanisms involved in patients whose disease is triggered by drugs or certain foodstuffs (LEWIS et al. 1989) remains largely speculative.

7.5 Treatment

Recognition of the association between HSV infection and recurrent erythema multiforme minor has had a major impact on treatment of the condition. Treatment with acyclovir during the prodromal stage has led to attacks either being aborted or markedly reduced in severity. Prophylactic acyclovir therapy is indicated in patients with severe or continuous recurrent erythema multiforme, and in particularly intractable cases azathioprine may also be required to supplement antiviral treatment (FARTHING et al. 1995). Symptomatic supportive treatment, including mouthwashes for mucosal involvement, may be indicated. The treatment of erythema multiforme can be summarised as follows:

- Acyclovir, supplemented with azathioprine in severe cases
- Supportive therapy
- Mouthwashes
- Prevention (prophylactic acyclovir, avoidance of triggers)

Patients with erythema multiforme major (Stevens-Johnson syndrome) suffer from more severe systemic upset than those with erythema multiforme minor. Intensive supportive treatment may be necessary, if mucosal lesions interfere with proper nutrition and skin involvement is sufficiently severe to raise the possibility of electrolyte loss and wound infection developing.

8 Lichen Planus

Although lichen planus is not a classic auto-immune disease characterised by the presence of circulating auto-antibodies, there is good evidence that it is immunologically mediated. An important clinical aspect of the disease is that it often causes desquamative gingivitis, which is clinically indistinguishable from that seen in MMP.

8.1 Epidemiology

A specific antigen has not been identified in lichen planus, and the disease usually develops spontaneously, although it may be precipitated by trauma, such as periodontal surgery (KATZ et al. 1988), and by a wide range of drugs (for a review, see SCULLY and EL-KOM 1985). The clinical features are strikingly similar to those seen in graft versus host disease (JUNGELL 1991), supporting the view that the disease results from cell-mediated immune response against an intra-epithelial antigen.

Lichen planus is one of the commonest mucocutaneous diseases, affecting 1% of the general population. It is generally a disease of the middle-aged (THORN et al. 1988), although atypical cases have been reported in children (MILLIGAN and GRAHAM-BROWN 1988).

There is an established risk of malignant transformation associated with oral lichen planus, with frequency rates between 0.4% and 12.3% (HOLMSTRUP et al. 1988). In their study of 611 Danish patients with lichen planus followed up for periods of up to 26 years, HOLMSTRUP et al. (1988) observed significantly more cases of oral cancer than would have been predicted by chance. It remains a matter of debate as to whether the lesions themselves are precancerous or whether mucosa affected by the disease is more susceptible to the effects of other carcinogens, but the practical management conclusion is that patients with lichen planus require long-term follow-up.

8.2 Oral Manifestations

There are six recognisable forms of lichen planus: (1) reticular or "classic", (2) papular, (3) plaque-like, (4) atrophic, (5) erosive or ulcerative and (6) bullous. Desquamative gingivitis is the result of gingival involvement in erosive lichen planus. In an extensive study of oral lesions in lichen planus, THORN et al. (1988) found that reticular lichen planus (Fig. 11) was the most common presentation of the disease, affecting over 90% of patients. Several forms of the disease were often found to coexist, with involvement of more than one site. Although site frequency was not reported in the paper by THORN et al. (1988), one third of their patients had gingival lesions (P. HOLMSTRUP, personal communication) at initial presentation, and a third of those showed remission of their gingival lesions during the course of the study. In contrast to cutaneous lichen planus, a prolonged clinical course is typical of the oral lesions and, whilst individual lesions do not remain static, oral mucosal involvement may persist for many years. Erosive lesions are the most persistent, and they also represent the most common gingival form of lichen planus, with extensive involvement of the attached gingiva in tooth-bearing areas giving rise to desquamative gingivitis. The lesions appear fiery red and are sore. As stated earlier, this clinical appearance may be indistinguishable from the

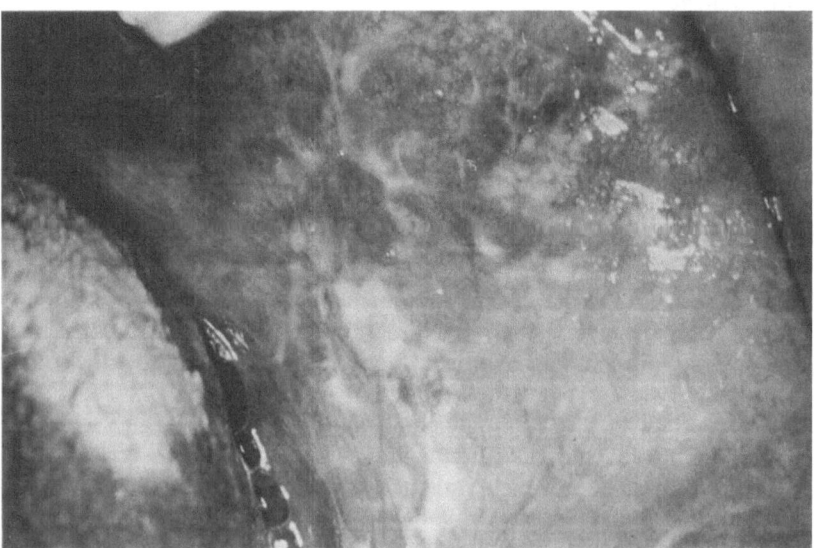

Fig. 11. Clinical photograph of classical reticular lichen planus involving the buccal mucosa. Lesions appear as white striations on an erythematous background, giving rise to a lace-like pattern of hyperkeratosis

desquamative gingivitis seen in MMP and, although careful clinical examination often reveals typical lesions of lichen planus at other sites, a biopsy and IF may be required for a definitive diagnosis.

8.3 Skin Lesions

The skin lesions in lichen planus typically appear as flat-topped violaceous papules, distributed in groups and principally affecting the flexor aspects of the wrists, the anterior surface of the lower legs, the lumbar region and the genitalia. Scratching or similar trauma may trigger the appearance of skin lesions, a characteristic termed the Koebner phenomenon, and this may lead to a linear clustering of the typical papules.

The skin lesions of lichen planus usually clear within 2 years (SCULLY and EL-KOM 1985) and have no reported malignant potential. Skin and oral lesions may co-exist, and around half of the patients with cutaneous lichen planus also have oral lesions. However, about one quarter have only oral lesions (JUNGELL 1991), which may be a reflection of the more prolonged clinical course of oral lesions than those affecting the skin.

8.4 Histopathological Features

Patients with lichen planus typically present with hyperkeratotic but atrophic epithelium and a dense lymphocytic infiltrate in the underlying connective tissue (Fig. 12). The inflammatory infiltrate is restricted to the upper corium, with an abrupt cut-off on its deep aspect, and the adjacent epithelium exhibits basal cell degeneration with an eosinophilic coagulum in the basement membrane associated with lymphocytic infiltration of the epithelium. The histopathological features of lichen planus can be summarised as follows:

- Epithelial atrophy with hyperkeratosis
- Loss of basal cell layer
- Civatte or colloid bodies
- Dense lymphocytic accumulation in upper dermis adjacent to epithelium

One of the shortcomings of many of the histopathological studies of lichen planus is that the amount of clinical information recorded is generally insufficient to establish the duration of lesions. Thus the results from investigations of "young" and "old" lesions have not been differentiated, and it is difficult to establish the pattern of evolution of the disease. It appears from immunocytochemical studies (FARTHING et al. 1990) that there is clustering of Langherhans cells within the epithelium associated with an increase in the number of intra-epithelial lymphocytes and with the accumulation of lymphocytes in the adjacent lamina propria. It is striking that the areas of hyperkeratosis are closely associated with the infiltration of the lower epithelial layers by lymphocytes. Hyalinised, eosinophilic Civatte

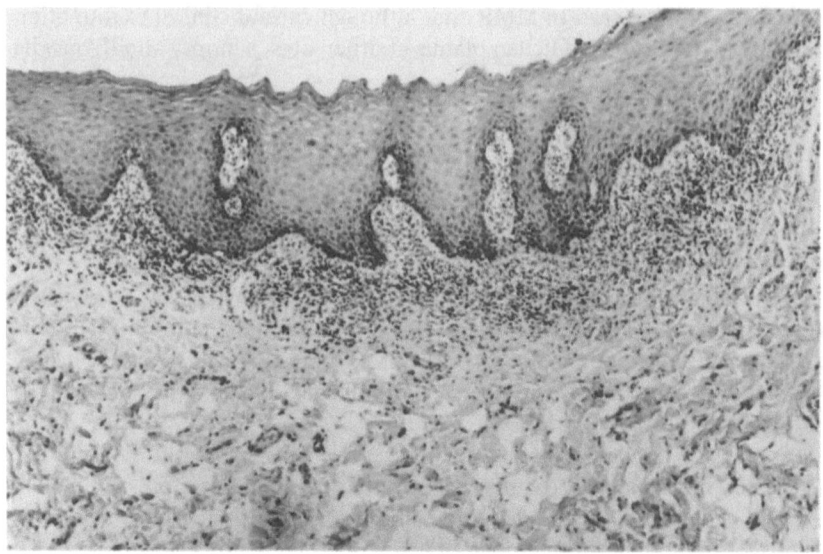

Fig. 12. Medium-power photomicrograph showing the typical features of lichen planus of the buccal mucosa. The epithelium exhibits a tendency to atrophy and is parakeratinised. A dense lymphocytic infiltrate is present in the upper part of the corium, with an abrupt cut-off on its deep aspect

bodies are occasionally present within the epithelium, and these are generally believed to be degenerate keratinocytes.

IF in lichen planus does not show characteristic features of the kind seen in either pemphigus or pemphigoid, but direct IF occasionally reveals accumulations of fibrin at the basement membrane zone, and Ig binding is associated with Civatte bodies (SCULLY and EL-KOM 1985).

8.5 Pathogenic Mechanisms

Although there has been a substantial amount of research into the pathogenic mechanisms involved in lichen planus, the mechanism by which keratinocyte damage is initiated remains obscure, and no lichen planus-specific antigen has been identified. Nevertheless, the processes by which lesions develop and persist have begun to emerge (FARTHING et al. 1990; WALSH et al. 1990; HEDBERG and HUNTER 1987; RICH and READE 1989; BOISNIC et al. 1990; FARTHING and CRUCHLEY 1989):

- Clustering and activation of Langerhans cells in epithelium.
- Keratinocytes express HLA-DR and intercellular adhesion molecule (ICAM)-1.
- Selective accumulation of cytotoxic/suppressor T cells within epithelium.
- Helper/inducer T cells persist in dermis.

- T cells are memory cells in both sites.
- Upregulation of ICAM-1 and E selectin expression on endothelial cells.

As described in Sect. 8.4, focal accumulations of Langerhans cells occur within the epithelium, expressing increased levels of HLA-DP and HLA-DQ (FARTHING et al. 1990), indicating that they are activated. The lymphocytes in the lamina propria are predominantly of the helper/inducer phenotype, but the lymphocytic infiltrate in the epithelium is the result of selective migration of cytotoxic/suppressor cells, which appear to accumulate in areas where there is selective expression of HLA-DR and ICAM-1 on keratinocytes. The lymphocytes in both epithelium and lamina propria are memory T cells, indicating that they are responding to a previously encountered or persistent antigen. The evidence is therefore strong that keratinocyte damage in lichen planus is lymphocyte mediated, but little is known of the mechanism by which it occurs. HLA-DR and ICAM-1 expression on keratinocytes is likely to be an important mechanism in lymphocyte accumulation, but again the trigger for their expression remains obscure.

In conclusion, whilst the mechanisms of cell damage in lichen planus can be explained, the true nature of the disease remains elusive. The true status of lichenoid drug symptoms remains to be established, and the mechanism by which malignant transformation occurs also demands further research.

8.6 Treatment

There is not at present a wholly effective treatment for lichen planus, especially in its erosive forms such as desquamative gingivitis. Topical steroids and intralesional steroid injections are the principal forms of treatment, but griseofulvin may also be effective in patients with erosive lesions. A proportion of patients with focal lichenoid reactions adjacent to amalgam restorations have been shown on patch testing to be allergic to mercury (LAINE et al. 1992). It has therefore been proposed in patients with such lesions that patch testing should be carried out and, if a positive result is obtained, the amalgam restorations be replaced. Other forms of treatment include mouthwashes and avoidance of irritants.

It seems probable that, once the real nature of lichen planus and its relationship to lichenoid eruptions have been elucidated, rational and effective treatments are likely to follow.

9 Conclusion

In spite of the similar clinical presentations of many of the mucocutaneous conditions described here, the molecular basis of their pathogenesis has been elucidated by recent research. It is to be hoped that this will lead to more precise clinical diagnosis and more rational strategies for treatment.

The process of accurate clinical diagnosis demands a thorough history of the duration, location and frequency of lesions, and it needs to be determined whether there are any specific triggers, such as medication or preceding herpes infection. Given the likely genetic susceptibility to a number of these diseases, the existence of a family history of the disease is particularly important. As well as establishing the characteristics of oral mucosal lesions, it is also crucial to ascertain whether other mucosal sites are affected and whether skin lesions are present. Ophthalmic examination is indicated in the case of MMP and similar diseases. Patch testing is indicated in lesions such as localised forms of lichen planus where a hypersensitivity reaction is suspected.

Routine histological examination is mandatory in the diagnosis of most of the diseases discussed in this chapter, taking care to include perilesional mucosa in the biopsy so that the diagnosis is not obscured by secondary inflammatory changes. The diagnosis of pemphigus and pemphigoid requires histopathological examination, and direct and indirect IF are important in these and similar diseases. In diseases such as those of the EB complex, ultrastructural examination is also indicated to determine the site and nature of the lesion.

There may remain some cases where a differential diagnosis cannot be resolved. However, the specific characterisation of the antigens involved in many of these diseases now raises the possibility of accurate diagnosis by immunoprecipitation of circulating antibodies or their detection using enzyme-linked immunosorbent assay (ELISA)-based systems. It is anticipated that within the next decade specific molecular diagnosis of this group of clinically similar mucocutaneous diseases should be possible.

References

Ahmed AR (1983) Clinical features of pemphigus. Clin Dermatol 1: 13–21

Ahmed AR, Hombal SM (1986) Cicatricial pemphigoid. Int J Dermatol 25: 90–96

Ahmed AR, Salm M (1983) Juvenile pemphigus. J Am Acad Dermatol 8: 799–807

Ahmed AR, Graham J, Jordan RE, Provost TT (1980) Pemphigus: current concepts. Ann Intern Med 92: 396–405

Amagai M, Klaus-Kovtun V, Stanley JR (1991) Autoantibodies against a novel epithelial cadherin in pemphigus vulgaris, a disease of cell adhesion. Cell 67: 869–877

Amagai M, Hashimoto T, Shimizu N, Nishikawa T (1994) Absorption of pathogenic autoantibodies by the extracellular domain of pemphigus vulgaris antigen (Dsg3) produced by Baculovirus. J Clin Invest 94: 59–67

Aslanzadeh J, Helm KF, Espy MJ, Muller SA, Smith TF (1992) Detection of HSV-specific DNA in biopsy tissue of patients with erythema multiforme by polymerase chain reaction. Br J Dermatol 126: 19–23

Bean SF (1974) Cicatricial pemphigoid: immunofluorescent studies. Arch Dermatol 110: 552–555

Bedane C, Prost C, Bernard P, Catanzano G, Bonnetblanc J-M, Dubertret L (1991) Cicatricial pemphigoid antigen differs from bullous pemphigoid antigen by its exclusive extracellular localization: a study by indirect immunoelectronmicroscopy. J Invest Dermatol 97: 3–9

Bernard P, Prost C, Lecerf V, Intrator L, Combemale P, Bedane C et al (1990) Studies of cicatricial pemphigoid autoantibodies using direct immunoelectron microscopy and immunoblot analysis. J Invest Dermatol 94: 630–635

Bernard P, Prost C, Durepaire N, Basset-Seguin N, Didierjean L, Saurat J-H (1992) The major cicatricial pemphigoid antigen is a 180-kD protein that shows immunologic cross-reactivities with the bullous pemphigoid antigen. J Invest Dermatol 99: 174–179

Beutner EH, Jordan RE (1964) Demonstration of skin antibodies in sera of pemphigus vulgaris patients by indirect immunofluorescence staining. Proc Soc Exp Biol 117: 505–510

Beutner EH, Lever WF, Witebsky E, Jordan RE, Chertock B (1965) Autoantibodies in pemphigus vulgaris. J Am Med Assoc 192: 682–688

Boisnic S, Frances C, Branchet M-C, Szpirglas H, Le Charpentier Y (1990) Immunohistochemical study of oral lesions of lichen planus: diagnostic and pathophysiologic aspects. Oral Surg 70: 462–465

Brice SL, Krzemien BS, Weston WL, Huff JC (1989) Detection of Herpes simplex virus DNA in cutaneous lesions of erythema multiforme. J Invest Dermatol 94: 183–197

Brice SL, Huff JC, Weston WL (1990) Erythema multiforme. Curr Probl Dermatol 1: 9–24

Bruckner-Tuderman L, Mitsuhashi Y, Schnyder UW, Bruckner P (1989) Anchoring fibrils and type VII collagen are absent from skin in severe recessive dystrophic epidermolysis bullosa. J Invest Dermatol 93: 3–9

Calvanico NJ, Martins CR, Diaz LA (1991) Characterisation of pemphigus foliaceus antigen from human epidermis. J Invest Dermatol 96: 815–821

Carter WG, Kaur P, Gil SG, Gahr PJ, Wayner EA (1990a) Distinct functions for integrins $\alpha 3$ $\beta 1$ in focal adhesions and $\partial 6$ $\beta 4$/bullous pemphigoid antigen in a new stable anchoring contact (SAC) of keratinocytes: relation to hemidesmosomes. J Cell Biol 111: 3141–3154

Carter WG, Wayner EA, Bouchard TS, Kaur P (1990b) The role of integrins $\alpha 2$ $\beta 1$ and $\alpha 3$ $\beta 1$ in cell-cell and cell-substrate adhesion of human epidermal cells. J Cell Biol 110: 1387–1404

Carter WG, Ryan MC, Gahr PJ (1991) Epiligrin, a new cell adhesion ligand for integrin $\alpha 3$ $\beta 1$ in epithelial basement membranes. Cell 65: 599–610

Correll RW, Schott TR (1985) Multiple painful vesiculo ulcerative lesions of the oral mucosa. J Am Dent Assoc 110: 765–766

Coulomb PA, Hulton ME, Letai A, Hevert A, Paller AS, Fuchs E (1991) Point mutations in human keratin 14 genes of epidermolysis bullosa simplex patients: genetic and functional analyses. Cell 66: 1301–1311

Cresswell SN, Black MM, Bhogal B, Skeete MVH (1981) Correlation of circulating antibody titres in pemphigus with disease activity. Clin Exp Dermatol 6: 477–483

Domloge-Hultsch N, Gammon WR, Briggaman RA, Gill SG, Carter WG, Yancey KB (1992) Epiligrin, a major human keratinocyte ligand is targeted by antibodies in patients with a form of cicatricial pemphigoid (abstract). J Invest Dermatol 98: 580

Eyre RW, Stanley JR (1987) Human autoantibodies against a desmosomal protein with a calcium-sensitive epitope are characteristic of pemphigus foliaceus patients. J Exp Med 165:1719–1724

Farthing PM, Cruchley AT (1989) Expression of MHC class II antigens (HLA DR, DP and DQ) by keratinocytes in oral lichen planus. J Oral Pathol Med 18: 305–309

Farthing PM, Matear P, Cruchley AT (1990) The activation of Langerhans cells in oral lichen planus. J Oral Pathol Med 19: 81–85

Farthing PM, Maragou P, Coates M, Tatnall F, Leigh IM, Williams DM (1995) Characteristics of the oral lesions in patients with cutaneous recurrent erythema multiforme. J Oral Pathol Med 24: 9–13

Fine RM, Weathers DR (1980) Desquamative gingivitis: a form of cicatricial pemphigoid. Br J Dermatol 102: 393–399

Fitzpatrick RE, Newcomer VD (1980) The correlation of disease activity and antibody titres in pemphigus. Arch Dermatol 116: 285–290

Fraser NG, Kerr NW, Donald D (1973) Oral lesions in dermatitis herpetiformis. Br J Dermatol 89: 439–450

Fry L, Seah PP (1974) Dermatitis herpetiformis: an evaluation of diagnostic criteria. Br J Dermatol 90: 137–146

Gammon WR, Briggaman RA, Woodley DT, Heald PW, Wheeler CE (1984) Epidermolysis bullosa acquisita - a pemphigoid-like disease. J Am Acad Dermatol 11: 820–832

Gebel K, Hornstein OP (1984) Drug-induced oral erythema multiforme. Dermatologica 168: 35–40

Giudice GJ, Emery DJ, Diaz LA (1992a) Cloning and primary structural analysis of the bullous pemphigoid autoantigen BP180. J Invest Dermatol 99: 243–250

Giudice GJ, Emery DJ, Jones JCR, Hopkinson SB, Zelickson B, Diaz LA (1992b) Protein domain organisation of the bullous pemphigoid-180 autoantigen (abstract). J Invest Dermatol 98: 580

Hashimoto T, Ogawa MM, Konohana A, Nishikawa T (1990) Detection of pemphigus vulgaris and pemphigus foliaceus antigens by immunoblot analysis using different antigen sources. J Invest Dermatol 94: 327–331

Hedberg NM, Hunter N (1987) The expression of HLA-DR on keratinocytes in oral lichen planus. J Oral Pathol 16: 31–35

Holmstrup P, Thorn JJ, Rindum J, Pindborg JJ (1988) Malignant development of lichen planus-affected oral mucosa. J Oral Pathol 17: 219–225

Hopkinson SB, Riddelle KS and Jones JCR (1992) Cytoplasmic domain of the 180-kD bullous pemphigoid antigen, a hemidesmosomal component: molecular and cell biologic characterisation. J Invest Dermatol 99: 264–270

Huff JC, Weston WL (1989) Recurrent erythema multiforme. Medicine 68: 133–140

Imber MJ, Murphy GF, Jordan RE (1987) The immunopathology of bullous pemphigoid. Clin Dermatol 5: 81–92

Ioannides D, Hytiroglou P, Phelps RG, Bystrin J-C (1991) Regional variation in the expression of pemphigus foliaceus, pemphigus erythematosus and pemphigus vulgaris antigens in human skin. J Invest Dermatol 96: 159–161

Ishida-Yamamoto A, McGrath JA, Chapman SJ, Leigh IM, Lane EB, Eady RAJ (1991) Epidermolysis bullosa simplex (Dowling Meara type) is a genetic disease characterised by an abnormal keratin-filament network involving keratins K5 and K14. J Invest Dermatol 97: 858–868

Iwasaki T, Welsh E, Kim JP, Wynn KC, Ryynanen J, Sollberg S et al (1992) Characterisation of type VII collagen from cultured WISH cells and normal and RDEB keratinocytes (abstract). J Invest Dermatol 98: 573

Jungell P (1991) Oral lichen planus. A review. Int J Oral Maxillofac Surg 20: 129–135

Kampgen E, Burg G, Wank R (1988) Association of herpes simplex virus-induced erythema multiforme with the human leukocyte antigen DQw3. Arch Dermatol 124: 1372–1375

Katz SI, Strober W (1978) The pathogenesis of dermatitis herpetiformis. J Invest Dermatol 70: 63–75

Katz J, Goultschin J, Benoliel R, Rotstein I, Pisanty S (1988) Lichen planus evoked by periodontal surgery. J Clin Periodontol 15: 263–265

Koch PJ, Goldschmidt MD, Zimbelmann R, Troyanovsky R (1992) Complexity and expression patterns of the desmosomal cadherins. Proc Natl Acad Sci USA 89: 353–357

Korman N (1988) Pemphigus. J Am Acad Dermatol 18: 1219–1238

Laine J, Kalimo K, Forssel H, Happonen R-P (1992) Resolution of oral lichenoid lesions after replacement of amalgam restorations in patients allergic to mercury compounds. Br J Dermatol 126: 10–15

Lane EB, Rugg EL, Navsaria H, Leigh IM, Heagerty AHM, Ishida-Yamamoto A et al (1992) A mutation in the conserved helix termination peptide of keratin 5 in hereditary skin blistering. Nature 356: 244–246

Laskaris G, Demetriou N, Angelopoulos A (1981) Immunofluorescent studies in desquamative gingivitis. J Oral Pathol 10: 398–407

Leigh IM, Mowbray JF, Levene GM, Sutherland S (1985) Recurrent and continuous erythema multiforme – a clinical and immunological study. Clin Exp Dermatol 10: 58–67

Leigh IM, Eady RAJ, Heagerty AHM, Purkis PE, Whitehead PA, Burgeson RE (1988) Type VII collagen is a normal component of epidermal basement membrane, which shows altered expression on recessive dystrophic epidermolysis bullosa. J Invest Dermatol 90: 639–642

Leonard JN, Wright P, Williams DM, Gilkes JJH, Haffenden GP, McMinn RMH et al (1984) The relationship between linear IgA disease and benign mucous membrane pemphigoid. Br J Dermatol 110: 307–314

Levene GM (1982) The treatment of pemphigus and pemphigoid. Clin Exp Dermatol 7: 643–652

Lewis MAO, Forsyth A, Gall J (1989) Recurrent erythema multiforme: a possible role of food-stuffs. Br Dent J 166: 371–373

Li K, Giudice GJ, Tamai K, Do HC, Sawamura D, Diaz LA and Uitto J (1992) Cloning of partial cDNA for mouse 180-kD bullous pemphigoid antigen (BPAG2), a highly conserved collagenous protein of the cutaneous basement membrane zone. J Invest Dermatol 99: 258–263

Lozada-Nur F, Silverman S (1980) Topically applied fluocinonide in an adhesive base in the treatment of oral vesiculo-erosive diseases. Arch Dermatol 116: 898–901

Lozada-Nur F, Gorsky M, Silverman S (1989) Oral erythema multiforme: clinical observations and treatment of 95 patients. Oral Surg 67: 36–40

Margolis RJ, Tonneson MG, Harrist TJ, Bhan AK, Wintroub BU, Mihm MC, Soter NA (1983) Lymphocyte subsets and Langerhans cells/indeterminate cells in erythema multiforme. J Invest Dermatol 81: 403–406

Michalaki H, Staquet M-J, Cerri A, Berti E, Roche P, Machado P et al (1992) Expression of the $\alpha6$ $\beta4$ integrin in lesional skin differentiates bullous pemphigoid from epidermolysis bullosa acquisita. J Invest Dermatol 98: 204–208

Milligan A, Graham-Brown RAC (1988) Lichen planus in children – a review of six cases. Clin Exp Dermatol 15: 340–342

Miura S, Smith CC, Burnett JW, Aurelian L (1992) Detection of viral DNA within skin of healed recurrent herpes simplex infection and erythema multiforme lesions. J Invest Dermatol 98: 68–72

Molin L (1987) Oral acyclovir prevents herpes simplex virus-associated erythema multiforme. Br J Dermatol 116: 109–111

Mutasim DF, Vaughan A, Farooqui J, Boissy R, Zu H (1992) Detection of pemphigoid antibodies by special immune fluorescence, immuno-blotting and immuno-electron microscopy in immunofluorescence negative bullous pemphigoid sera (abstract). J Invest Dermatol 98: 589

Nisengard RJ, Rogers RS (1987) Treatment of desquamative gingival lesions. J Periodontol 58: 167–172

Nowak AJ (1988) Oropharyngeal lesions and their management in epidermolysis bullosa. Arch Dermatol 124: 742–745

Peng T, Nisengard RJ, Levine MJ (1986) Gingival basement membrane antigens in desquamative lesions of the gingiva. Oral Surg Oral Med Oral Pathol 61: 584–589

Person JR, Rogers RS (1977) Bullous and cicatricial pemphigoid: clinical histopathologic and immunopathologic correlations. Mayo Clin Proc 52: 54–64

Pisanti S, Sharar Y, Kaufman E, Posner LN (1974) Pemphigus vulgaris: incidence in Jews of different ethnic groups according to age, sex and initial lesion. Oral Surg Oral Med Oral Pathol 38: 382–387

Raque CJ, Stein KN, Samitz MH (1970) Pemphigus vulgaris involving the oesophagus. Arch Dermatol 102: 371–373

Regauer S, Seiler GR, Barrandon Y, Easley KW, Compton CC (1990) Epithelial origin of cutaneous anchoring fibrils. J Cell Biol 111: 2109–2115

Rich AM, Reade PC (1989) A quantitative assessment of Langerhans cells in oral mucosal lichen planus and leukoplakia. Br J Dermatol 120: 223–228

Ruoslahti E, Pierschbacher MD (1987) New perspectives in cell adhesion: RGD and integrins. Science 238: 491–496

Scully C, El-Kom M (1985) Lichen planus: review and update on pathogenesis. J Oral Pathol 14: 431–458

Silverman S, Gorsky M, Lozada-Nur F, Liu A (1986) Oral mucous membrane pemphigoid: a study of sixty five patients. Oral Surg Oral Med Oral Pathol 61: 233–237

Takeichi M (1991) Cadherin cell adhesion receptors as a morphogenetic regulator. Science 251: 1451–1455

Thorn JJ, Holmstrup P, Rindum J, Pindborg JJ (1988) Course of various clinical forms of oral lichen planus. A prospective follow-up study of 611 patients. J Oral Pathol 17: 213–218

Tonneson MG, Harrist TJ, Wintroub BU, Mihm MC, Soter NA (1983) Erythema multiforme: microvascular damage and infiltration of lymphocytes and basophils. J Invest Dermatol 80: 282–286

Uitto J and Christiano AM (1992) Molecular genetics of the cutaneous basement membrane zone. J Clin Invest 90: 687–692

Venning VA, Frith PA, Bron AJ, Millard PR, Wojnarowska F (1988) Mucosal involvement in bullous and cicatricial pemphigoid: a clinical and immunopathological study. Br J Dermatol 118: 7–15

Walsh LJ, Savage NW, Ishii T, Seymour GJ (1990) Immunopathogenesis of oral lichen planus. J Oral Pathol Med 19: 389–396

Williams DM (1989) Vesiculo bullous mucocutaneous disease: pemphigus vulgaris. J Oral Pathol Med 18: 544–553

Williams DM (1990) Vesiculo bullous mucocutaneous disease: benign mucous membrane and bullous pemphigoid. J Oral Pathol Med 19: 16–23

Williams DM, Leonard JN, Wright P, Gilkes JJH, Haffenden GP, McMinn RMH et al (1984) Benign mucous membrane (cicatricial) pemphigoid revisited: a clinical and immunological reappraisal. Br Dent J 157: 313–316

Wojnarowska F, Whitehead P, Leigh IM, Bhogal BS, Black MM (1991) Identification of the target antigen in chronic bullous disease of childhood and linear IgA disease of adults. Br J Dermatol 124: 157–162

Woodley DT, Burgeson RE, Lunstrum G, Bruckner-Tuderman L, Reese MJ, Briggaman RA (1988) Epidermolysis bullosa acquisita antigen is the globular carboxyl terminus of type VII procollagen. J Clin Invest 81: 683–687

Wright JT, Fine JD, Johnson L (1993) Hereditary epidermolysis bullosa: oral manifestations and dental management. Pediatr Dent 15: 242–247

Yurchenco PD, Cheng Y-S, Colognato H (1992) Laminin forms an independent network in basement membranes. J Cell Biol 117: 1119–1133

Zaim MT, Giorno RC, Golitz LE, Kunke KS, Huff JC (1987) An immunopathological study of herpes-associated erythema multiforme. J Cutan Pathol 14: 257–262

Zegarelli DJ, Zegarelli EV (1977) Intraoral pemphigus vulgaris. Oral Surg Oral Med Oral Pathol 44: 384–393

New Aspects of Oral Viral Diseases

C. SCULLY

Current Topics in Pathology
Volume 90, G. Seifert (Ed.)
© Springer-Verlag Berlin Heidelberg 1996

1 Introduction

The past decade has seen intense and increasing interest in the oral health care consequences of viral infection, particularly the possible relationships between viruses and oral diseases – especially malignant neoplasms, the possible infectivity of saliva and oral secretions and, latterly, the oral consequences of infection with the human immunodeficiency viruses (HIV).

Apart from HIV, most viruses known to cause significant oral disease are DNA viruses, all capable of latency and of being reactivated to cause shedding and disease, not least by loss of immune competence. These infections thus figure large in causing the oral lesions in HIV-infected and other immunocompromised individuals and in being potential sources of infection. Amongst such infective agents, the most important are the herpesviruses and papillomaviruses. These are discussed in this chapter, which is focused on the developing understanding over the decade up to 1995 of the relationship between viruses and oral mucosal lesions (Table 1).

Space here precludes coverage of the more tenuous relations of viruses with oral and salivary gland disease, of salivary carriage of viruses, and of hepatitis, HIV, human T cell leukaemia virus (HTLV)-I, HTLV-II, measles, mumps, rubella and other viruses. Possible virally induced mucosal disorders such as Kawasaki's disease (mucocutaneous lymph node syndrome) and possible relationships between hepatitis viruses and other oral disease, such as that between hepatitis C and Behcet's syndrome, hepatitis C and oral cancer, and hepatitis C and lichen planus, are not discussed here; details can be found elsewhere (SCULLY et al. 1990, 1991; SCULLY and BAGG 1992; SCULLY and SAMARANAYAKE 1992; SCULLY 1993, 1995; PEDERSEN et al. 1993; NAGAO et al. 1995).

There are at least seven, now possibly eight known herpesviruses (Table 2) and, of these, oral lesions have been firmly attributed to at least five, namely herpes simplex viruses (HSV) types 1 and 2, varicella zoster virus (VZV), Epstein-Barr virus (EBV) and cytomegalovirus (CMV). All can cause a primary infection which is generally subclinical, and all remain latent thereafter and can be reactivated,

Table 1. Viral infections with oral manifestations

Virus implicated	Major proven oral manifestations
Herpes simplex-1	Herpetic stomatitis
	Herpes labialis
	Recurrent intra-oral ulcers
	Erythema multiforme
Herpes simplex-2	Herpetic stomatitis
	Herpes labialis
	Erythema multiforme
Herpes varicella zoster	Pain and ulceration
Epstein-Barr virus	Ulceration
	Lymphomas
	Palatal petechiae
	Hairy leukoplakia
Cytomegalovirus	Ulceration
Human herpesvirus-6	?
Human herpesvirus-7	?
Kaposi's sarcoma herpesvirus	? Kaposi's sarcoma
Human papillomaviruses	Papillomas, verruca vulgaris, condyloma acuminatum focal epithelial hyperplasia
Molluscum contagiosum	Labial papules
Orf	Labial nodule
Measles	Koplik's spots
Rubella	Palatal petechiae
Mumps	Sialadenitis
Coxsackie/echo viruses	Ulceration
Human immunodeficiency viruses	Fungal infections
	Viral infections
	Auto-immune disease (e.g. petechiae)
	Tumours

Table 2. Human herpesviruses

Herpesviruses	Abbreviation
1 Herpes simplex type 1	HSV-1
2 Herpes simplex type 2	HSV-2
3 Varicella zoster virus	VZV
4 Epstein-Barr virus	EBV
5 Cytomegalovirus	CMV or HCMV
6 Human herpesvirus-6	HHV-6
7 Human herpesvirus-7	HHV-7
8 Kaposi's sarcoma herpesvirus	KSHV

sometimes with resultant disease. Some herpesviruses are oncogenic. In the immunocompromised host, virus infection or reactivation can cause severe and sometimes even fatal disease.

There are over 70 human papillomaviruses known (HPV), some of which cause oral lesions alone, some also lesions affecting skin or other mucosae (Table 3). Most HPV cause benign lumps such as papillomas or warts, but the possible

Table 3. Human papillomavirus-induced cutaneous and mucosal lesions

HPV type	Clinical features
1a,b,c	Deep plantar warts
2a–e	Common warts (verruca vulgaris) Mosaic plantar warts Oral verrucous carcinoma Oral warts
3a,b	Flat warts (juvenile warts) Warts in EV (non-malignant)
4	Small palmar and plantar warts Oral warts
5a,b	Warts in EV (malignant) Skin carcinoma (in immunosuppressed patients)
6a–f	Vulvar carcinoma Laryngeal papillomas Genital condyloma Buschke-Lowenstein tumour Cervical intra-epithelial neoplasia Oral papillomas/condylomas
7	Common warts (Butcher's warts) Oral warts (in immunosuppressed patient)
8	Warts in EV Squamous cell carcinoma in EV
9	Warts in EV (non-malignant)
10a,b	Flat warts
11a,b	Oral papillomas/condylomas Laryngeal papillomas Laryngeal carcinomas Cervical intra-epithelial neoplasia Genital warts Penile carcinoma
12	Warts in EV
13a,b	Focal epithelial hyperplasia (Heck's disease)
14a,b	Warts in EV Squamous cell carcinoma in EV
15	Warts in EV (non-malignant)
16	Carcinoma of oesophagus Carcinoma of larynx Oral carcinoma Genital condyloma Cervical intra-epithelial neoplasia Bowenoid papulosis Carcinoma of cervix Carcinoma of penis Carcinoma of anus Lung carcinoma
17a,b	Warts in EV Squamous cell carcinoma in EV

Table 3. *Continued*

HPV type	Clinical features
18	Carcinoma of cervix Carcinoma of penis
19	Warts in EV
20	Warts in EV Squamous cell carcinoma in EV
21–25	Warts in EV
26	Verruca vulgaris (in immunosuppressed patients)
30	Laryngeal carcinoma Cervical intra-epithelial neoplasia
31	Carcinoma of cervix
32	Focal epithelial hyperplasia (Heck's disease) Oral papilloma
33	Cervical intra-epithelial neoplasia Carcinoma of cervix Tonsillar carcinoma
34	Non-genital Bowens disease Cervical intra-epithelial neoplasia
35	Cervical intra-epithelial neoplasia Carcinoma of cervix
36	Warts in EV Actinic keratosis
37	Keratoacanthoma
38	Melanoma
39	Bowenoid papulosis Cervical intra-epithelial lesion Cervical carcinoma
40	Laryngeal carcinoma
41	Vulvar papilloma Cervical intra-epithelial lesion
42	Flat condylomas (Bowenoid lesions)
43/44	Low-grade epithelial dysplasias of genital epithelium
45	Cervical intra-epithelial neoplasia Cervical carcinoma
46/47	Warts in EV
48	Squamous cell carcinoma in EV
49/50	Warts in EV
51/52	Cervical intra-epithelial neoplasia Carcinoma of cervix
53	Cervical intra-epithelial neoplasia
54	Genital condyloma
55	Bowenoid papulosis
56	Cervical intra-epithelial neoplasia Carcinoma of cervix

Table 3. *Continued*

HPV type	Clinical features
57	Cervical intra-epithelial neoplasia Nasal papilloma Oral papilloma
58	Cervical intra-epithelial lesion
59	Skin warts
60	Cervical intra-epithelial lesion
61	Vaginal intra-epithelial lesion
62	Vaginal intra-epithelial lesion
63	Skin warts (foot)
64	Vaginal intra-epithelial lesion
65	Skin warts (finger)
66	Carcinoma of cervix
67	Vulval intra-epithelial lesion
68	Vulval intra-epithelial lesion
69	Cervical intra-epithelial lesion
70	Papilloma of vulva
71	Vaginal intra-epithelial lesion

EV, epidermodysplasia verruciformis. After DE VILLIERS 1989 and ZUR HAUSEN and DE VILLIERS 1994.

association of these viruses with oral carcinoma is the focus of intense attention and is therefore discussed in some detail below.

2 Herpesviruses and Herpes-like Viruses

2.1 Herpes Simplex Viruses

HSV are definitely the causal agents of a range of orofacial lesions, including primary herpetic stomatitis, recurrent herpes labialis and recurrent intra-oral infections. HSV is also implicated in many instances of recurrent erythema multiforme. HSV might play a role in some cranial neuropathies, Behcet's syndrome, and other oral ulcers and oral squamous carcinoma.

There are two subtypes, HSV-1 and HSV-2, sharing considerable homology. Different strains are found in different geographical regions, and some strains vary in, for example, their neuro-invasive qualities (SAKAOKA et al. 1987; BERGSTROM and LYCKE 1990). HSV subtypes and strains can be differentiated by DNA restriction-endonuclease analysis (herpesvirus fingerprinting).

Enclosing the HSV DNA genome is a protein capsid, and the whole is enclosed in a lipid-containing envelope derived from the nuclear membrane of the host cell.

This envelope contains glycoproteins (gp), some of which are responsible for HSV infectivity: for example, gpB and gpC may be responsible for attachment to cell surface receptors.

Recent advances in the understanding of HSV epidemiology, pathogenesis and treatment are reviewed elsewhere (COREY and SPEAR 1986; WILDY 1985; SCULLY 1989, 1995; SCULLY et al. 1991; MILLER and REDDING 1992; SCULLY and SAMARANAYAKE 1992; VESTEY and NORVAL 1992; SYRJANEN 1992).

2.1.1 Natural History of Infection

HSV binds by envelope glycoproteins to epithelial cell surface receptors which are heparan sulphate proteoglycans (WUDUNN and SPEAR 1989). The nucleocapsid is then released into the cell cytoplasm. The nucleocapsid releases HSV DNA, which reaches the cell nucleus.

Alpha genes ("immediate early" or IE genes) are then expressed, followed by beta genes ("early" or E genes), which produce regulatory proteins and enzymes needed for DNA replication. The virus thus shuts down most cell protein synthesis while initiating viral gene transcription. Later, the gamma genes ("late" or L genes) that specify HSV structural proteins are expressed (O'HARE and HAYWARD 1985). As each category of gene is expressed, the former is turned off. The HSV genome is then replicated, structural proteins synthesised and nucleocapsids assembled (appearing as nuclear inclusion bodies), and these pass through the nuclear membrane (thereby acquiring the envelope) into the cytoplasm and thence to the cell surface. The cell typically dies as the virus is released to spread to adjacent cells, and intra-epithelial vesiculation results from this cytopathic effect.

HSV also infects the trigeminal nerve, where it remains latent in the ganglion and can be reactivated, sometimes with clinical recurrent infection (STRAUS et al. 1985).

2.1.2 Epidemiology of Infection

Neonates are often protected by maternal antibodies to HSV that have crossed the placenta. Oral HSV infection is seen mainly in pre-school children, most commonly in lower socio-economic classes (ADES et al. 1989). By the age of 15 years, 50% of the population has been infected by HSV-1 (CHRISTENSON et al. 1992), and by adult life some 63% have antibody evidence of infection by HSV-1 (BLACKWELDER et al. 1982). Infections are, however, now seen increasingly in older children and adults in developed countries.

HSV-1 is usually responsible for herpetic stomatitis, but HSV-2 may also cause oral lesions (LOWHAGEN et al. 1990; GUINAN et al. 1985; SACKS 1984; STRAND et al. 1986; COREY 1988; LAFFERTY et al. 1987). There may be concurrent oral and genital infections with either HSV-1 or HSV-2 or both, but previous oral HSV-1 infection may protect to some extent against genital infection with HSV-2, probably by means of a common mucosal antibody response (ASHLEY et al. 1994).

2.1.3 Transmission

A total of 5%–8% of children and 2%–10% of adults periodically shed infectious HSV in saliva even in the absence of clinical lesions (Overall 1984). Shedding is more common in immunocompromised subjects. Infection is contracted from HSV lesions or infected secretions such as saliva (Spruance 1984). Failure to follow cross-infection control procedures in oral health care facilities may lead to spread of infection to staff (Rowe et al. 1982; Perl et al. 1992) or to patients (Manzella et al. 1984; Perl et al. 1992).

2.1.4 Clinical Features of Oral Primary Infections

Many primary infections with HSV are subclinical or pass unrecognised. Stomatitis and pharyngitis are the most frequent clinical manifestations of primary oral infection (McMillan et al. 1993). The clinical picture is fairly distinct, with mouth ulcers, gingivitis, fever and cervical lymphadenopathy. The saliva contains large quantities of HSV. In children, there are occasionally extra-oral manifestations such as rashes (Scully 1985). The illness tends overall to be more severe in adults.

Chronic and progressive oral HSV infection may be seen in immuno-compromised individuals (Corey and Spear 1986; Grattan et al. 1986), including those with HIV infection (Jones et al. 1992; discussed elsewhere), while those with atopic eczema may develop widespread skin and sometimes visceral infection (eczema herpeticum).

2.1.5 Immunology

Intact epithelium constitutes the main defence against HSV infection, though humoral and cellular responses directed against cell surface viral glycoproteins are also important. The latter is the most important mechanism for recovery and subsequent control of HSV infection (Wildy and Gell 1985; Kohl 1985; Rouse 1985).

Antibodies also mediate viral neutralisation and antibody-dependent cellular cytotoxicity (ADCC). Responses to IE, E and L proteins (structural and non-structural proteins), especially to the IE proteins ICP4 and ICP0, are seen early in primary infection.

2.1.6 Latency

Latent infections are persistent infections where the viral genome is present but the gene expression is limited and no infectious virus is produced. The mechanisms are fully reviewed elsewhere (Roizman and Sears 1987; Banks and Rouse 1992). HSV resides in neuronal cells such as the trigeminal ganglion. HSV DNA can also be found in some clinically normal oral epithelium (Cox et al. 1993).

Latent virus expresses early replicative functions, but there is a block in HSV transcription and neither late viral antigens nor free virus can be detected (STANBERRY 1986). Furthermore, the neurones in which HSV is latent express no major histocompatitbility antigens (MHC) antigens and thus, even were viral antigens to be produced, they could not be presented to T lymphocytes. HSV glycoprotein gPG can bind complement component C3b and thereby impede the alternative complement pathway, offering another mechanism of evading immune attack.

Finally, though the mechanisms are unclear, it is clear that herpesviruses can be immunosuppressive and that HSV (probably via a viral glycoprotein) can impair a range of immune functions, including functions of natural killer (NK) cells, neutrophils and macrophages (BANKS and ROUSE 1992). Herpesvirus infections can thus exacerbate the immune defect in HIV and other infections.

2.1.7 Reactivation

Trigger factors appear to operate either via derepression of the latent viral genes or deregulation of immune surveillance mechanisms. Genetic factors must also be at play, as only about one third of non-immunocompromised patients have clinical recurrences.

Triggers for HSV reactivation include trauma (BARKVOLL and ATTRAMADOL 1987), including that of dental extraction, facial fractures and of decompression of the trigeminal nerve (KAMEYAMA et al. 1988, 1989), ultraviolet light (SPRUANCE 1985), fever or immunosuppression (HILL 1985; GREENBERG et al. 1987) and radiotherapy (REDDING 1990). Other factors that are often stated to be associated with recurrent herpetic infection include menstruation and other hormonal changes, but there appear to be no studies that confirm this.

Although it is often suggested that stress can also lead to recurrent infections, few studies have been done, and their results are inconsistent, though it has been reported that levels of serum antibody to HSV-1 are elevated in medical students during and just before examinations (GLASER et al. 1985, 1987), in separated and divorced men (KIECOLT-GLASER et al. 1988) and in individuals living near the Three Mile Island nuclear plant in the United States (MCKINNON et al. 1989). Though the relationship between stress, immune function and various infectious diseases is an area of much current interest (COHEN and WILLIAMSON 1991), the association between recurrent infections by HSV-1 and psychological stress remains to be proved.

Associations of recurrences of HSV infection with HLA-A1, HLA-B5 and HLA-DR1 and a decreased frequency of HLA-B35 have been shown, but other reported HLA associations are equivocal (LEGENDRE et al. 1982; GALLINA et al. 1985; JABBAR et al. 1991).

Reactivation of HSV is more common than clinical recurrence (HARBOUR et al. 1983) and still occurs in the presence of high titres of neutralising specific antibody. There is some evidence that prostaglandin E_2 may, by depressing ADCC and production of interleukin-2, reactivate HSV (BLYTH and HILL 1984).

Immunoglobulin G (IgG) antibodies to internal capsid protein and a range of structural proteins (gB, gD, VP19, VP20 and VP23), but not IE proteins, are found in recurrences (Wildy 1986; Kuhn et al. 1987). An increased titre of antibody to gD is associated with reduced recurrences of HSV, while deficient antibody to VP66 is associated with increased disease severity (Bernstein et al. 1987).

The protective role of cellular immune responses is emphasised by the frequent and severe episodes of HSV infection seen in patients with defective cellular immunity. Multiple immunocyte populations, including various T cell subsets (especially cytotoxic T cells), macrophages, NK cells and natural cytotoxic cells, are involved (Rouse 1985; Rager-Zisman et al. 1987).

Recurrences are presumably because of transient immunodepression with reduced natural cytotoxic cell activity, altered neutrophil motility and lymphoproliferative responses and reduced levels of some lymphokines, such as leucocyte migration inhibition factors and immune interferon (Green et al. 1985).

Clinical lesions in reactivated HSV infection are usually at the mucocutaneous junction on the lips (herpes labialis). Why, in otherwise healthy patients, recurrent HSV infections are usually labial and not intra-oral is unclear, but may relate to oral protective factors such as salivary IgA or lysozyme.

If intra-oral lesions arise in normal subjects, they are typically on the palate or gingiva. In immunocompromised subjects, intra-oral lesions are usually progressive linear ulcers, often on the tongue (Grossman et al. 1993), and may be related to reduced ADCC activity.

There is increasing evidence of intra-oral recurrences, notably as chronic ulcers in the mouth, especially in leukaemic or other immunocompromised persons (Greenberg et al. 1987a,b; Barrett 1986, 1987; Cohen and Greenberg 1985; Montgomery et al. 1986; Bergmann et al. 1990). Recurrence rates of oral HSV infections are unclear and figures vary from 16% to 45%.

2.1.8 Diagnosis of Infections

Many primary infections by HSV-1 can be diagnosed by clinical examination, and no laboratory diagnostic tests are necessary. However, in cases of immunocompromised individuals having lesions with an atypical appearance, laboratory testing can be valuable.

The most useful specimen consists of fluid from an intact vesicle or lesion, since this has a very high concentration of virus particles. The fluid can be adsorbed onto a cotton swab, provided that the swab is kept in viral transport medium and arrives at the laboratory within a few hours (Gonik et al. 1991).

The standard technique for HSV diagnosis of inoculation of a specimen onto susceptible cells examined daily for a cytopathic effect or the use of specific antisera can take several days, but there are now more rapid and more acceptable methods available.

HSV on oral swabs (or that that has started to grow in cell culture) can be detected by immunological methods to demonstrate viral antigens (Fox et al. 1987; Lipson et al. 1991), giving a diagnosis within 5h of the specimen arriving at the laboratory, with a sensitivity of 88%–99% and a specificity of 90%–100% (Verano and Michalski 1990; MacPhail et al. 1995). However, these rapid methods require up to 100 times more virus in the specimen that do conventional methods and, with specimens from asymptomatic persons, the sensitivity may drop to below 60% (VERANO and MICHALSKI 1990).

Simple diagnostic kits that may be used directly in the dental office are now available. Examples are the Kodak SureCell assay (FERRIS and FISHER 1992) and SYVA MicroTrak (MACPHAIL et al. 1995). These give a result within 15 min, but suffer from the same disadvantages of sensitivity and specificity as the laboratory-based rapid methods, and the shelf-life of the kits is usually short (only a few months). For vesicular lesions due to HSV, the sensitivity has been reported to be as high as 100%, but when infections are at a non-vesicular stage the sensitivity drops to as low as 76% (DORIAN et al. 1990) or even lower (ZIMMERMAN et al. 1991). Thus a negative result should be confirmed by a standard laboratory culture.

Other rapid laboratory methods use DNA hydridisation, but reported sensitivities are as low as 25% (SEAL et al. 1991). The polymerase chain reaction (PCR), however, is proving a reliable and sensitive rapid method for detecting HSV on smears, though it is not diagnostically superior to viral culture (NAHASS et al. 1992).

2.1.9 Management

2.1.9.1 Primary Stomatitis. HSV-induced oral lesions are managed mainly with supportive treatment, particularly maintenance of fluid intake, antipyretics, analgesics and topical antiseptics to prevent bacterial superinfection. Antivirals are

Table 4. Indications for acyclovir therapy

Type of infection	Route and dosage[a]
Mucocutaneous HSV in an immunocompromised patient	200–400 mg orally five times/day or 5 mg/kg intravenously every 8 h for 7–10 days[b] 5% cream topically every 6 h for 7 days
HSV encephalitis	10 mg/kg intravenously every 8 h for 10–14 days[c]
Neonatal HSV	10 mg/kg intravenously every 8 h for 10–14 days[c]
Varicella in normal host	20 mg/kg orally four times/day for 5 days (maximal dose 800 mg/day)
Varicella in an immunocompromised patient	10 mg/kg intravenously every 8 h for 7–10 days[c]
Herpes zoster in a normal host	800 mg orally five times/day for 7 days
Herpes zoster in an immunocompromised patient	10 mg/kg intravenously every 8 h for 7–10 days

Modified from WHITLEY and GNANN (1992).
HSV, herpes simplex virus.
[a] The doses are for adults with normal renal function unless otherwise stated.
[b] A dose of 250 mg/m² body surface area should be given to children under 12 years of age.
[c] A dose of 500 mg/m² body surface area should be given to children under 12 years of age.

Table 5. Antiviral therapy of oral herpes simplex virus (HSV) infection

Disease	Otherwise healthy patient	Immunocompromised patient
Primary herpetic gingivostomatitis	Consider oral acyclovir 100–200 mg five times a day[a]	Acyclovir 250 mg/m^2 intravenously every 8 h or 400 mg orally five times a day
Recurrent herpetic lesions, e.g. herpes labialis	Acyclovir 5% cream	Consider systemic acyclovir as above, depending on risk to patient of infection

[a] See text for details.

indicated predominantly for immunocompromised patients or where there are frequent severe recurrences or complications (Tables 4, 5). Acylovir, active against HSV thymidine kinase, is still the antiviral of most proven efficacy and safety.

Non-immunocompromised patients with primary HSV stomatitis generally present for treatment with lesions in a late stage of development, and the general view is that acyclovir is then unlikely to be of especial value, *may* elicit resistant HSV, and is therefore not indicated (Table 4).

2.1.9.2 Recurrences. Acyclovir 5% cream may shorten or abort recurrences of herpes labialis (Gibson et al. 1986), but must be applied in the early prodromal phase to have effect in the immunocompetent patient. Use later in the disease is unlikely to be beneficial and is possibly contraindicated, bearing in mind the theoretical possibility of producing viral resistance (Table 5).

Oral acyclovir has been shown to produce marginal improvement in herpes labialis and suppresses recurrences (Raborn et al. 1987). Long-term suppressive therapy using 200 mg acyclovir orally four times a day may significantly suppress recurrences; though associated with no important side effect (Raborn et al. 1988), it should be avoided in pregnancy.

Acyclovir also appears to be clinically beneficial in treatment of herpetic whitlows (Laskin 1985), eczema herpeticum (Taieb et al. 1985), herpetic encephalitis (Whitley et al. 1986) and post-herpetic erythema multiforme (Lynn et al. 1987).

Because reactivation of HSV is a major cause of morbidity in immunocompromised patients, producing prolonged pain and occasionally mucocutaneous or visceral dissemination, systemic acyclovir can then be of substantial value (Gluckman et al. 1983). Viral shedding, pain and duration of lesions are substantially reduced using acyclovir, either intravenously at a dose of 250 mg/m^2 body surface area every 8 h or orally 400 mg five times a day (Shepp et al. 1985). However, treatment of established lesions in immunocompromised patients is less satisfactory than prophylaxis, and it has been suggested that prophylaxis might actually minimise, rather than increase, the risk of acyclovir resistance. Acyclovir has been advocated for prophylaxis in immunocompromised adults using an oral dose of 200 mg three to four times daily (Mindel 1991) or acyclovir topically.

Acyclovir resistance is now becoming a clinical problem, however (Epstein and Scully 1991). Crumpacker (1988) found that 7% of HSV isolates were acyclovir resistant, mostly those from immunocompromised hosts. Significant clinical infections with acyclovir-resistant HSV are now being reported with increasing frequency (WESTHEIM et al. 1987; SCHINAZI et al. 1986), particularly in patients with leukaemia, after tissue and organ transplants and in those with HIV disease (SCHINAZI et al. 1986; NORRIS et al. 1987; ERLICH et al. 1989; YOULE et al. 1988; MACPHAIL et al. 1989).

Most acyclovir-resistant HSV isolates are thymidine kinase deficient (CRUMPACKER 1988) but are, fortunately, still sensitive to foscarnet (trisodium phosphonoformate hexahydrate) (YOULE et al. 1988; MACPHAIL et al. 1989). Foscarnet inhibits HSV-specific DNA polymerase and has low toxicity to mammalian cells (RINGDEN et al. 1986).

2.1.10 Erythema Multiforme

Erythema multiforme is a recurrent condition characterised by a rash, oral and labial erosions and conjunctivitis in various combinations, which may be precipitated by a range of factors, particularly drugs and micro-organisms. Most cases have thus far been regarded as idiopathic, since no precipitant was known, though the association of some erythema multiforme with HSV has always been well recognised (GRIMWOOD et al. 1983; LOZADA-NUR and SHILLITOE 1985; HUFF and WESTON 1989). However, a history of HSV infection often precedes recurrent erythema multiforme (LEIGH et al. 1985); HSV antigens have now been found in circulating immune complexes (KAZMIEROWSKI et al. 1982; ORTON et al. 1984) and can sometimes be demonstrated in cutaneous (ORTON et al. 1984) and oral lesions (MALMSTROM et al. 1990), even though HSV cannot be regularly cultured or identified electron-microscopically (LEIGH et al. 1985; HUFF and WESTON 1989). HSV DNA has now been demonstrated in lesional tissue by in situ hybridization (BRICE et al. 1989), and PCR has now shown HSV DNA to be present in up to 80% of cases (ASLANZADEH et al. 1992; BRICE et al. 1989; DARRAGH et al. 1991; WESTON et al. 1992; MIURA et al. 1992). It is clear, therefore, that much of what has been regarded as idiopathic recurrent erythema multiforme is, in fact, HSV related.

A combination of immune reactions, particularly immune complex formation to HSV, probably cause this type of erythema multiforme rather than any epidermotropic viral effect of HSV (LEADING ARTICLE 1989). Individuals who have the genetic background of HLA-B15 (DUVIC et al. 1983) and HLA DQw3 (KAMPGEN et al. 1988) appear to be predisposed to HSV-induced erythema multiforme; there are as yet no defined immune response differences between those who do and those who do not develop erythema multiforme (BRICE et al. 1993).

Antivirals such as acyclovir can control recurrences of HSV-related erythema multiforme (MOLIN 1987; GREEN et al. 1985; LEMAK et al. 1986), though, interestingly, HSV DNA remains in the skin despite continuous acyclovir therapy (MIURA et al. 1992). In severe cases, corticosteroids may also be indicated (DETJEN et al. 1992), or levamisole may be of value (LOZADA-NUR et al. 1992).

2.1.11 Lichen Planus

HSV DNA may sometimes be found in lichen planus, but HSV is not necessarily causal (COX et al. 1993).

2.1.12 Keratoses

Again, HSV DNA may be found in keratoses (COX et al. 1993), but the association may not be causal.

2.1.13 Oral Carcinoma

The current evidence highlights the role of papillomaviruses rather than HSV in oral carcinoma, as discussed later. HSV-1 is nevertheless clearly oncogenic. HSV is capable of transforming cells *in vitro*, provided cytolysis is inhibited (DUFF and RAPP 1971; RAPP 1981), by factors such as ultraviolet light (RAPP 1981) and certain chemicals (HIRSCH et al. 1984). In some *in vitro* systems such as SV40-transformed hamster embryo cells, HSV is more effective than some chemical carcinogens in amplifying SV40 DNA sequences (SCHLEHOFER et al. 1983; MATZ et al. 1984), acting via HSV-encoded DNA polymerase (MATZ et al. 1984, 1985). Several reports indicate that HSV acts synergistically with chemical carcinogens in causing oncogenic transformation (JOHNSON 1982; KOCERA et al. 1983; PARK et al. 1991), and it is now clear that HSV is synergistic with tobacco-specific nitrosamines in cell transformation.

In vitro HSV induces chromosomal aberration, mutations and gene amplification, and in the hamster cheek pouch model of dimethylbenzanthracene-induced carcinogenesis it enhances *erbB1* oncogene amplification and overexpression (OH et al. 1989), a feature that coincides with the appearance of malignancy. HSV also binds to the receptor for basic fibroblast growth factor, and this interaction might conceivably activate *myc* and other oncogenes.

Animal studies suggest that HSV may be a co-carcinogen with tobacco or other chemicals (HIRSCH et al. 1984; PARK et al. 1986; LARSSON et al. 1989; OH et al. 1989) and that immunisation against HSV prevents the co-carcinogenic activity of HSV with dimethylbenzanthracene (PARK et al. 1990). Substantial evidence suggests, therefore, that HSV might under particular circumstances be oncogenic.

Studies of the association of HSV with oral carcinoma have shown interesting results. A number of studies have shown changes in levels of serum antibodies to HSV patients with oral carcinoma (LARSSON et al. 1991; VASUDEVAN et al. 1991; SHILLITOE et al. 1982, 1983; KUMARI et al. 1985). For example, serum IgA antibodies to HSV-1-induced antigens may be increased in tobacco smokers, whether they have oral carcinoma or not, but the increases in smokers without tumours are less than in those with carcinomas.

There is a higher reactivity to the HSV IE protein ICP4 in patients with oral cancer, suggesting a different course of an earlier herpetic infection, with a prolonged exposure to IE proteins of HSV as a consequences of smoking

(LARSSON et al. 1991). Smoking may act, at least in part, by suppressing NK cell activity, which is involved in control of HSV. Indeed, there are close relationships between NK cell activity and antibody production to HSV in patients with carcinoma of the head and neck (SCHANTZ et al. 1986). Systemic factors often associated with oral carcinoma, such as alcohol and liver disease, might also impair NK cell activity.

Examination of oral carcinoma tissues for HSV viral "footprints" has given interesting, but equivocal results, though failure to demonstrate HSV products does not, of course, exclude a "hit and run" mechanism. HSV antigens have been shown in carcinomas in some, but not all studies. Our demonstration, using *in situ* hybridisation, of RNA complementary to HSV DNA in biopsy specimens from oral carcinoma but not from autologous, clinically normal oral mucosa suggested an association of HSV with oral carcinoma (SCULLY et al. 1982; EGLIN et al. 1983), and others have since demonstrated HSV-1 DNA in oral carcinoma tissue (VASUDEVAN et al. 1991). However, this is not *proof*, since hybridisation could be revealing segments of normal host nucleic acid with homology to part of the HSV genome.

Therefore, the evidence for an association of oral carcinoma with HSV, though stronger than for other herpesviruses or adenoviruses, is not unequivocal. However, carcinogenesis is not a single-step procedure with a single aetiology, and it has been suggested that HSV may act synergistically with HPV in carcinogenesis. With regards to cervical carcinoma, epidemiological evidence indicates that this may be possible and, in experimental situations, it has been demonstrated that keratinocytes immortalised by HPV-16 DNA are tumourigenic in nude mice following transfection with HSV DNA (IWASAKA et al. 1988; DiPAOLO et al. 1990).

Further studies are needed to investigate the role of HSV in oral carcinogenesis. The possible association of HSV with carcinoma is discussed fully elsewhere (PARK et al. 1992; SCULLY 1983, 1992; SCULLY et al. 1991; SCULLY and SAMARANAYAKE 1992; SHILLITOE 1991; LARSSEN et al. 1991).

2.1.14 Aphthae

The controversial possible association of HSV with aphthae and Behcet's syndrome is discussed elsewhere (SCULLY et al. 1991; SCULLY 1993; PEDERSEN et al. 1993).

2.2 Herpes Varicella Zoster Virus

VZV, sometimes termed herpesvirus-3, can cause chickenpox (varicella) or shingles (zoster) (STRAUS et al. 1988; HYMAN 1987; SCULLY and SAMARANAYAKE 1992; SCULLY, 1995).

There appears to be only one type of VZV. The virus contains five glycoproteins, of which the main ones are gpI, gpII and gpIII (DAVISON et al. 1986), antibodies against these glycoproteins having neutralizing activity (GROSE and LITWIN 1988; BRUNELL et al. 1987).

2.2.1 Varicella (Chickenpox)

2.2.1.1 Immunopathogenesis. VZV infects mainly via the respiratory tract and, after a viraemia, may produce mucocutaneous lesions. Most infections are subclinical, but chickenpox is the clinical manifestation of primary infection with VZV. It is seen predominantly in children, usually in late winter and spring. There appears to be an increasing incidence of chickenpox both in adult immigrants from the developing world and in immunocompromised patients.

The oropharynx is a site for early replication of VZV. The virus then spreads to sensory nerve ganglia, where it becomes latent. Immunity to VZV is mainly cellular. Cytotoxic T cells and ADCC mechanisms appear to be protective, as is interferon, and, where these mechanisms are impaired, there may be severe disease and recurrence (SCULLY, 1995; SCULLY and SAMARANAYAKE 1992).

Infection with VZV usually confers life-long protection except in some immunocompromised patients.

2.2.1.2 Clinical Features. The incubation period is 14–21 days. Many primary infections are subclinical or pass unnoticed, but chickenpox may present with malaise, anorexia, irritability and fever followed by vesicles and mouth ulcers mainly on the palate and tongue. There is a rash affecting the scalp and then the face, neck and trunk. Lesions are seen at all stages in development, from itchy, red macules to papules (1–4 mm in diameter), vesicles, pustules and scabs (i.e. the rash is centripetal, and it crops).

2.2.1.3 Diagnosis. Diagnosis of chickenpox is clinical, and only enterovirus infections and a few other viral infections need to be excluded. A Tzanck smear from a lesion, culture or electron microscopy can be useful where the diagnosis is in doubt, but PCR detection of VZV DNA is superior (NAHASS et al. 1992).

2.2.1.4 Complications. Most patients recover spontaneously in 2–3 weeks, but a few, especially pregnant women, develop complications such as pneumonia (PREBLUD, 1986; PREBLUD et al. 1984). Varicella during pregnancy also poses a risk to the fetus, which may be born with cicatricial scarring and limb deformities and may subsequently also suffer zoster as a child.

Immunocompromised patients can develop widespread and severe disease. Such patients are covered with poxes which also affect oral and other mucosae, liver and spleen.

Reye's syndrome, characterised by central nervous system (CNS) symptoms, cerebral oedema and fatty degeneration of the liver, may follow varicella if there is salicylate use: VZV appears to be a factor in 16%–28% of cases.

2.2.1.5 Management. Varicella is benign in otherwise healthy persons, and only supportive management is required. However, antivirals such as acyclovir may be indicated if the patient is immunocompromised. Passive immunisation with varicella zoster immunoglobulin (VZIg) can also modify or prevent varicella in these groups, and a safe and effective varicella vaccine is also now available (GERSHON et al. 1990; ISSACS and MENSER 1990).

2.2.2 Zoster (Shingles)

During chickenpox, VZV ascends to the dorsal root ganglion cells, where it becomes latent. When reactivated, VZV is transported via sensory nerve axons to the skin and/or mucosa and may produce zoster.

2.2.2.1 Epidemiology. Zoster affects up to 20% of all individuals at some stage in life, but is most common in the elderly and in the immunocompromised. A total of 75% of those affected are more than 45 years old, and some 50% of immunocompromised persons suffer at least one attack of zoster. Occasionally, there are recurrent attacks of zoster in healthy persons, but this is far less common than in immunocompromised persons (SCULLY, 1995).

2.2.2.2 Clinical Features and Diagnosis. Most zoster affects elderly patients, usually in the thoracic (56%) or head and neck (13%) regions. In the head and neck region, ophthalmic zoster is about 20 times more common than zoster in other trigeminal divisions, and it threatens the eye.

The rash of zoster resembles that of chickenpox in its development, but it is restricted to a dermatome, i.e. the area of skin (and mucosa) supplied by a sensory nerve. The rash is typically unilateral and in a band-like distribution, hence the terms zoster (Greek) or shingles (Latin), meaning "belt". Macules progress through papules and small vesicles to produce pustules by 3–4 days. If the maxillary or mandibular divisions of the trigeminal nerve are involved, mouth ulceration is usually seen (MILLAR and TROULIS, 1994).

Severe pain often precedes, accompanies and follows the rash of herpes zoster, sometimes persisting for months or years (post-herpetic neuralgia). The pain may simulate toothache. Some 70% of those with zoster, mostly the elderly, have pain persisting after the rash heals, usually for about 1 month, which is the definition of post-herpetic neuralgia. Nearly 30% have neuralgia persisting for up to 6 months, and some longer. Post-herpetic neuralgia may be aggravated by temperature changes and tends to be worse at night, but usually slowly improves and resolves over 1 year or so. Only 2%–5% have pain lasting 1 year or more (WOOD 1991).

The nature of post-herpetic neuralgia varies between patients, but two main types have now been distinguished. The first is a constant pain, and the other a paroxysmal pain, stimulating idiopathic trigeminal neuralgia. Either may be triggered by touching the area.

2.2.2.3 Variants and Complications. Zoster is occasionally bilateral (HILL and LAMEY, 1986) or may be generalised (this is usually in the immunocompromised). Very occasionally, oral lesions alone are seen in mandibular or maxillary zoster.

Zoster occasionally occurs without a rash (zoster sine herpete) (BARRETT et al. 1993). Necrosis of jaw bone and, if zoster affects a child, dental hypoplasia and retarded tooth eruption may be seen (SMITH et al. 1984).

2.2.2.4 Herpes Zoster in the Immunocompromised Patient.

Zoster is common in immunocompromised patients, especially in those with Hodgkin's lymphoma, particularly where there has been radio- or chemotherapy, and in HIV disease. In patients with HIV infectio, zoster can be severe and may be predictive of the development of acquired immunodeficiency syndrome (AIDS) (MELBYE et al. 1987).

Morbidity is high in immunocompromised patients, with persistent zoster lesions, significant tissue destruction, scarring, viral dissemination and more severe post-herpetic neuralgia. The rates of post-herpetic neuralgia in immunocompromised patients range from 18% to 45%, about the same as rates in immunocompetent patients (WOOD, 1991). Chronic zoster and persistent CNS infection with progressive encephalopathy may ocasionally develop (MANDAL 1987; RYDER et al. 1986).

2.2.2.5 Diagnosis of Oro-facial Zoster.

Diagnosis of zoster is usually clinical and made on the basis of the severe unilateral pain, the unilateral rash restricted to a dermatome, and unilateral mouth ulcers. A Tzanck smear, culture, electron microscopy or serology are very occasionally required for diagnosis (SZAKI et al. 1990; TOVI et al. 1985).

Occasionally, cutaneous recurrent HSV lesions or enterovirus lesions occur in one dermatome and simulate zoster. Hand, food and mouth disease, measles and Rickettsial pox very rarely need to be considered in the differential diagnosis.

2.2.2.6 Management.

An underlying immune defect should be excluded, but zoster is more commonly simply a consequence of old age.

Treatment is mainly supportive but, in ophthalmic zoster, it is important to seek an early specialist opinion because of the danger to sight. Antivirals such as acyclovir may also be needed, particularly in immunocompromised patients. Oral acyclovir given not later than 72h after rash onset in a dose of 800mg five times daily for 7-10 days hastens resolution of lesions and reduces both the acute pain and the incidence and duration of post-herpetic neuralgia (CROOKS et al. 1991). Zoster-immune globulin may also help to control lesions in immunocompromised patients.

Analgesics are indicated to control the pain in zoster, but post-herpetic neuralgia may prove refractory to even potent analgesics. Corticosteroids given in the acute phase may be of some value in preventing the development of pain. Amantadine given in acute zoster or levodopa may be of value in controlling herpetic neuralgia, but tricyclics or an anticonvulsant such as sodium valproate or carbamazepine is usually preferred (LEADING ARTICLE 1990; LOESER 1986). Topical capsaicin, an antagonist of substance P, is of unproven value, but shows promise. EMLA cream may be of some analgesic value (STOW et al. 1989).

Transcutaneous nerve stimulation or ethyl chloride sprays may relieve the pain. Very ocasionally, neurosurgery is indicated; one procedure (dorsal root entry zone coagulation, the Nashold procedure) may produce at least short-term benefit.

2.2.2.7 Aphthae. There may be a slight rise in VZV antibody titres in patients with aphthae (PEDERSEN and HORNSLETH 1993). The speculative association of VZV with aphthae is discussed elsewhere (PEDERSEN et al. 1993; PEDERSEN 1989).

2.2.2.8 Oral Carcinoma. There is, at least on serological evidence, no association between VZV and oral carcinoma (LARSSON et al. 1991).

2.3 Epstein-Barr Virus

EBV is a herpesvirus that infects and replicates in oral and oropharyngeal epithelium and infects, activates and can immortalize B lymphocytes (SCULLY and SAMARANAYAKE 1992; SCULLY 1995).

In developing countries, most children have been infected by EBV, usually asymptomatically, by the age of 18 months. In developed countries, there are two peaks of prevalence of EBV infection, one in pre-school children and the other in teenagers and adolescents (EVANS 1982).

The virus causes the clinical syndrome of infectious mononucleosis, mainly in adolescents of higher socio-economic groups, but it is implicated in a range of other disorders.

2.3.1 Virology

EBV consists mainly of a nucleocapsid and an envelope with external glycoprotein spikes containing mainly (gp350/220). EBV genes code nuclear antigens (EBNA) and latent membrane proteins (LMP), as well as others.

At least two EBV types have been identified on the basis of their *Bam*H1 WYH gene, which encodes EBNA-2A (see below). These types, known as EBV-A (or EBV-1) and EBV-B (or EBV-2), are closely related and differ mainly in genes related to the cycle of latent infection. The types are distinguished mainly by the variant of EBNA-2 that they express: EBV-A expresses EBNA-2A, and EBV-B expresses EBNA-2B. They also differ in EBNA-3A, EBNA-3B and EBNA-3C (ROWE et al. 1989; SAMPLE et al. 1990) and in LMP-1 (WALLING et al. 1994; MILLER et al. 1994). Both EBV types are seen worldwide, but EBV-A is the main type in the West, and EBV-B the main type in Africa (SIXBEY et al. 1989).

EBV-A is more prevalent in higher socio-economic classes (YAO et al. 1991). However, immunodeficient individuals, especially those with HIV disease, show more infection with EBV-B or dual infections (SIXBEY et al. 1989; SCULLEY et al. 1990).

2.3.2 Immunopathogenesis of Infection

EBV binds to receptors mainly on epithelial cells and B lymphocytes. Lingual epithelium has been shown to have receptors for EBV (Corso et al. 1989; TALACKO et al. 1991), as have cervical, salivary and lacrimal epithelia. The EBV receptors are identical to receptors for the complement component C3d and are sometimes known as C3dR, CR2 or CD21. The EBV receptor binds to the EBV gp350/220. EBV infects mainly the basal and intermediate layers of epithelium, where it remains latent and, as the epithelial cells differentiate and move towards the luminal surface, the receptor is lost. This whole area is thoroughly reviewed elsewhere (WOLF et al. 1993).

When EBV infects B lymphocytes, some B cells produce EBV early antigen (EA) and viral capsid antigen (VCA) and undergo lysis, but other B cells carry EBV as a latent infection for the rest of the cell's life and express nuclear antigens. Eight genes are expressed: six EBNA and two LMP. The functions of only some antigens are known, but it is clear that EBNA-2 and LMP-1 induce cell proliferation, probably either by stimulating oncogenes or inactivating tumour suppressor genes. EBNA-2 appears to be involved in cell transformation, and LMP interacts with vimentin of the cytoskeleton, acting as an oncogene. EBV can also up-regulate the oncogene *bcl-2* (HENDERSON et al. 1991) and can degrade the tumour suppressor gene product *p53* (FARRELL et al. 1991). *Bcl-2* up-regulation stops programmed cell death (apoptosis) and activates CD23 (see below) and the adhesion molecules lymphocyte function-associated antigen (LFA)-1, intercellular adhesion molecule (ICAM)-1 and LFA-3. LMP can induce phenotypic changes in epithelial cells. EBNA-2, -3 and -6 and LMP are target molecules for T lymphocyte killing.

EBV-infected B cells move into the G_1 phase of the cell cycle and begin to express a surface receptor termed CD23 (blast-2), which is a receptor for B cell growth factors and can stimulate the growth of EBV-transformed cells. EBV infection also induces new antigens such as CD30, against which T lymphocytes and NK cells can respond.

Membrane antigens (MA) are expressed only later in EBV infection; one such antigen is detectable only by a T lymphocyte response and is thus termed LYDMA (lymphocyte-detectable membrane antigen). Another, termed gp340, is a principal target for neutralising antibodies. As discussed above, adhesion molecules (LFA-1, ICAM-1 and LFA-3) are also expressed.

EBV infection thus gives rise to two main consequences. Firstly, activated T cells, mainly suppressor (Ts) and cytotoxic (Tc) cells appear in the peripheral blood as atypical mononuclear cells (Downey cells), hence "mononucleosis". Secondly, B lymphocytes, polyclonally activated by EBV, can produce multiple antibodies, including some auto-antibodies and also antibodies reacting to other species (heterophile antibodies). The latter can react with sheep (or cow or horse) erythrocytes, and this forms the basis of the heterophile antibody test (Paul-Bunnell-Davidsohn test).

Immune defences, predominantly T cells, NK cells and other cytotoxic cells, and interferon lyse B cells infected with EBV. Then, some 2 weeks after infection, suppressor T cells appear, which suppress heterophile and other antibody production by B cells and suppress the T cell lymphoproliferative responses, thus causing a mild, transient immune defect.

2.3.3 Clinical Features of Primary Infection

The incubation period is 30–49 days (mainly 15–25 days). In young children, EBV infection is often asymptomatic or may produce pharyngitis or tonsillitis. In adolescents or adults, EBV typically produces a glandular fever syndrome (infectious mononucleosis) in about 50% of those infected. Sore throat, fever, lymph node enlargement and profound malaise are the main features.

The saliva contains EBV. Oral lesions are seen in about 32% of patients and are the first sign in about half of these. Cervical lymph node enlargement, pharyngitis, creamy white confluent tonsillar exudate, faucial oedema, palatal petechiae, pericoronitis and occasional oral ulceration or acute ulcerative gingivitis are seen. Candidosis may appear if there is significant immune suppression consequent upon the EBV infection.

2.3.4 Diagnosis

Investigations may well be indicated, since similar glandular fever-like syndromes can be caused by HIV, human (HCMV), toxoplasmosis, and human herpesvirus-6. Diphtheria may enter into the differential diagnosis of the faucial exudate.

A blood film in infectious mononucleosis shows mononucleosis and atypical lymphocytes (Downey cells); these are large cells with pale-blue vacuolated cytoplasm and an elongated or dented nucleus with coarse chromatin. However, Downey cells, which have T suppressor–cytotoxic activity, are not specific to infectious mononucleosis.

Serodiagnosis is more helpful. Most patients have heterophile antibodies, which are IgM antibodies that appear early in the incubation period, persist for up to 1 year, are detectable by the Paul-Bunnell or Monospot tests and are positive only in infectious mononucleosis. IgG and IgM antibodies to VCA with no antibodies to EBNA is the typical serological pattern.

Throat swabs may be required to exclude diphtheria.

2.3.5 Management

Supportive care and rest are indicated. Acyclovir is of little overall benefit in management of infectious mononucleosis. If there is pharyngeal oedema, systemic corticosteroids may be indicated.

2.3.6 Complications of Infection

Most patients recover uneventfully, but post-viral fatigue is common. Occasionally, pharyngeal oedema can threaten the airway, and a range of auto-immune and other complications can arise. Neurological complications, splenic rupture or serious liver disease and Reye's syndrome are rare.

Lymphoproliferative disorders may occur, especially in immunocompromised patients, in HIV disease and in the rare X-linked Duncan's lymphoproliferative syndrome.

2.3.6.1 Chronic Infection. EBV may cause unusual or protracted chronic illness with vague malaise, fever, weight loss, hepatosplenomegaly, lymphadenopathy and other features (LEADING ARTICLE 1985; BEAUPARLANT et al. 1994). However, it is unclear whether EBV is responsible for the chronic fatigue syndrome (CFS), since features of this are very varied and often non-specific.

It is likely that CFS represents a spectrum of illness with various aetiologies such as enteroviruses or possibly human herpesvirus-6.

2.3.7 Latency and Reactivation

EBV remains latent mainly in salivary glands. It can be latent in apparently healthy oral mucosa (LONING et al. 1987; GROSS et al. 1988; SNIJDERS et al. 1990; MADINIER et al. 1992), and in the West this is mainly either EBV-A (50%) or EBV-B (41%), though a minority (9%) have both types (SIXBEY et al. 1989). EBV also remains latent in B cells in some long-term carriers and appears to avoid immune detection (YAO et al. 1989). EBV-infected B cells may occasionally transform to lymphoma; the EBNA-2 gene is directly involved, but additional factors such as environmental mutagens or mitogens (for example, malaria infection) or cytogenic errors are probably also involved.

Immunosuppression is the only stimulus to EBV reactivation that has been well described; immunosuppressed patients shed EBV in the oropharynx, and it is found in saliva (YAO et al. 1991; ALSIP et al. 1988; DIAZ-MITOMA et al. 1990; PREIKSAITIS et al. 1992). The *Bam*HI Z EBV replication activator (ZEBRA) protein is involved in the switch from viral latency to the productive cycle (MATHEW et al. 1994).

2.3.8 Hairy Leukoplakia

Hairy leukoplakia (HL) is a white lesion in the mouth originally described in individuals infected with HIV. HL has been considered virtually pathognomonic of HIV infection and a good indicator of impending AIDS (REICHART et al., 1989; but see below). The lesions of HL are corrugated or have a shaggy or "hairy" appearance, are usually found on the lateral margins of the tongue, are mostly without symptoms and have no known pre-malignant potential (GREENSPAN et al. 1984; GREENSPAN and GREEN 1989; GREEN et al. 1989; SCULLY et al. 1989).

Histological features include hyperparakeratosis, hyperplasia and ballooning of prickle cells with depletion of Langerhan's cells (DANIELS et al. 1987; KANAS et al. 1988; SCIUBBA et al. 1989) and with only a sparse inflammatory cell infiltrate in the lamina propria (EVERSOLE et al. 1986). Ultrastructural features are discussed elsewhere (BELTON and EVERSOLE 1986; KANAS et al. 1988). Electron-microscopic examination of cytological smears (EPSTEIN et al. 1995) may be diagnostically superior to Papanicolaou (PAP)-stained smears (MIGLIORATI et al. 1993; LUMERMAN et al. 1990; FRAGA-FERNANDEZ and VICANTI-PLAZA 1992).

EBV has been shown to be present in HL. Electron microscopy, immunostaining, and Southern blot and *in situ* hybridization for EBV DNA shows EBV in the upper spinous layers of the epithelium (SCIUBBA et al. 1989; GROSS et al. 1988; SYRJANEN et al. 1988; GREENSPAN et al. 1984, 1985; EVERSOLE et al. 1988; SCIUBBA and SCHWARTZ, 1987; LONING et al. 1987; SUGIHARA et al. 1990; MABRUK et al. 1994, 1995). Viral proteins characteristic of the replicative phase can be found (YOUNG et al. 1991). EBV receptors on the parakeratinised oral mucosae (CORSO et al. 1989), such as on the lateral margin of the tongue, appear to explain the site predilection for HL, but EBV DNA is also present in some sites where no HL is clinically evident (ZHANG et al. 1988; NAHER et al. 1991). The decrease in epithelial Langerhan's cells might be a sequel of, or might predispose to, viral infection (DRIJKONINGEN et al. 1988). EBV regulation, at least in B lymphocytes, is known to be disturbed in HIV infection (BIRX et al. 1986). The exact site of EBV latency in the epithelium is unclear (BECKER et al. 1991; NIEDOBITEK et al. 1991). EBV-1 or EBV-2 or both may be found, and co-infection and recombination are common (WALLING et al. 1992, 1994, 1995). The EBV in patients from the West usually appear to lack EBNA-2 or are present as EBNA-2-defective variants which may escape T cell attack (GILLIGAN et al. 1990; PATTON et al. 1990; WALLING et al. 1994) or may result in the unusual course of this infection. LMP are expressed (GILLIGAN et al. 1990; THOMAS et al. 1991; SANDVEJ et al. 1992).

Further evidence for a causal role for EBV in HL is the regression of HL on treatment with antivirals which block EBV replication, such as acyclovir (FRIEDMAN-KIEN, 1986; USCHENDORF et al. 1988; RESNICK et al. 1988; FICARRA et al. 1988) or ganciclovir (NEWMAN and POLK, 1987), and the failure to resolve with antifungals (FICARRA et al. 1988), despite the frequent presence of candida species. HL in HIV-infected individuals may also occasionally improve spontaneously or with zidovudine (BROCKMEYER et al. 1989; KESSLER et al. 1988; PHELAN and KLEIN, 1988). However, HL is usually without symptoms and, though it may be the source of concern to the patient, its treatment is rarely indicated.

Thus it appears that HL is associated with EBV and is not uncommon in HIV-infected individuals. However, recent work indicates that the situation is more complex than formerly supposed. Firstly, oral white lesions other than HL can occasionally be seen in HIV-infected subjects, and these may have some of the histological features typical of HL, especially the hyperparakeratosis (GREEN et al. 1989; EVERSOLE et al. 1986); however, they are typically EBV DNA negative, though it seems likely that EBV DNA will be found in some, in view of its evident latency in oral and oropharyngeal mucosa (SIXBEY et al. 1984; JALAL et al. 1992; MABRUK et al. 1995). Secondly, it is increasingly evident, and not surprising, that lesions clinically and histologically similar to HL can be seen in patients with HIV infection (BREHMER-ANDERSSON et al. 1994). Finally, HL may be seen in patients immunocompromised for reasons other than HIV infection, such as those undergoing bone marrow (EPSTEIN et al. 1988, 1991, 1993; BIREK et al. 1989), renal (ITIN et al. 1988; SYRJANEN et al. 1989; GREENSPAN et al. 1989; MACLEOD et al. 1990; KANITAKIS et al. 1991), heart (SCHMIDT-WESTHAUSEN et al. 1990, 1991) or liver transplants (SCHMIDT-WESTHAUSEN et al. 1993), in myelodysplasia (FICARRA et al. 1991), ulcerative colitis (FLUCKIGER et al. 1994) and Wegener's granulomatosis (WALLING et al. 1995) and in patients on systemic corticosteroids (SCHIODT et al. 1995). HL has even been seen in apparently healthy HIV-seronegative subjects (EISENBERG et al. 1992), though in others their HIV status could not be absolutely assured (GREENSPAN and GREEN, 1989).

Thus it appears that HL is not absolutely specific for HIV, but rather a manifestation of chronic immunosuppression, and it is occasionally seen in apparently immunocompetent persons. In immunocompromised patients, the occurrence of HL is not always related to the CD4 lymphocyte count (REICHART et al. 1989; SCHMIDT-WESTHAUSEN et al. 1993).

HL does not appear to be potentially malignant and the EBNA-2 defect may explain this, since that gene is required for transformation. Nevertheless, there may be an association between HL and the subsequent development of malignant lymphoproliferative diseases (MOORE et al. 1991).

2.3.9 Lymphoproliferative Diseases

EBV infection can lead to a number of lymphoproliferative diseases in which transformation-associated EBV genes such as LMP-1 can be found (YOUNG et al. 1989).

2.3.9.1 Burkitt's Lymphoma. Burkitt's lymphoma (BL) is a highly malignant B lymphocyte lymphoma found endemically in equatorial Africa and in Papua New Guinea. It was the first human tumour known to be associated with a virus. African BL is found in areas where there is hyperendemic malaria, and it accounts for about 50% of childhood malignancies in Africa. Sporadic cases are found elsewhere and in HIV disease.

2.3.9.1.1 Epidemiology. BL is virtually unknown in infancy. The peak incidence in African BL is in the 4- to 7-year age-group, and 80% of patients fall in the 3- to 12-year age-group. There is male to female predominance of 2:1 to 4:1. Jaw involvement is most common in the younger age-groups. Most patients in Africa have been African; elsewhere there is no notable racial predilection.

2.3.9.1.2 Pathogenesis. EBV was first found in explants of BL following the search for an infectious agent suggested by the unique geographic distribution of African BL. Virus particles are not seen in tumour biopsy material; presumably, tissue culture releases a block that inhibits expression of latent EBV.

The first direct evidence of viral-specific material in these tumours was provided by the discovery of MA on freshly biopsied tumour cells and of EBNA in at least 90% of cells, though EBNA-2 and LMP appear to be down-regulated (ROWE et al. 1987). EBV DNA is almost invariably detectable in biopsy material. These studies demonstrate that the EBV genome is present and expressed in the tumour cells in African BL. Further evidence of an oncogenic role of the virus is afforded by the demonstration of the ability of EBV to transform B lymphocytes *in vitro* and induce tumours in primates. The titres of serum antibodies directed against EBV antigens are increased in patients with Burkitt's lymphoma; anti-EBNA are present with very high titres of IgG anti-VCA and antibody to membrane antigen (anti-MA). Anti-EA (R) also appears.

However, EBV infection alone is clearly insufficient for tumour production, since many apparently normal individuals are infected with EBV without any malignant sequelae and, in American BL, EBV DNA is usually absent. Genetic, life-style or environmental factors must be involved. Malaria and chromosome abnormalities have been implicated as co-factors. Malaria may influence the immune response to EBV, and such patients may also be immunocompromised secondary to malnutrition. Chromosomal changes are also involved.

The first step in development of the lymphoma seems to be the induction of polyclonal B cell immortalisation by EBV, followed by promotion mediated by environmental factors, such as malaria (which stimulates further proliferation of B cells), and, finally, chronic B cell proliferation. Specific chromosome defects, which appear to occur randomly during the latter stage, result in a reciprocal 8–14 chromosomal translocation, the *myc* oncogene coming to be placed next to the immunoglobulin gene locus and subsequently be stimulated, leading to dysregulation of cell growth resulting in the lymphoma. EBV in B cells appears to elude virus-specific T cell recognition (ROONEY et al., 1985).

2.3.9.1.3 Clinical Features. BL is typically multifocal, affecting the jaws, bone marrow, post-orbital region and gastro-intestinal tract and, in girls, breasts and ovaries.

Approximately 50% of children with African BL present with jaw tumours, but in non-African cases only about 5% have jaw lesions (PATTON et al., 1990). The maxilla is mainly affected, and tumours are mainly in the molar–premolar region. Lesions in the mandible develop in the posterior body. Some 40% have multiple jaw tumours.

Dental findings include sudden, painless loosening of teeth, premature tooth eruption or displacement of teeth. Interestingly, labial anaesthesia is rare, though cranial nerve palsies due to intracranial disease are common. Radiography shows breaks in, or loss of the lamina dura, small discrete jaw radiolucencies and possibly widening of the periodontal ligament space. However, root resorption is rare (HOPP et al. 1982).

Salivary gland involvement is seen clinically in about 4% of patients, but three times as many have histological involvement. Cervical lymphadenopathy is common (AKINWANDE et al. 1986; MOSADOMI 1984).

2.3.9.1.4 Diagnosis. The clinical features of BL in a patient from an endemic area are usually suggestive, but a biopsy is needed. The histological appearance is of a poorly differentiated lymphocytic lymphoma composed mainly of surface IgM-positive B cells. Large lymphocytes with irregularly shaped (cleaved) nucleoli and cytoplasm confined to the cell periphery are present, with scattered, large, pale-staining macrophages giving a distinctive "starry sky" appearance.

2.3.9.1.5 Management. BL is sensitive to cyclophosphamide and, though a single dose may be sufficient to cause tumour regression, this drug is often used in combination with vincristine, methotrexate and corticosteroids. Local surgery or radiotherapy may help debulk a tumour. Survival rates exceed 50% and are best in younger children treated early and having minimal tumour burden.

2.3.9.2 Non-Hodgkin's Lymphomas. Non-Hodgkin's lymphomas (NHL) are being increasingly seen since the advent of the AIDS epidemic (KARP and BRODER, 1991). Approximately 3% of HIV-infected persons have NHL at the onset of AIDS, and projections suggest that many more will later develop NHL (GAIL et al. 1991). Indeed, one autopsy study showed NHL in 20% of HIV-infected patients (WILKES et al. 1988). Lymphomas have emerged as an increasingly common cause of death in AIDS; patients often present at an advanced stage, with extranodal involvement, and respond poorly to chemotherapy (MYSKOWSKI et al. 1990; CARBONE et al. 1991).

EBV is associated with about one half of the NHL in HIV disease (LENOIR and DELECLUSE, 1989). The onset of lymphomas in HIV disease is preceded by persistent generalised lymphadenopathy (PGL) in one third of cases, and therefore enlargment of pre-existent palpable lymph nodes is always an indication for a biopsy to exclude malignant lymphoma. Most NHL in AIDS are high-grade B cell malignancies, particularly diffuse large cell lymphomas and immunoblastic lymphomas, but primary lymphomas of the brain, especially BL, are also common (BERAL et al. 1991; CARBONE et al. 1991). At initial presentation, the lymphomas in AIDS are typically widely disseminated, with extranodal involvement in 65%–98% of patients. The CNS is commonly involved, presenting either as leptomeningeal lymphoma in patients with systemic disease or primary HIV-related lymphoma in the CNS, and gastro-intestinal tract involvement is seen in 7%–45% (ZIEGLER et al. 1984; KARP and BRODER 1991).

Oral NHL are now a recognised, but uncommon complication of HIV infection, typically observed as a rapidly growing mass in the fauces, gingiva or elsewhere, as an ulcer or as tooth mobility (ZIEGLER et al. 1984; LOZADA-NUR et al. 1984; LEESS et al. 1987; HOMMEL et al. 1987; BRAHIM et al. 1988; KAUGARS and BURNS, 1989; GREEN and EVERSOLE, 1989; RUBIN et al. 1989; MITCHELL et al. 1989; SODERHOLM et al. 1990; GROOT et al. 1990; COLMENERO et al. 1991; CARBONE et al. 1991; LANGFORD et al. 1991; DONKOR et al. 1991). Oral lymphomas in HIV disease may be associated with EBV (GREEN and EVERSOLE, 1989).

2.3.9.3 Other Diseases

2.3.9.3.1 Mid-line Granuloma. EBV has been associated with mid-line granuloma (VILDE et al. 1985; HARABUCHI et al. 1990), now known to be a lymphoma.

2.3.9.3.2 Hodgkin's Disease. Hodgkin's disease (HD) occurs in two peaks, at around age 25 years and at around 70 years, the younger type being found in lower socio-economic conditions. EBV serum antibody titres are higher in lymphocyte depletion and mixed cellularity types of HD, and EBV RNA and LMP have now been detected in some HD (YOUNG et al. 1989).

2.3.9.3.3 Duncan's Disease. Patients with the X-linked lymphoproliferative syndrome (Duncan's disease), if exposed to EBV, may develop a spectrum of disorders ranging from fatal infectious mononucleosis to acquired hypo-gammaglobulinaemia following infectious mononucleosis, or lymphoma (PURTILO 1980; PURTILO and SAKAMOTO 1981; PURTILO et al. 1982; SAEMUNDSEN et al. 1981).

2.3.9.3.4 Lymphomatoid Granulomatosis. Lymphomatoid granulomatosis is an unusual entity which is characterised by a mixed mononuclear cell infiltrate and areas of necrosis with atypical lymphoreticular cells and which, in some 20%–50% of cases, progresses to malignant lymphoma.

Several cases of lymphomatoid granulomatosis have been seen in AIDS patients as oral ulcers (MONTILLA et al. 1987; LIN-GREENBERG et al. 1990). EBV infection has been implicated in HIV-related lymphomatoid granulomatosis (MITTAL et al. 1990).

2.3.9.3.5 Thymic Lymphoma. EBV may be involved in thymic lymphoma (LEYVRAZ et al. 1985; DIMERY et al. 1988).

2.3.9.3.6 Hairy Cell Leukaemia. EBV has also been implicated in hairy cell leukaemia, a rare form of leukaemia (WOLF et al. 1990).

2.3.9.3.7 Sjogren's Syndrome. Sjogren's syndrome (SS) is a B cell lymphoprolifera-tive disorder that may lead to lymphoma and has occasionally closely followed primary EBV infection (WHITTINGHAM et al. 1985) PFUGFELDER et al. 1987; GASTON et al. 1991), suggesting that EBV may be one factor initiating SS. The possible association of EBV with SS is discussed elsewhere (MAITLAND and SCULLY, 1994; MIYASAKA et al. 1994). EBV RNA may be associated with the auto-antigens SS-A (Ro) and SS-B (La) found in SS (LERNER et al. 1981). EBV DNA and EBV EA may be found in SS-affected salivary tissue (MARIETTE et al. 1991; SAITO et al. 1989; KARAMERIS et al. 1992; DEACON et al. 1991, 1992; MAITLAND et al. 1995; DISS et al. 1995), though others have not found EBV EA (SYRJANEN et al. 1990). EBV DNA appears to be found in salivary glands in amounts greater than in other auto-immune diseases or normal salivary glands in some studies (MARIETTE et al. 1991; SCHUURMAN et al. 1989; SAITO et al. 1989; KARAMERIS et al. 1992), but not in others (DEACON 1991, 1992; MAITLAND et al. 1995). The detection of EBV DNA, however, appears dependent on the methodol-ogy, with, for example, PCR detecting EBV DNA in some samples which appear EBV negative by *in situ* hybridisation (MARIETTE et al. 1991; SYRJANEN et al. 1990).

The salivary glands are therefore a possible site of latency of EBV (and other viruses), although the findings neither confirm nor refute a direct association of HCMV or EBV with SS. It may be that the clinical picture termed SS is the common end-result of various aetiological factors and that different viruses might be a trigger in genetically susceptible patients or may simply be reactivated and non-causal (Fox et al., 1991). Indeed, a wide range of viruses, including HCMV, EBV, hepatitis C virus and, more recently, various retroviruses, have been implicated in SS. A salivary gland syndrome resembling SS has also been described in HIV patients (SCHIODT et al. 1989) and in those infected with HTLV-1 (SHATTLES et al. 1992; TERADA et al. 1994; SUMIDA et al. 1994).

Thus, although EBV and several other herpesviruses may latently infect salivary glands, any individual or collective role for these viruses or other agents singly or multiply in the disease remains to be confirmed.

2.3.9.3.8 Salivary Gland Tumours. EBV appears unrelated to the pathogenesis of most salivary gland neoplasms, with the possible exception of lymphoepithelial carcinoma (RAAB-TRAUB et al. 1991; HSU et al. 1994), though EBV DNA was found in all five salivary gland tumours (undefined) in one study (TYAN et al. 1993).

2.3.10 Carcinomas

2.3.10.1 Nasopharyngeal Carcinoma. EBV is also associated with undifferentiated nasopharyngeal carcinomas (FREEMAN et al. 1994; NASRIN et al. 1994), though environmental factors (probably nitrosamines from smoked fish), and genetic factors are important. There is familial clustering of cases and an association with certain HLA haplotypes in Chinese patients, particularly A2 and the antigen Singapore-2. However, no association with HLA types has been demonstrated in Tunisian patients with nasopharyngeal carcinoma. In causasoids, HLA-A2 appears to be protective (BURT et al. 1994).

The serology of nasopharyngeal carcinoma is somewhat similar to that of BL, with very high titres of IgG anti-VCA and anti-MA, but with high anti-EBNA and the presence of IgA anti-VCA. Anti-VCA and anti-EA of the IgA class may be predictive of the development of nasopharyngeal carcinoma. Furthermore, the anti-EA of nasopharyngeal carcinoma patients is of a different type (anti-D) from that found in BL (anti-R).

EBV DNA has repeatedly been shown to be present in tumour tissue from nasopharyngeal carcinoma and is also found in tumours from widely differing geographical areas, but only in undifferentiated anaplastic tumours, in the epithelium rather than in lymphoid tissues. EBNA-1, LMP-1 and LMP-2A/2B have also been detected (YOUNG et al. 1988; LIEBOWITZ 1994).

2.3.10.2 Oral Carcinoma. The association of EBV with anaplastic nasopharyngeal carcinoma is well established, and the oncogenicity of EBV is not in doubt. EBV DNA has been detected in oral carcinomas by some (MAO and SMITH, 1993; TYAN et al. 1993; HORIUCHI et al., 1995), but EBV DNA and antigens have not been demonstrated by others in oral carcinoma tissue or in carcinoma cell lines (KARJA et al. 1988; TALACKO et al. 1991; YIN et al. 1991).

2.3.10.3 Antral Carcinoma. In one very small series of three tumours, all contained EBV DNA (TYAN et al. 1993).

2.3.10.4 Adult Rhabdomyoma. EBV has been discounted in the aetiology of adult rhabdomyoma (CLEVELAND et al. 1994).

2.3.10.5 Aphthae. EBV appears unrelated to the aetiology of aphthae (PEDERSEN et al. 1993).

2.4 Human Cytomegalovirus

HCMV is a ubiquitous herpesvirus. It is emerging as an important opportunistic pathogen in immunocompromised individuals, particularly those infected with HIV; it is now apparent that HCMV may cause oral ulceration in immunocompromised subjects, and it may play a role in other diverse conditions in these and other patients (FORBES 1989; EPSTEIN and SCULLY 1994).

Sometimes termed human herpesvirus-5, or beta herpesvirus, HCMV is indistinguishable by electron microscopy from HSV and VZV. There are several strains of HCMV, but these do not appear distinct to particular syndromes (SCULLY and SAMARANAYAKE 1992; EPSTEIN and SCULLY 1994; SCULLY 1995).

2.4.1 Epidemiology

HCMV infection is much more common than identifiable clinical disease, with serological evidence of previous infection in up to 80% by adult life (BELSHE 1984; BERRY et al. 1988; Ho, 1990). HCMV infection is endemic worldwide. In developing countries, HCMV infection is usually acquired in early childhood, but in the developed world many escape infection in childhood, and then sexual transmission plays a greater role. In the United Kingdom, by 35 years of age about 50% of the population have antibody to HCMV (BELSHE 1984; BERRY et al. 1988; FORBES 1989; Ho, 1990).

HCMV is readily transmitted in infected blood and tissues and can be transmitted sexually (EPSTEIN and SCULLY, 1994; SPECTOR et al. 1984; ADLER et al. 1982). Maternal antibodies appear not to protect infants, who can be infected via genital HCMV or virus in breast milk (STAGNO et al. 1980).

2.4.2 Immunopathogenesis

HCMV can infect all nucleated cells and, after infection, these cells express IE and E HCMV antigens and can then become the target for cytotoxic T lymphocytes. HCMV infects salivary acinar cells, and ductal epithelial cells are especially infected, particularly those in the major salivary glands and proximal renal tubules. HCMV appears to induce a series of cellular responses that characteristically cause cell enlargement (*cytomegalo*) with intranuclear inclusions; hence the formerly used term, cytomegalic inclusion disease (ALBRECHT et al. 1990). HCMV also infects phagocytes and via these and other routes can spread throughout the body.

T lymphocytes play a major role in immune surveillance; CD8 and, in salivary glands CD4 cells, are protective in concert with γ-interferon (LUCIN et al. 1992). Humoral immune responses to HCMV may also to some extent be protective. IgM-specific antibodies appear early in HCMV infection, peak at 2–4 weeks and are usually undetectable within 16 weeks. IgG antibodies peak at 1–2 months. Immunocompromised subjects who have defective cellular immunity and no IgM anti-HCMV antibodies are at risk of disseminated HCMV infections.

A gene similar to that coding cellular MHC class 1 antigens is found in HCMV, and this may be involved in viral attachment and may also interfere with immune responses (WILEY 1988; GRIFFITHS and GRUNDY 1988). HCMV can probably also interfere with complement activation, antigen recognition and inflammatory cell function (BANKS and ROUSE 1992). HCMV is immunosuppressive (ROOK 1988) and thus, like other herpesviruses, may be able to modulate the course of other infections, such as HIV.

2.4.3 Clinical Features of Primary Infection

Most primary infections with HCMV are asymptomatic or cause only mild, flu-like symptoms, but over 90% of those infected have subclinical hepatitis. Infection of otherwise healthy young infants rarely causes obvious clinical illness, but infection in older children may manifest with anicteric hepatitis, respiratory disease or a mononucleosis-like syndrome with a negative heterophile antibody test (Paul-Bunnell test) and little in the way of tonsillitis, lymphadenopathy or splenomegaly. Otherwise healthy adolescents and adults can also present with infection which, after an incubation of 4–8 weeks, appears as a glandular fever-like syndrome that is Paul-Bunnell negative, or they may have blood dyscrasias (usually thrombocytopenia or haemolytic anaemis) or, rarely, pneumonia or encephalitis (BELSHE 1984; HO, 1984; SCULLY and SAMARANAYAKE 1992; EPSTEIN and SCULLY 1994).

2.4.4 Latency

HCMV remains latent after the primary infection mainly in oropharyngeal and renal epithelial cells. Lymphocytes and monocytes have also been implicated as sites of latency (HO 1982), and there may, in fact, be multiple sites of latency. HCMV may be harboured with no ill effects, but reactivation is common, with viral shedding, and disease may result, especially in immunocompromised subjects. HCMV appears in the blood, oropharyngeal secretions, saliva, urine, breast milk, tears, sputum, faeces and genital fluids of infected individuals (EPSTEIN and SCULLY 1994), and there may be chronic shedding of the virus, particularly from immunocompromised subjects.

2.4.5 Infection in Pregnancy

The fetus is susceptible at any stage of pregnancy and, though HCMV infection or reactivation in the mother is often asymptomatic, HCMV infection may be transmitted to the foetus and produces damage (PECKHAM 1991; STAGNO and

WHITLEY 1985). Indeed, HCMV now causes more congenital abnormalities and mental handicap in Western countries than does rubella, though only 0.5% live births are infected and only 5%–10% of HCMV-infected fetuses are severely damaged (PECKHAM 1991; BEST 1987; STAGNO and WHITLEY 1985).

The resultant clinical picture in an HCMV-infected fetus may include low birth weight, prematurity, purpura, anaemia, jaundice, microcephaly/hydro-cephaly, cerebral calcification, cataracts, chorioretinitis, micro-ophthalmia and pneumonitis. Liver disease, microcephaly and mental handicap are the main defects. There may incidentally also be hypoplasia in the deciduous dentition. A further 10%–15% of those infected but without obvious abnormalities at birth may later show hearing loss or a degree of mental handicap (STAGNO and WHITLEY 1985).

Lymphocytes from mothers in whom HCMV infects the fetus appear to be impaired in their *in vitro* responses to HCMV antigens (OKABE et al. 1983; PASS et al. 1983).

2.4.6 Infection in Immunocompromised Patients

Primary or reactivated HCMV infections are extremely common in immunocompromised patients, especially bone marrow or organ transplant patients and those with HIV disease (JACOBSEN and MILLS 1988; SUTTMANN et al., 1988). HCMV is also the most common viral infectious complication in patients after tissue transplantation and is a cause of significant morbidity and mortality in many immunocompromised patients (BELSHE 1984; HO, 1982; BERRY et al. 1988; SPECTOR et al. 1984; JACOBSEN and MILLS 1988).

2.4.6.1 Bone Marrow Transplantation. HCMV reactivation or re-infection is seen in more than 75% of HCMV-seropositive patients who receive bone marrow transplants (WINSTON et al. 1982; HERSMAN et al. 1982; MEYERS and THOMAS 1988). The incidence of serious infection is even higher if the transplant recipients are HCMV seronegative but their donor seropositive, i.e. where there is primary HCMV infection in the bone marrow recipient (HERSMAN et al. 1982; MEYERS and THOMAS 1988).

Together with HSV, HCMV is implicated in about one quarter of cases of oesophagitis following bone marrow transplantation and, with the control of HSV by acyclovir, HCMV infections may be expected to increase in proportion (MEYERS and THOMAS 1988). Ulcerations due to HCMV have now been identified at all levels in the gastro-intestinal tract, including the oral cavity, as discussed below.

2.4.6.2 Organ Transplantation. There is HCMV infection in up to 96% of patients having solid organ transplantation such as renal, liver or cardiac transplants (RUBIN and TOLKOFF-RUBIN 1984; GENTRY and ZELUFF 1988; RUBIN 1988), usually within the first 4 months after transplantation (GENTRY and ZELUFF 1988; RUBIN 1988).

HCMV infection may produce a mononucleosis syndrome and/or progressive multi-system disease and, following cardiac transplantation, it is the single most common cause of morbidity and mortality, usually from pneumonia (GENTRY and ZELUFF 1988).

2.4.6.3 Human Immunodeficiency Virus Disease.

Patients with HIV disease are often infected with HCMV and carry several strains of HCMV (SPECTOR et al. 1984; JACOBSEN and MILLS 1988; DREW et al. 1982; LEPORT et al. 1987; POLK et al. 1987), including in their saliva (LUCHT et al. 1993). HCMV infection may also lead to a range of clinical manifestations from a mononucleosis syndrome (LEPORT et al. 1987), to pneumonitis, hepatitis, chorioretinitis, CNS infection (POLK et al. 1987; GOTTLIEB et al., 1981; LERNER and TAPPER 1984) and gastro-intestinal ulceration (including oral ulcers; see later), and may be lethal (MACHER et al. 1983). Indeed, HCMV infection is a predictor of AIDS in those infected with HIV (POLK et al. 1987).

HCMV appears to assume increased pathogenicity in HIV disease and may interact with HIV (HIRSCH et al. 1984), as well as exacerbating the immune defect, like many herpesvirus infections (MERIGAN 1981), causing suppression of NK cell and cytotoxic T lymphocyte function.

Thus there are good theoretical and practical reasons for attempting to prevent and for treating HCMV infections in immunocompromised persons.

2.4.6.4 Gastro-intestinal and Oral Ulceration Related to HCMV Infection in Immunocompromised Patients.

Oesophageal ulcers have been the principle clinical lesions of infection with HCMV in some immunocompromised individuals (TOGHILL and McGAUGHEY 1972; ST. ONGE and BEZAHLER 1982; VILLAR et al. 1984; MYERSON et al. 1984; RABENECK et al. 1990) and have been the presenting feature in some HIV-infected subjects (RABENECK et al. 1990). The ulceration appears to result from vasculitis (RUBIN 1988). Diagnostic criteria have varied, but ulcerations have usually been attributed to HCMV when viral inclusions have been present in cells in adjacent connective tissue and HCMV has been isolated from the lesions.

HCMV-related oral ulcers have also been reported in immunocompromised patients (MYERSON et al. 1984; JONES et al. 1993), sometimes with underlying osteomyelitis (JONES et al. 1993; BERMAN and JENSEN 1990). Inclusions suggestive of HCMV infection may be seen in the endothelium subjacent to the ulcers, although in these cases no direct infection of the epithelium by HCMV has been proved.

Pharyngeal (LALWANI and SNYDERMAN 1991) and oral ulcerations (ANDRIOLO et al. 1986; KANAS et al. 1987; CLICK et al. 1991; LANGFORD et al. 1990; JONES et al. 1992, 1993; SCHUBERT et al. 1993) due to HCMV have also now been described in patients with HIV disease, the diagnosis of HCMV usually being based upon light or electron microscopic demonstration of intranuclear and cytoplasmic HCMV inclusions. HCMV inclusions are eosinophilic, and intracytoplasmic inclusions stain with Gomori's methenamine silver or with periodic acid–Schiff.

In four cases of HCMV-associated oral ulcers in HIV-infected patients who had disseminated HCMV infection, tissue HCMV inclusions were seen on light microscopy and the diagnosis was confirmed by immunohistochemistry and in situ DNA hybridisation. HCMV was detected principally in endothelial cells or perivascular and subepithelial connective tissue. HCMV antigen was detected in occasional epithelial cells. Activated T lymphocytes were identified in the tissue, and high titres of serum HCMV antibodies were present (LANGFORD et al. 1990). In other cases, HCMV was also confirmed immunohistochemically or by in situ DNA hybridisation in some cases (JONES et al. 1992, 1993).

It is tempting to speculate that some other aphthous-type oral ulcers disease may be HCMV related, but this needs further investigation (see below).

2.4.7 Diagnosis

Serology and a full blood picture are usually indicated, inorder to exclude other causes of glandular fever-like syndromes, especially EBV or HIV. Enzyme-linked immunosorbent assay (ELISA) for IgM HCMV is the most widely accepted specific diagnostic assay at present (ROOK, 1988) but, in practice, serology is currently under-used for specific diagnosis (SCULLY and SAMARANAYAKE 1992; EPSTEIN and SCULLY 1994; BELSHE 1984; HO 1982).

Viral culture of body fluids or tissues has been the "gold standard" for diagnosis of infection. However, as viral shedding may occur in the absence of clinical disease, it may not necessarily indicate a pathogenic role for HCMV. Direct techniques in tissue studies *may be* more specific. Tissue biopsy may show the typical histopathological changes of HCMV infection, with enlarged cells and inclusion bodies (Cowdry type A) in nuclei and cytoplasm. However, biopsy is not usually indicated, and it is more reasonable to examine for HCMV antigens in infected cells or secretions by immunostaining using specific monoclonal antibodies such as in detection of EA fluorescent foci (DEAFF) or the leucocyte antigen detection (LAD) test. HCMV nucleic acids can also be sought by *in situ*, dot blot or Southern blot hybridization or by PCR, techniques now increasingly used for diagnosis (MANGANO et al., 1992; WARREN et al., 1992; SHUSTER and BENEKE, 1985). PCR, in particular, is proving extremely useful (WARREN et al. 1992; GREENBERG et al. 1995) and can facilitate rapid diagnosis.

2.4.8 Possible Associations with Other Conditions

2.4.8.1 Kaposi's Sarcoma. Epidemiological data – particularly the high prevalence of Kaposi's sarcoma (KS) in homosexuals and reports of cases of KS in homosexuals who were not HIV antibody positive after 8–10 years – suggested that KS in HIV disease might be associated with a transmissible agent other than HIV (ARCHER et al. 1989; BERAL et al. 1990; FRIEDMAN-KIEN et al. 1990; HAVERKOS et al. 1990; MARQUART et al. 1991). HCMV was one candidate, but it may only have been an opportunistic infection within the KS tissue, as may mycoplasma or other agents

(MARQUART and OEHLSCHLAEGEL 1985; Lo et al. 1989). HCMV can be latent in endothelium even in non-HIV-infected persons and may thus be an incidental finding in the lesions of KS (BELSHE 1984; Ho 1982).

Recent findings of a novel herpesviruses in KS further discount a role for HCMV (see below).

2.4.8.2 Oral Carcinoma. There is, at least on serological evidence, no association between HCMV and oral carcinoma (Larsson et al. 1991).

2.4.8.3 Salivary Gland Disease. HCMV is an interesting virus because it was first recognised in salivary glands as the "salivary gland inclusion virus". Nevertheless, it has not been proved to cause salivary gland disease. It has been reported that salivary gland tumours can be induced experimentally by mouse CMV (LAMEY et al., 1982). CMV has induced adenocarcinomas in mice, but several of the animals had been irradiated or received anti-lymphocytic serum, and thus immune or other factors may have been at play. HCMV is also a possible candidate virus for involvement in human salivary gland tumours, though HCMV has not been cultured from salivary tumours (LAMEY et al. 1982) and HCMV antigens are not found (Fox et al. 1986), but, again, this does not necessarily exclude involvement. HCMV DNA could be present without antigen expression.

HCMV may also be implicated in SS. Some serological studies have shown normal serum titres of HCMV antibodies in SS (SCULLY 1989), but others have shown raised titres (SHILLITOE and ALSPAUGH 1985; THOM et al. 1988), suggesting there may be viral reactivation. "Virus-like" structures have been seen by electron microscopy in minor salivary glands and other tissues in SS, but have not been shown to be viral, and immunostaining has failed to demonstrate HCMV antigens. These structures may be associated in some way with the abnormal immunoglobulin synthesis seen in SS.

HCMV DNA has been found by us in SS salivary tissue, but it is also found in non-specific sialadenitis (MAITLAND et al. 1995). Furthermore, the lymphomas complicating SS appear not to contain HCMV DNA (Fox 1989). An aetiological link between IICMV and SS thcrcforc hao little oupport, deepite suggestions of some viral link (FLESCHER and TALAL 1991).

HCMV might also be implicated in xerostomia in HIV disease, and although one study showed no relation (LUCHT et al. 1993), there was a strong correlation between the presence of HCMV in saliva and xerostomia in another study (GREENBERG et al. 1995), and HCMV has also been implicated in submandibular sialadenitis, which was responsive to ganciclovir in one patient with AIDS (PIALOUX et al. 1991).

2.4.8.4 Behcet's Syndrome and Aphthae. There may be reactivation of HCMV, but there are no consistent antibody responses to HCMV in aphthae (PEDERSEN 1989; PEDERSEN and HORNSLETH 1993); HCMV is not detectable in lesions (OGAWA et al. 1990) and, in Behcet's syndrome, HCMV serum antibodies are not increased (HAMZAOUI et al., 1990), making a regular association between HCMV and these conditions unlikely. However, perhaps up to 10% of oral ulcers contain HCMV (LEIMOLA-VIRTANEN et al. 1995).

2.4.8.5 Graft Versus Host Disease. The possible association between HCMV and graft versus host disease (GVHD) is discussed at length elsewhere (APPLETON and SUILAND 1993).

2.4.9 Prophylaxis and Treatment

Passive immunisation using specific immunoglobulin with high-titre, anti-HCMV antibody may provide a degree of protection against primary infection in seronegative subjects who are accidentally exposed to HCMV. No reliably effective vaccine is available against HCMV.

Unfortunately, acyclovir is not reliably effective in treating active HCMV infection (MEYERS 1989; SELBY et al. 1989), presumably because HCMV lacks thymidine kinase (MEYERS 1989). Acyclovir may have some activity against HCMV reactivation. Low doses of acyclovir – $250\,mg/m^2$ t.i.d. (SARAL et al. 1981) or $5\,mg/kg$ b.i.d. (HANN et al. 1983) – have not, however, proved reliably effective in prevention of HCMV reactivation after bone marrow transplantation, though one study reported that oral acyclovir (200 mg, q.i.d.) significantly reduced HCMV shedding (GLUCKMAN et al. 1983) and high-dose acyclovir ($450\,mg/m^2$, p.i.d.) prevented HCMV reactivation (MEYERS et al. 1988).

The principle anti-viral against HCMV is ganciclovir (2-hydroxy-1-(hydroxymethyl)-ethoxymethyl guanine) (DHPG) (BALFOUR and ENGLUND 1989; FIELD et al. 1983; DE CLERC 1988). Unfortunately, bone marrow suppression results in up to 50% of those treated with ganciclovir (HANN et al. 1983; BALFOUR and ENGLUND 1989; REED et al. 1990), and there may also be other adverse effects, such as fever, rashes, nausea, vomiting, CNS toxicity and hepatotoxicity. Ganciclovir is therefore indicated mainly for serious HCMV infections (LASKIN et al. 1987) such as retinitis. Ganciclovir is effective treatment for HCMV retinitis in AIDS (BRYSON 1988) and for HCMV pneumonitis in solid organ transplantation (MAI et al. 1989), but not in bone marrow transplantation patients (REED et al. 1990).

Unfortunately, HCMV may become ganciclovir resistant (ERICE et al. 1989). Foscarnet (phosphonoformate) inhibits HCMV DNA polymerase but, unfortunately, renal toxicity is seen in up to half of the patients (BRYSON, 1988; FARESE et al. 1990), and nausea, malaise, vomiting, fatigue, headache, other CNS toxicity, haematologic toxicity and hepatotoxicity may be seen. Foscarnet is nevertheless currently the only really effective treatment for ganciclovir-resistant HCMV infections (SCULLY 1995).

2.5 Human Herpesvirus-6

Human herpesvirus-6 was initially identified a decade ago and thought to be a human B cell lymphotropic virus (HBLV) restricted to lymphoproliferative disorders (SALAHUDDIN et al. 1986). It is now known to be the causal agent of a rash, exanthem subitum (YAMANISHI et al. 1988; UEDA et al. 1989), and may be associated with GVHD (YOSHIKAWA et al. 1991). Most children develop antibody before the age of 1 year, indicative of previous infection (TAKASHASHI et al. 1988). Two variants of human herpesvirus-6, A and B, have been identified (ABLASHI et al. 1993).

Human herpesvirus-6 is commonly found in saliva (PIETROBONI et al. 1988; Fox et al. 1990; GOPAL et al. 1990; HARNETT et al. 1990; KIDO et al. 1990; LEVY et al. 1990), especially in immunocompromised patients, but it is not known to be associated with aphthae (PEDERSEN et al. 1993) or any specific oral disease. One recent study has indicated a high prevalence of serum antibodies to human herpesvirus-6 in patients with oral carcinoma compared with controls, though the significance of these observations is unclear and the findings are not specific (VASUDEVAN et al. 1991).

Finally, this is another sialotropic herpesvirus that should be considered in SS (KRUEGER et al. 1990). Raised serum antibody levels to human herpesvirus-6 have been found in SS (ABLASHI et al. 1989; BIBERFELD et al. 1988), and human herpesvirus-6 DNA has been found in salivary glands (KRUEGER et al. 1990; HADDAD et al. 1992). It has also been detected in lymphomas in SS (Fox et al. 1990; ABLASHI et al. 1991). However, causal relationships have yet to be established.

2.6 Human Herpesvirus-7

Human herpesvirus-7 resembles human herpesvirus-6, but is a separate entity (FRENKEL et al. 1990). It is found in saliva of children and adults, rarely of infants (HIDAKA et al. 1993; BLACK et al. 1993). Infection appears to be typically acquired between the ages of 2 and 5 years (WYATT et al. 1991). A pathogenic role remains to be established.

2.7 Kaposi's Sarcoma Herpesvirus (Human Herpesvirus-8)

Herpesvirus-like DNA sequences resembling, but distinct from, EBV have been demonstrated in tissue from KS of the endemic, sporadic and AIDS-related types (CHANG 1994; SCHALLING et al. 1995), from skin carcinoma in immunosuppressed patients (RADY et al. 1995) and from abdominal B cell lymphomas in AIDS (CESARMAN et al. 1995). Tentatively termed KS herpesvirus (KSHV), this agent has been found in all lesions and from all sites studied and has been found in blood but not throat swabs; it was not found in non-KS tissue (SU et al. 1995; HUANG et al. 1995; AMBROZIAK et al. 1995; MOORE and CHANG 1995; BOSHOFF et al. 1995; DUPIN et al. 1995; COLLANDRE et al. 1995). Whether this agent is present in other disorders is, as yet, unclear (LEVY et al. 1990).

3 Papillomaviruses

Papillomaviruses are epitheliotropic DNA viruses that have early genes E1–E7, late genes L1 and L2 and a long control region, the upstream regulatory region (URR). They can induce hyperplastic, papillomatous and verrucous lesions in the stratified squamous epithelia of skin and mucosae in a wide range of hosts. Interest in them has been reawakened because of a possible malignant potential, including in relation to oral carcinoma, and because DNA technology has allowed for studies (CHANG et al. 1991; SCULLY et al. 1985, 1988; DE VILLIERS, 1989a; SCULLY and SAMARANAYAKE 1992; SCULLY 1995; SYRJANEN and SCULLY, in press).

Papillomaviruses are classified according to their host range and the relatedness of their nucleic acids, and each is first named according to its natural host, e.g. cottontail rabbit (or Shope) papillomaviruses (CRPV), bovine papillomaviruses (BPV) and human papillomaviruses (HPV).

Papillomaviruses isolated from the same species are subclassified into papillomavirus types according to their nucleotide sequence homology. Any new isolate which has less than 50% cross-hybridisation to previously typed viruses by reassociation kinetics is designated as a new type and numbered in order of discovery. However, if the nucleotide homology exceeds 50%, the virus is considered as a subtype, and if it is close to 100%, with only a few nucleotide differences, it is considered as a variant of the same viral type. More recently, the definition of a new virus type has been modified to rely on the nucleotide sequence of specific viral genes, namely E6, L1 and URR.

3.1 Human Papillomavirus Infection

HPV comprise the largest group of papillomaviruses, 73 types had been identified by 1995 (DE VILLIERS 1989a; ZUR HAUSEN and DE VILLIERS 1994). The Papillomavirus Nomenclature Committee agreed at the 1991 Papillomavirus Workshop that, for a novel HPV isolate to be recognised as a new HPV type, its entire genome must be cloned and the nucleotide sequence of the E6, L1 and URR genes should demonstrate less than 90% nucleotide sequence identity with established papillomavirus types.

HPV gain access by direct implantation through breaches in the epithelium. They are shed in cells from the superficial epithelium. HPV induce lesions in many body sites, including the skin and mucosae of the mouth, urethra, larynx, trachea, bronchus, nasal cavity/paranasal sinuses, oesophagus, ano-genital tract, urethra and conjunctivae (CHANG et al. 1992; BRANDSMA and ABRAMSON 1989; YOUNG et al. 1989). Perhaps as importantly, HPV DNA has also been recently demonstrated in *normal* tissues adjacent to HPV lesions in the genital and upper aerodigestive tract, in normal genital mucosa (YOUNG et al. 1989), newborn foreskin and 'by us and others' in normal oral mucosa (see below).

Early studies sought HPV antigens, but HPV are now detected in lesions mainly by examination for HPV DNA (SYRJANEN 1990; SCULLY and SAMARANAYAKE 1992). PCR is the most sensitive test, while Southern blot hybridisation is the most specific detection method.

HPV are now recognised to fall into several general groups. HPV-1, HPV-2, HPV-3 and HPV-4 are seen mainly in cutaneous warty lesions. Another group, comprising HPV-5, HPV-8, HPV-10, HPV-12, HPV-14 and HPV-17, is associated with the unusual cutaneous disorder epidermolysis verruciformis, a disease in which patients have life-long warts, which in some instances, especially in lesions exposed to ultraviolet light, transform to carcinomas. Another group, comprising HPV-6, HPV-11, HPV-16, HPV-18, HPV-31, HPV-35 and others (see below), is associated with mucosal warts or carcinomas, especially in the ano-genital region. Of these, HPV-6 and HPV-11 only have a low risk of association with carcinoma Finally some HPV have very restricted and specific associations for example, HPV-13 and HPV-32 have only been found in oral lesions.

3.1.1 Ano-genital Infections

Infections with "genital" HPV types (mainly HPV-6, -11 and -16) appear to be widespread, but are often clinically inapparent and are sometimes transmitted transplacentally, at birth (SEDLACEK et al. 1989; TSENG et al. 1992), sexually (LEY et al. 1991; MURETTO and FERENCZY 1992), by auto-inoculation or by other unidentified routes (PAO et al. 1992). Up to 35% of subjects up to 40 years of age shed HPV ano-genitally (SCHIFFMAN 1994).

Viral DNA is found in over 90% of cervical carcinomas. Convincing experimental data support the concept that specific "high-risk" types of HPV (HPV-16, -18, -31, -33, -35, -39, -45, -51, -52 and -56) are causally involved in the pathogenesis of ano-genital cancer, particularly cancer of the cervix (SHILLITOE 1991; SYRJANEN and SCULLY, in press).

3.1.2 Latent and Subclinical Oral Infections

By Southern blot hybridisation, from 15.1% (KELLOWSKI et al. 1992) to over 40% (MAITLAND et al., 1989) of biopsies from clinically normal oral mucosa from adults can be shown to contain HPV DNA, and the PCR technique has increased the detection of HPV DNA in the former study to 21.8% (KELLOWSKI et al., 1992a). HPV DNA can also be shown by PCR in exfoliated normal oral squamous cells (JALAL et al. 1992).

It is clear, therefore, that HPV DNA can be present in normal oral tissues in up to one third or more of the population, and the evidence suggests that the mucosa may act as a reservoir for new HPV infections and/or as a source of recurring HPV lesions. The source of infection is unclear. A study on oral HPV infection in women with past or present genital HPV infection (KELLOWSKI et al. 1990, 1992b) using dot blot hybridisation on exfoliated oral squames showed only a 3.8% HPV DNA prevalence, almost certainly an underestimation of the true HPV prevalence because basal layer cells cannot be collected in this way.

The term subclinical papillomavirus infection was originally applied to lesions in the uterine cervix that were not visible on clinical inspection but showed histological changes similar to those found in flat warts (SYRJANEN 1989). Though such cervical lesions can be visualised under the colposcope by the application of acetic acid, similar lesions cannot be seen in the mouth (KELLOWSKI et al. 1990). Unfortunately, the term subclinical has been extensively misused in the current literature; it should be reserved exclusively for the epithelial changes, no matter how minor, that do not fulfil the criteria of classical, clinically manifest HPV lesions (SYRJANEN et al. 1989). These epithelial changes are discussed below.

3.1.3 Human Papillomavirus-Related Oral Lesions

HPV are clearly implicated in the aetiology of oral squamous cell papillomas, genital warts in the oral cavity (condyloma acuminata), common warts (verrucae vulgaris) in the oral cavity and focal epithelial hyperplasia. HPV have also been demonstrated in a variety of other benign oral lesions, papillary hyperplasia, fibrous hyperplasia, lichen planus and leukoplakia by histopathological, ultrastructural, immunohistochemical and DNA hybridisation studies, though these may not be causal associations (CHANG et al. 1991; SCULLY et al. 1988). Indeed, HPV DNA has also been found in congenital white sponge naevus (COX et al. 1992) and in some odontogenic cysts that have had no apparent connection with the oral cavity (COX et al. 1991).

Among the known HPV types, HPV-1, -2, -4, -6, -7, -11, -13, -16, -18, -32 and -57 have been found in different types of oral lesions. Of these, HPV-13 and HPV-32 seem to be exclusively confined to one specific oral lesion, i.e. focal epithelial hyperplasia (CHANG et al. 1991; SCULLY et al. 1988; DE VILLIERS 1989; GARLICK et al. 1989).

3.1.4 Squamous Cell Papilloma

Oral squamous cell papilloma is a relatively common, benign tumour which can occur at any age and is typically found on the palate. HPV aetiology has been proved by showing HPV particles, HPV antigens and HPV DNA, mainly from HPV-6 and HPV-11, in up to 80% of the lesions studied (DE VILLIERS, 1989; YOUNG and MIN 1991). Papillomas may also occasionally contain HPV-2, -13, -16, -32 and HPV-31/33/35 DNA (LONING et al. 1985; NAGHASHFAR et al. 1985; SYRJANEN et al. 1987; EVERSOLE and LAIPIS 1988; YOUNG and MIN 1991).

3.1.5 Condyloma Acuminatum

There have been only occasional case reports of oral condyloma acuminatum. They are usually multiple small, white or pink nodules with a surface more cauliflower-like than that of papillomas. Differentiation from squamous cell papillomas is difficult and largely academic. Evidence for an HPV aetiology of oral condylomas has been provided by the electron microscopic demonstration of HPV particles, immunohistochemical studies demonstrating HPV antigens and DNA studies showing HPV DNA mainly from HPV-6 and HPV-11, but also occasionally HPV-2, in up to 85% of these lesions (SYRJANEN et al. 1986; EVERSOLE et al. 1987).

The histology and the HPV types are thus similar both in oral papillomas and condylomas.

3.1.6 Common Wart (Verruca Vulgaris)

Occasional case reports have described common warts in the oral cavity usually as firm, whitish, sessile, circumscribed, exophytic lesions on the lips, with hyperkeratinisation of the superficial epithelia and elongation of the rete rides which, at the margins, usually bend inward toward the centre of the lesion. HPV-6, -11 and -16 and cutaneous HPV types, e.g. HPV-1, -2, -4 and -7, have been found in oral common warts in some studies (NAGASHEAR et al. 1985; ADLER-STORTHZ et al. 1986; ZEUSS et al. 1991; EVERSOLE et al. 1987). Indeed, HPV-2 and HPV-4 have been detected in more than 55% of oral warts (DE VILLIERS 1989), and HPV-57 DNA has also recently been demonstrated in the majority of oral verrucae (DE VILLIERS et al. 1989; PADAYACHEE 1994).

It is probably appropriate that the term oral wart should be restricted to lesions associated with the cutaneous HPV types while, if the mucosal HPV types (6 and 11) are found, the lesions are really oral condylomata or papillomas. This distinction has implications in tracing the source of HPV infection, i.e. oro-genital contact versus oro-cutaneous contact.

3.1.7 Focal Epithelial Hyperplasia

Focal epithelial hyperplasia, or Heck's disease, is a benign lesion of the oral mucosa originally thought to be restricted to certain ethnic groups, particularly Inuits and natural Indians from North and South America. These lesions, however, have subsequently been found, albeit rarely, in many other ethnic groups around the world.

Focal epithelial hyperplasia is a manifestation of HPV infection in the oral cavity in individuals with a specific genetic predisposition, as is the case in epidermodysplasia verruciformis lesions of the skin, described above. Papillomavirus particles and HPV antigens have been repeatedly observed in focal epithelial hyperplasia lesions, and it is now evident that more than 90% of biopsies from the hyperplasia contain HPV-13 and/or -32 DNA (BEAUDENON et al. 1987; GARLICK et al. 1989; HENKE et al. 1989).

3.1.8 Oral Warty Lesions

HPV-7, -13, -18 and -32 have been found in oral warty lesions in HIV infection (GREENSPAN et al. 1988). HPV may also be present in the oral mucosa in HIV infection in the absence of clinical disease (SNIJDERS et al. 1990), as they may be in otherwise healthy persons.

3.1.9 Diagnosis of Human Papillomavirus-Induced Lesions

Until quite recently, HPV diagnosis was based exclusively on the morphological criteria seen on histopathology, because HPV cannot be cultivated and diagnostic serology has not been widely available. The morphological change particularly characteristic of HPV infection is koilocytosis, in which keratinocytes typically in the intermediate layer of the epithelium are hyperchromatic, with slightly irregular nuclei surrounded by a distinct cytoplasmic clear zone (halo). At the margins of the halo, the cytoplasm is condensed and usually exhibits an amphophilic-staining pattern. Koilocytic cells are still regarded as the most reliable morphological criteria for diagnosis of HPV infection (SYRJANEN, 1989). However, there can be difficulties in the distinction between true koilocytes and other vacuolised cells, and this is important, especially in the oral cavity, where different types of vacuolised cells unrelated to infection are not infrequently seen (KELLOWSKI et al. 1990). Another cytological change frequently associated with HPV infection is the presence of parakeratotic (dyskeratotic) cells either singly or in clusters. Both the koilocytotic and dyskeratotic keratinocytes frequently show bi- or multinucleation (SYRJANEN 1989).

Various HPV antigens can be detected immunocytochemically, but the most *reliable* method so far to diagnose HPV infection is to detect HPV nucleic acid in the lesion by hybridisation methods or gene amplification. These techniques have now largely replaced immunocytochemistry, and there are several commercial kits available for diagnosis in biopsies based on *in situ*, dot blot, or Southern blot hybridization methods. PCR is the only method which can also be used to reliably detect latent HPV infections in oral squames rather than biopsies (SYRJANEN 1990; JALAL et al., in press).

3.1.10 Management of Human Papillomavirus-Related Oral Lesions

Surgery is the usual management of HPV-related lesions, but retinoids may be effective (BURG and SOBETZKO 1990) and interferon may be used.

3.1.11 Relation to Other Oral Diseases

3.1.11.1 Lichen Planus. Oral lichen planus specimens may show positive immunostaining for HPV structural proteins (KASHIMA et al. 1990), and *in situ* hybridization has shown HPV-11, -16 and HPV-16-related virus (SYRJANEN et al. 1986; MAITLAND et al. 1987; Cox et al. 1993); however, for the reasons discussed above, the presence of HPV in oral lichen planus lesions does not prove an aetiological link. Other investigators have not found HPV in lichen planus (YOUNG and MIN 1991).

3.1.11.2 Oral Leukoplakia (Keratosis). Though some have not found HPV DNA in keratoses (YOUNG and MIN, 1991), HPV-suggestive changes have been noted in some lesions and, subsequently, HPV antigens and DNA from HPV-2, -6, -11 and -16 have been found by several groups (SYRJANEN et al. 1986; GREER et al. 1990; KASHIMA et al. 1990; ABDELSAYD 1991). Indeed, we and others have shown that HPV-16 and HPV-16-related sequences can be detected in more than 80% of keratoses (KASHIMA et al. 1990; SYRJANEN et al. 1988; MAITLAND et al. 1989). Nevertheless, the presence of HPV in *normal* oral mucosa casts serious doubt on any regular causal relationship, though HPV-2 and -6 DNA have been found in smokeless tobacco-related keratoses (GREER et al. 1987, 1990), and HPV-16 is strongly associated with proliferative verrucous leukoplakia (PALEFSKY et al. 1995; SHROYER and GREER 1991).

Recent studies have discounted the presence of HPV in HL (SYRJANEN et al. 1989; FICARRA et al. 1988; ALESSI et al. 1990), and it now appears certain that HL is related to EBV (see p. 47).

3.1.11.3 Verrucous Carcinoma. Oral verrucous carcinoma is clearly aetiologically linked with tobacco consumption and betel chewing (CHANG et al. 1991). However, viral involvement in verrucous carcinomas has long been suspected at other body sites (e.g. larynx and the ano-genital area), and the morphological features in oral verrucous carcinoma of papillomatosis, dyskeratosis and koilocytosis support an HPV aetiology (CHANG et al. 1990). Despite this, early studies found no or only weak evidence for HPV in oral verrucous carcinoma (YOUNG and MIN, 1991; ADLER-STORTHZ et al. 1986; JOHNSON et al. 1991). However, recent work has demonstrated HPV-6, HPV-11 (SHROYER et al. 1993), HPV-18 (NOBLE-TOPHAM et al. 1993) and HPV-2 (CHANG et al. 1992) in oral verrucous carcinoma.

3.1.11.4 Squamous Cell Carcinoma. Oral squamous cell carcinoma is clearly aetiologically linked with tobacco and/or alcohol use. A substantial portion of these tumors, however, also contain HPV sequences, often of the "high-risk" group (Table 6). The rate of HPV detection varies in reports based on clinical material from oral squamous cell carcinoma from 0% to 94% (Table 6), but the ability to detect HPV is strongly dependent on the sensitivity of the method used, as well as the representativeness of the sample analysed, and is higher in most of the more recent studies (KASHIMA et al. 1990; WATTS et al. 1991; WOODS et al. 1993; COX et al. 1993; MILLER et al. 1994; OSTWALD et al. 1994). Oral squamous cell carcinoma biopsies, when analysed by *in situ* hybridisation and PCR, disclosed HPV-11, -16 or -18 DNA sequences in 10%–60% (CHANG et al. 1990; TSUCHIYA et al. 1991; SHINDOH et al. 1992; TYAN et al. 1993; WOODS et al. 1993; OSTWALD et al. 1994; MILLER et al. 1994). An HPV-16-related virus was found by us in about 40% (MAITLAND et al. 1989). HPV DNA sequences may also be found in leucocytes from patients with oral carcinoma (HONIG et al. 1995).

Most carcinoma-derived cell lines contain integrated HPV DNA genomes, the integrations causing disruptions and deletions within the early viral genes, whereas in benign lesions HPV DNA is present almost exclusively as free, mono-meric or oligomeric episomes.

Table 6. Frequency of human papillomavirus (HPV) nucleic acid detection in oral squamous carcinomas

Sample size	Frequency (%)	HPV types	DNA detection method	Reference
7	43	1–19, 21–25	Southern blot	DE VILLIERS 1985
6	50	11, 16	Southern blot	LONING et al. 1985
5	80	6, 11, 16, 18	In situ	DEKMEZIAN et al. 1987
13	39	6/11, 16/18	Dot blot	LONING et al. 1987
51	12	6, 11, 13, 16, 18, 30	In situ	SYRJANEN et al. 1988
36	14	11, 16, 18	Southern blot	BRANDSMA and ABRAMSON 1989
7	28	16, 18	PCR-dot blot	KIYABU et al. 1989
15	46	16	Southern blot	MAITLAND et al. 1987
17	77	6, 11, 16, 18	Southern blot	CHANG et al. 1989
8	50	16	PCR	MAITLAND et al. 1989
40	6	6, 11, 16, 18	In situ	CHANG et al. 1990
40	27	6, 11, 16, 18	PCR	CHANG et al. 1990
50	6	6, 11, 16, 18, 31, 33, 35	In situ	GREER et al. 1990
10	10	16	In situ and PCR	SHROYER and GREER 1991
24	13	6/11, 16/18	Southern blot	TSUCHIYA et al. 1991
23	68	6/11, 16/18	Southern blot	WATTS et al. 1991
23	94	6, 11, 16, 18	PCR	WATTS et al. 1991
39	49	4, 16, 18	PCR/Southern blot	YEUDALL and CAMPO 1991
17	0	16/18, 31/33/35	In situ	YOUNG and MIN 1991
17	18	16	PCR/Southern blot	BRACHMAN et al. 1992
118	25	6, 16	PCR/Southern blot	MADDEN et al. 1992
24	33	16	PCR	SHINDOH et al. 1992
8	50	16	Southern blot	COX et al. 1993
30	14	16	PCR/In situ	FRAZER et al. 1993
9	11	16	PCR	TYAN et al. 1993
18	77	Various	PCR/Southern blot	WOODS et al. 1993
27	22	16/18	PCR/Southern blot	ANDERSON et al. 1994
64	25	Various	PCR/Southern blot	BRANDWEIN et al. 1994
30	67	16/18	PCR	MILLER et al. 1994
26	62	6/11, 16, 18	PCR/Southern blot	OSTWALD et al. 1994

PCR, polymerase chain reaction.

HPV can, with chemical carcinogens, transform oral keratinocytes (SHIN et al. 1994). Interestingly, only the HPV types closely associated with malignancies have immortalising activities; the benign HPV types are unable to function in this way (WOODWORTH et al. 1989). Transformation studies with oncogenic HPV DNA has localised the transforming activity mainly to the E6 and E7 genes. However, despite the central role of these early HPV genes, malignant transformation appears to require additional factors such as co-infection with HSV or HCMV, exposure to tobacco alcohol, glucocorticoids or other hormones, or possibly other co-factors (SYRJANEN and SCULLY, in press; WOODWORTH et al. 1989; MITRANI-ROSENBAUM et al. 1989; PATER et al. 1990).

Although the E7 protein alone has transforming and immortalising activities in rodent cells, cooperation between E6 and E7 appears to be both necessary and sufficient for the efficient immortalisation of primary human genital keratinocytes. Sequence rearrangements in URR may also be responsible for the oncogenicity of specific HPV types (KITASATO et al. 1994). The E5 gene may also be involved, since the E5 protein alters responses of the cell receptor tyrosine kinases (MARTIN et al. 1989) and can thus modulate epidermal growth factor receptor (EGFR) activity. Protein (oncoproteins) encoded by the E6 and E7 genes from "high cancer risk" HPV types are able to interfere with some cellular growth-regulatory proteins (WERNESS et al. 1990; MUNGER et al. 1989). The E6 oncoprotein can bind to and interfere with the p53 tumour suppressor gene product (WERNESS et al. 1990). The E7 oncoprotein can bind to and interfere with the retinoblastoma tumour suppressor gene product pRB (MUNGER et al. 1989). The importance of the E6–p53 and E7–pRB interactions is substantiated by the observation that there is a correlation between the ability of the HPV genes to bind these cell growth-regulatory proteins and the oncogenicity of the HPV type. High risk-type viruses HPV-16 and HPV-18 E6 proteins can associate with p53, whereas no complex can be detected with HPV-6 or HPV-11 ("low-risk") E6 proteins (WERNESS et al. 1990). E7 proteins from the oncogenic HPV types of 16 and 18 bind pRB more strongly than does E7 from the benign HPV types 6 and 11 (MUNGER et al. 1989). Only a few studies exist on HPV E6 or E7 gene expression in carcinomas originating from head or neck region, but tonsillar carcinomas express high levels of HPV-16/E6/E7 transcripts which originate from integrated as well as episomal HPV DNA (SNIJDERS et al. 1992).

These interactions provide at least a theoretical model as to how HPV might be involved in carcinogenesis. Normal p53 seems to act as a tumour suppressor because it functions as a guardian of the genome, thus maintaining its integrity. Damage to cellular DNA leads to accumulation of p53 and to cessation of cell proliferation, providing time for the cell DNA repair mechanisms to act. If the repair fails, p53 can trigger cell "suicide" through apoptosis. Those cells that carry a mutation in p53 or carry an oncogenic virus may become genetically unstable, which can lead to other mutations and chromosome aberrations and finally to selection of malignant cell clones. Interestingly, we and others have demonstrated p53 mutations in oral carcinomas (SOMERS et al. 1992; SAKAI and TSUCHIDA 1992; GUSTERSON et al. 1991; FIELD et al. 1991, 1992; WARNAKULASURIYA and JOHNSON 1992; OGDEN et al. 1992; MATTHEWS et al. 1993). It has been shown that *cervical* carcinoma cell lines which are HPV negative have a mutation in either p53 or RB gene; HPV-positive carcinomas have been shown to express wild-type p53 and pRB (MUNGER et al. 1989; SCHEFFNER et al. 1990). The hypothesis is that the inactivation of normal function of p53 (SCHEFFNER et al. 1990) or pRB (or the related p107) proteins is a critical step in squamous cell carcinogenesis.

H-*ras* oncogene mutation also appears correlated with HPV in oral carcinoma (ANDERSON et al. 1994), and it is clear that some HPV can interact with various transcription factors, especially NF-1 (nuclear factor-1), API (includes oncogenes *jun* and *fos*) (BERNARD and APT, 1994), protein phosphatase 2A (PP2A) and others (ZUR HAUSEN and DE VILLIERS 1994).

Recently, the possible aetiological role of HPV infection in the pathogenesis of oral pre-cancer lesions and cancer has been supported by the discovery of HPV-suggestive lesions in oral pre-cancer specimens as well as by DNA hybridisation studies disclosing HPV-11, -16 and -18 DNA (CHANG et al. 1991; SCULLY et al. 1988; CHANG et al. 1990; SYRJANEN et al. 1988; OSTWALD et al. 1994).

3.1.11.5 Spindle Cell Carcinoma. Interestingly, spindle cell oral carcinomas appear not to contain HPV (LARSEN et al. 1994).

3.1.11.6 Nasopharyngeal Carcinoma. HPV-11 and HPV-16 may be detected in nasopharyngeal carcinoma (TYAN et al. 1993; HORDING et al. 1994).

3.1.12 Conclusion

HPV are present in oral squamous cell carcinomas and fulfil most of the criteria needed for oncogenicity, but their role in oral cancer still needs further elaboration. HPV may be implicated in oral carcinogenesis, though the evidence is as yet less convincing than it is for other mucosal carcinomas (YEUDALL 1992). Newer techniques of nucleic acid technology will undoubtedly reveal a clearer picture of this rapidly expanding field of research.

References

Abdelsayd RA (1991) Study of human papillomavirus in oral epithelial dysplasia and epidermoid carcinoma in the absence of tobacco and alcohol use. Oral Surg Oral Med Oral Pathol 71: 730–732

Ablashi DV, Agut H, Berneman Z et al (1993) Human herpesvirus 6 variants – a nomenclature. Arch Virol 129: 363–366

Ablashi DV, Josephs SF, Buchbinder A et al (1988) Human B lymphotropic virus (human herpes-virus-6). J Virol Methods 21: 29–48

Ablashi DV, Salahuddin SZ, Josephs SG et al (1991) Human herpesvirus 6 (HHV-6). In Vivo 5: 193–199

Ades AE, Peckham CS, Dale GE, Best JM, Jeansson S (1989) Prevalence of antibodies to herpes simplex virus type 1 and 2 in pregnant women and estimated rates of infection. Epidemiol Commun Health 43: 53–60

Adler SP, Chandrika T, Lawrence L, Baggett J (1982) Cytomegalovirus infections in neonates acquired by blood transfusion. Pediatr Infect Dis 2: 114–118

Adler-Storthz K, Newland JR, Tessin BA, Yeudall WA, Shillitoe EJ (1986a) Identification of human papillomavirus types in oral verruca vulgaris. J Oral Pathol 15: 230–233

Adler-Storthz K, Newland JR, Tessin BA, Yeudall WA, Shillitoe EJ (1986b) Human papillomavirus type 2 DNA in oral verrucous carcinoma. J Oral Pathol 15: 472–475

Akinwande J, Odukoya O, Nwoku AL, Taiwo EO (1986) Burkitt's lymphoma of the jaws in Lagos: 10 year review. J Maxillofac Surg 14: 323–328

Albrecht T, Boldogh I, Fons M, Abubakar S, Deng CZ (1990) Cell activation signals and the pathogenesis of human cytomegalovirus. Intervirology 31: 68–75

Alessi E, Berti E, Cusini M et al (1990) Oral hairy leukoplakia. J Am Acad Dermatol 22: 79–86

Alsip GR, Ench Y, Sumaya CV, Boswell RN (1988) Increased Epstein-Barr virus DNA in oropha-ryngeal secretions from patients with AIDS, AIDS-related complex, or asymptomatic hu-man immunodeficiency virus infections. J Infect Dis 157: 1072–1076

Ambroziak JA, Blackbourn DJ, Herndier B et al (1995) Herpesvirus-like sequences in HIV-infected and uninfected Kaposi's sarcoma patients. Science 268: 582–583

Anderson JA, Irish JC, McLachlin CM, Ngan BY (1994) H-ras oncogene mutation and human papillomavirus infection in oral carcinomas. Arch Otolaryngol Head Neck Surg 120: 755–760

Andriolo M, Wolf JW, Rosenberg JS (1986) AIDS and AIDS-related complex: oral manifestations and treatment. J Am Dent Assoc 113: 586–589

Appleton AL, Sviland L (1993) Pathogenesis of GVHD: role of herpesviruses. Bone Marrow Transplant 11: 349–355

Archer CB, Spittle MF, Smith NP (1989) Kaposi's sarcoma in a homosexual – 10 years on. Clin Exp Dermatol 14: 233–236

Ashley R, Wald A, Corey L (1994) Cervical antibodies in patients with oral herpes simplex virus type 1 (HSV-1) infection: local anamnestic responses after genital HSV-2 infection. J Virol 68: 5284–5286

Aslanzadeh J, Helm KF, Espy MJ, Muller SA, Smith TF (1992) Detection of HSV-specific DNA in biopsy tissue of patients with erythema multiforme by polymerase chain reaction. Br J Dermatol 126: 19

Balfour HH Jr, Englund JA (1989) Antiviral drugs in pediatrics. Am J Dis Child 143: 1307–1316

Banks TA, Rouse BT (1992) Herpesviruses: immune escape artists? Clin Infect Dis 14: 933–941

Barkvoll P, Attramadal A (1987) Recurrent herpes labialis in a military brass band. Scand J Dent Res 95: 256–258

Barrett AP (1986) A long-term prospective clinical study of orofacial herpes simplex virus infections in acute leukaemia. Oral Surg Oral Med Oral Pathol 61: 149–152

Barrett AP (1987) A long-term prospective clinical study of oral complications during conventional chemotherapy for acute leukemia. Oral Surg Oral Med Oral Pathol 63: 313–316

Barrett AP, Katelaris CH, Morris JG, Schifter M (1993) Zoster sine herpete of the trigeminal nerve. Oral Surg Oral Med Oral Pathol 75: 173–175

Beaudenon S, Praetorius F, Kremsdorf D et al (1987) A new type of human papillomavirus associated with oral focal epithelial hyperplasia. J Invest Dermatol 88: 130–135

Beauparlant P, Alfieri C, Joncas JH (1994) Radioimmunoprecipitation in the diagnosis of chronic active Epstein-Barr virus infection. J Med Virol 42: 241–246

Becker J, Leser U, Marschall M et al (1991) Expression of proteins encoded by Epstein-Barr virus trans-activator genes depends on the differentiation of epithelial cells in oral hairy leukoplakia. Proc Natl Acad Sci USA 88: 8332–8336

Belshe RB (ed) (1984) Textbook of human virology. PBS, Littleton

Belton CM, Eversole LR (1986) Oral hairy leukoplakia: ultrastuctural features. J Oral Pathol 15: 493–499

Beral V, Peterman TA, Berkelman RL, Jaffe HW (1990) Kaposi's sarcoma among persons with AIDS: a sexually transmitted infection? Lancet 335: 123–138

Beral V, Peterman T, Berkelman R, Jaffe HW (1991) AIDS-associated non-Hodgkin's lymphoma. Lancet 337: 805–809

Bergmann OJ, Mogensen SC, Ellegaard J (1990) Herpes simplex virus and intraoral ulcers in immunocompromised patients with haematologic malignancies. Eur J Clin Microbiol Infect Dis 9: 184–190

Bergstrom T, Lycke E (1990) Neuroinvasion by herpes simplex virus. An in vitro model for characterisation of neurovirulent strains. J Gen Virol 71: 405–410

Berman S, Jensen J (1990) Cytomegalovirus induced osteomyelitis in a patient with the acquired immunodeficiency syndrome. South Med J 83: 1231–1232

Bernard HV, Apt D (1994) Transcriptional control and cell type specificity of HPV gene expression. Arch Dematol 130: 210–215

Bernstein DI, Stanberry LR, Harrison CJ et al (1987) Antibody response to herpes simplex glycoprotein D: effects of acyclovir and relation to recurrence. J Infect Dis 156: 423–429

Berry NJ, Burns DM, Wannamethee G et al (1988) Seroepidemiologic studies on the acquisition of antibodies to cytomegalovirus, herpes simplex virus, and human immunodeficiency virus among general hospital patients and those attending a clinic for sexually transmitted diseases. J Med Virol 24: 385–393

Biberfeld P, Petren AL, Eklund A et al (1988) Human herpesvirus 6 (HHV-6, HLBV) in sarcoidosis and lymphoproliferative disorders. J Virol Methods 21: 49–59

Birek C, Patterson B, Maximiw WC, Minden MD (1989) EBV and HSV infections in a patient who had undergone bone marrow transplantation: oral manifestations and diagnosis by in situ nucleic acid hybridization. Oral Surg Oral Med Oral Pathol 68: 612–617

Birx DL, Robert RR, Taroto G (1986) Defective regulation of Epstein-Barr virus infection in patients with acquired immunodeficiency syndrome (AIDS) or AIDS-related disorders. N Engl J Med 314: 874–879

Black JB, Inoue N, Kite-Powell K, Zaki S, Pellett PE (1993) Frequent isolation of human herpesvirus 7 from saliva. Virus Res 29: 91–98

Blackwelder WC, Dolin R, Mittal KK, McNamara PM, Payne FJ (1982) A population study of herpes virus infections and HLA antigens. Am J Epidemiol 115: 569–576

Blyth WA, Hill TJ (1984) Establishment, maintenance and control of herpes simplex virus (HSV1) latency. In: Rouse B, Lopez T (eds) Immunobiology of herpes simplex virus infection. CRC Press, Boca-Raton, pp 9–32

Boshoff C, Whitby D, Hatziioannou T et al (1995) Kaposi sarcoma associated herpesvirus in HIV-negative Kaposi sarcoma. Lancet 345: 1043–1044

Brachman DG, Graves D, Vokes E, Beckett M, Haraf D, Montag A, Dunphy E, Mick R, Yandell D, Weichselbaum RR (1992) Occurrence of p53 gene deletions and human papilloma virus infection in human head and neck cancer. Cancer Res 52: 4832

Brahim JS, Katz RW, Roberts MW (1988) Non-Hodgkin's lymphoma of the hard palate mucosa and buccal gingival associated with AIDS. J Oral Maxillofac Surg 46: 328–330

Brandsma JL, Abramson AL (1989) Association of papillomavirus with cancers of the head and neck. Arch Otolaryngol Head Neck Surg 115: 621–625

Brehmer-Andersson E, Lucht E, Lindskog S, Ekman M, Biberfeld P (1994) Oral hairy leukoplakia: pathogenetic aspects and significance of the lesion. Acta Derm Venereol 74: 81–89

Brice SL, Krzemien D, Weston WL et al (1989) Detection of herpes simplex virus DNA in cutaneous lesions of erythema multiforme. J Invest Dermatol 93: 193

Brice SL, Stockert SS, Bunker JD, Bloomfield D, Huff JC, Norris DA, Weston WL (1993) The herpes-specific immune response of individuals with herpes-associated erythema multiforme compared with that of individuals with recurrent herpes labialis. Arch Dermatol Res 285: 193–196

Brockmeyer NH, Kreuzfelder E, Mertins L, Daecke D, Boos M (1989) Zidovudine therapy of asymptomatic HIV 1-infected patients and combined zidovudine-acyclovir therapy of HIV 1-infected patients with oral hairy leukoplakia. J Invest Dermatol 92: 647

Brunell PA, Novelli VM, Keller PM, Ellis RW (1987) Antibodies to the three major glycoproteins of varicella-zoster virus: search for the relevant host immune response. J Infect Dis 156: 430–436

Bryson YJ (1988) Promising new antiviral drugs. J Am Acad Dermatol 18: 212–218

Burg G, Sobetzko R (1990) Oral florid papillomatosis: is etretinate therapy indicated? Hautarzt 41: 314–316

Burt RD, Vaughan TL, Nisperos B, Swanson M, Berwick M (1994) A protective association between the HLA-A2 antigen and nasopharyngeal carcinoma in US caucasians. Int J Cancer 56: 465–467

Carbone A, Tirelli U, Vaccher E et al (1991) A clinico-pathologic study of lymphoid neoplasias associated with human immunodeficiency virus infection in Italy. Cancer 68: 842–852

Cesarman E, Chang Y, Moore PS, Said JW, Knowles DM (1995) Kaposi's sarcoma-associated herpesvirus-like DNA sequences in AIDs-related body-cavity-based lymphomas. N Engl J Med 332: 1186–1191

Chang KW, Chang CS, Lai KS, Chou MJ, Choo KB (1989) High prevalence of human papillomavirus infection and possible association with betel quid chewing and smoking in oral epidermoid carcinomas in Taiwan. J Med Virol 28: 57–61

Chang F, Kosunen I, Kosma VM, Syrjanen S, Lahtinen J, Syrjanen K (1990a) Verrucous carcinoma of the anus containing human papillomavirus type 16 DNA detected by in situ hybridization, a case report. Genitourin Med 66: 342–345

Chang F, Syrjanen S, Nuutinen J, Karja J, Syrjanen K (1990b) Detection of human papillomavirus (HPV) DNA in oral squamous cell carcinomas by in situ hybridization and polymerase chain reaction. Arch Dermatol Res 282: 493–497

Chang F, Syrjanen S, Kellokoski J, Syrjanen K (1991) Human papillomavirus (HPV) infections and their associations with oral disease. J Oral Pathol Med 20: 305–317

Chang F, Syrjanen S, Mang L, Syrjanen K (1992) Infectious agents in the etiology of esophageal cancer. Gastroenterology 103: 1336–1348

Chang Y (1994) Identification of herpesvirus-like DNA sequences in AIDS-associated Kaposi's sarcoma. Science 266: 1865–1869

Chang Y, Cesarman E, Pessin MS et al (1994) Identification of herpesvirus-like DNA sequences in AIDS-associated Kaposi's sarcoma. Science 266: 1865–1869

Choo QL, Kuo G, Weiner AJ, Overby LR, Bradley DW, Houghton M (1989) Isolation of a cDNA clone derived from a blood-borne non-A, non-B viral hepatitis genome. Science 244: 359–362

Christenson B, Bottiger M, Svensson A, Jeansson S (1992) A 15-year surveillance study of antibodies to herpes simplex virus type 1 and 2 in a cohort of young girls. J Infect 25: 147–154

Cleveland DB, Chen SY, Allen CM, Ahing SI, Svirsky JA (1994) Adult rhabdomyoma: a light microscopic, ultrastructural, virologic, and immunologic analysis. Oral Surg Oral Med Oral Pathol 77: 147–153

Cohen S, Williamson GM (1991) Stress and infectious disease in humans. Psychol Bull 109: 5–24

Cohen SG, Greenberg MS (1985) Chronic herpes simplex virus infection in immunocompromised patients. Oral Surg Oral Med Oral Pathol 59: 465–471

Collandre H, Ferris S, Grau O et al (1995) Kaposi's sarcoma and new herpesvirus. Lancet 345: 1043

Colmenero C, Gamallo G, Pintado V, Patron M, Sierra J, Valencia E (1991) AIDS related lymphoma of the oral cavity. Int J Oral Maxillofac Surg 20: 2–6

Corey L (1988) First episode, recurrent, and asymptomatic herpes simplex infections. J Am Acad Dermatol 18: 169–172

Corey L, Spear PG (1986) Infections with herpes simplex viruses. N Engl J Med 314: 686–691, 749–757

Corso B, Eversole LR, Hutt-Fletcher L (1989) Hairy leukoplakia: Epstein-Barr virus receptors on oral keratinocyte plasma membranes. Oral Surg Oral Med Oral Pathol 67: 416–421

Cox MF, Eveson J, Maitland N, Scully C (1991a) Human papillomavirus type 16 DNA in an odontogenic keratocyst. J Oral Pathol Med 20: 143–145

Cox MF, Scully C, Maitland NJ (1991b) Viruses in the aetiology of oral cancer? Examination of the evidence. Br J Oral Maxillofac Surg 29: 381–387

Cox MF, Eveson J, Porter SR, Maitland NJ, Scully C (1992) Human papilloma virus type 16 DNA in oral white sponge naevus. Oral Surg Oral Med Oral Pathol 73: 476–478

Cox MF, Maitland NJ, Scully C (1993) Human herpes simplex-1 and papillomavirus type 16 homologous DNA sequences in normal, premalignant and malignant oral mucosa. Oral oncology. Eur J Cancer 29B: 215–220

Crooks RJ, Jones DA, Fiddian AP (1991) Zoster-associated chronic pain: an overview of clinical trials with acyclovir. Scand J Infect [Suppl] 78: 62–68

Crumpacker CS (1988) Significance of resistance of herpes simplex virus to acyclovir. J Am Acad Dermatol 18: 190–195

Daniels TE, Sylvester RA, Silverman S, Dolando V, Talal N (1974) Tubuloreticular "virus-like" structures within labial salivary glands in patients with Sjogren's syndrome. Arthritis Rheum 17: 593–597

Daniels TE, Greenspan D, Greenspan JS (1987) Absence of Langerhans's cells in oral hairy leukoplakia, an AIDS-associated lesion. J Invest Dermatol 87: 178–182

Darragh TM, Egbert BM, Berger TG, Yen TS (1991) Identification of herpes simplex virus DNA in lesions of erythema multiforme by the polymerase chain reaction. J Am Acad Dermatol 24: 23

Davison AJ, Edson CM, Ellis RW et al (1986) New common nomenclature for glycoprotein genes of varicella-zoster virus and their glycosylated products. J Virol 57: 1195–1197

De Clerc QE (1988) Antiviral chemotherapy today and tomorrow. Ann Intern Med 139: 84–86

Deacon EM, Mathews JB, Potts AJC, Hamburger J, Bevan IS (1991) Detection of Epstein-Barr virus antigens and DNA using immunocytochemistry and polymerase chain reaction: possible relationship with Sjogren's syndrome. J Pathol 163: 351–360

Deacon LM, Shattles WG, Mathews JG, Young LS, Venables JW (1992) Frequency of EBV-DNA detection in Sjogren's syndrome. Am J Med 92: 453–454

Dekmezian RH, Batsakis JG, Goepfert H (1987) In situ hybridization of papillomavirus DNA in head and neck squamous cell carcinomas. Arch Otolaryngol Head Neck Surg 113: 819

Detjen PF, Patterson R, Noskin GA, Phair JP, Loyd SO (1992) Herpes simplex virus association with recurrent Stevens-Johnson syndrome. Arch Intern Med 152: 1513–1516

De Villiers EM (1989a) Heterogeneity of the human papillomavirus group. J Virol 65: 4898–4903

De Villiers EM (1989b) Papilloma viruses in cancers and papillomas of the aerodigestive tract. Biomed Pharmacother 43: 31–36

De Villiers EM, Hirsch-Benham A, Von Knebel-Doebertiz C et al (1989) Two newly identified human papillomavirus types (HPV 40 and 57) isolated from mucosal lesions. Virology 171: 248–253

Diaz-Mitoma F, Ruiz A, Flowerdew G et al (1990) High levels of Epstein-Barr virus in the oropharynx: a predictor of disease progression in human immunodeficiency virus infection. J Med Virol 31: 69–75

Dimery IW, Lee JS, Blick M, Pearson G, Spitzer G, Hong WK (1988) Association of the Epstein-Barr virus with lymphoepithelioma of the thymus. Cancer 61: 2475–2480

DiPaolo JA, Woodworth CD, Popescu NC, Koval DL, Lopez JV, Doniger J (1990) HSV-2-induced tumorigenicity in HPV-16-immortalized human genital keratinocytes. Virol 177: 777–779

Diss TC, Wotherspoon AC, Speight P, Pan L, Isaacson PG (1995) B-cell monoclonality, Epstein Barr Virus and t(14;18) in myoepithelial sialadenitis and low-grade B-cell MALT lymphoma of the parotid gland. Am J Surg Pathol 19: 531–536

Donkor P, Punnia-Moorthy A, Painter DM (1991) A case of AIDS presenting as intra-oral malignant lymphoma. Aust Dent J 36(1): 22–28

Dorian KJ, Beatty E, Atterbury KD (1990) Detection of herpes simplex virus by the Kodak Sure Cell herpes test. J Clin Microbiol 28: 2117–2119

Drew WL, Miner RC, Ziegler JL et al (1982) Cytomegalovirus and Kaposi's sarcoma in young homosexual men. Lancet 2: 125–127

Drijkoningen M, De Wolf-Peeters C, Degreef H, Desmet V (1988) Epidermal Langerhans cells, dermal dendritic cells, and keratinocytes in viral lesions of skin and mucous membranes, an immunohistochemical study. Arch Dermatol Res 280: 220

Duff RG, Rapp F (1971) Oncogenic transformation of hamster embryo cells after exposure to herpes simplex virus type 2. Nature 233: 48–50

Dupin N, Gradadam M, Calvez V et al (1995) Herpesvirus like DNA sequences in patients with Mediterranean Kaposi's sarcoma. Lancet 345: 761–762

Duvic M, Reisner EG, Dawson DV, Ciftan E (1983) HLA-B15 association with erythema multiforme. J Am Acad Dermatol 8: 493

Eglin RP, Scully C, Lehner T, Ward-Booth P, McGregor IA (1983) Detection of RNA complementary to herpes simplex virus DNA in human oral squamous cell carcinoma. Lancet ii: 766–768

Eisenberg E, Krutchkoff D, Yamase H (1992) Incidental oral hairy leukoplakia in immunocompetent persons. Oral Surg Oral Med Oral Pathol 74: 332–333

Epstein JB, Scully C (1991) Herpes simplex virus in immunocompromised patients: growing evidence of drug resistance. Oral Surg Oral Med Oral Pathol 72: 47–50

Epstein JB, Scully C (1993) Cytomegalovirus: a virus of increasing relevance to oral medicine and pathology. J Oral Pathol Med 22: 348–353

Epstein JB, Priddy RW, Sherlock CH (1988) Hairy leukoplakia-like lesions in immunosuppressed patients following bone marrow transplantation. Transplantation 46: 462–464

Epstein JB, Sherlock CH, Greenspan JS (1991) Hairy leukoplakia-like lesions following bone marrow transplantation. AIDS 5: 101–102

Epstein JB, Wolber RA, Sherlock CH (1992) Cytomegalovirus-induced gingival hyperplasia following cardiac transplantation. Ann Intern Med 116: 1034

Epstein JB, Sherlock CH, Wolber RA (1993) Hairy leukoplakia after bone marrow transplantation. Oral Surg Oral Med Oral Pathol 75: 690–695

Epstein JB, Fatahzadeh M, Matisic J, Anderson G (1995) Exfoliative cytology and electron microscopy in the diagnosis of hairy leukoplakia. Oral Surg Oral Med Oral Pathol Oral Radiol Endod 79: 564–569

Erice A, Chou S, Biron KK, Stanat SC, Balfour HH, Jordan MC (1989) Progressive disease due to ganciclovir-resistant cytomegalovirus in immunocompromised patients. N Engl J Med 320: 289–293

Erlich KS, Mills J, Chatis PS, et al (1989) Acyclovir-resistant herpes simplex virus infections in patients with the accquired immunodeficiency syndrome. N Engl J Med 320: 293–296

Evans AS (1982) The transmission of EB viral infections. In: Hooks J, Jordan G (eds) Viral infections in oral medicine. Elsevier, Amsterdam, p 211

Eversole LR, Laipis PJ (1988) Oral squamous papillomas: detecton of HPV DNA by in situ hybridization. Oral Surg Oral Med Oral Pathol 65: 545–550

Eversole LR, Jacobsen P, Stone CE, Freckleton V (1986) Oral condyloma planus (hairy leukoplakia) among homosexual men: a clinico-pathologic study of 36 cases. Oral Surg Oral Med Oral Pathol 61: 249–255

Eversole LR, Laipis PJ, Merrell P, Choi E (1987) Demonstration of human papillomavirus DNA in oral condyloma acuminatum. J Oral Pathol 16: 266–272

Eversole LR, Stone CE, Beckman AM (1988) Detection of EBV and HPV-DNA sequences in oral "hairy" leukoplakia by in situ hybridisation. J Med Virol 26: 271–277

Farese RV, Schambelan M, Hollander H, Stingari S, Jacobson MA (1990) Nephrogenic diabetes insipidus associated with foscarnet treatment of cytomegalovirus retinitis. Ann Intern Med 112: 955–956

Farrell PJ, Allan GJ, Shanahan F et al (1991) p53 is frequently mutated in Burkitt's lymphoma cell lines. EMBO J 10: 2879–2887

Ferris DG, Fischer PM (1992) Elementary school student's performance with two ELISA test systems. JAMA 268: 766–770

Ficarra G, Barone R, Gaglioti D, Milo D, Riccardi R, Romagnoli P, Zorn M (1988a) Oral hairy leukoplakia among HIV-positive intravenous drug abusers: a clinicopathologic and ultrastructural study. Oral Surg Oral Med Oral Pathol 65: 421–426

Ficarra G, Barone R, Gaglioti D (1988b) Oral hairy leukoplakia among HIV positive intravenous drug abusers: a clinicopathologic and ultrastructural study. Oral Surg Oral Med Oral Pathol 65: 421–426

Ficarra G, Miliani A, Adler-Storthz K et al (1991) Recurrent oral condylomata acuminata and hairy luekoplakia: an early sign of myelodisplastic syndrome in an HIV-seronegative patient. J Oral Pathol Med 20: 398–402

Field AK, Davies ME, Dewitt C et al (1983) 9-({2-9hydroxy-1-hydroxymethyl)ethoxymethyl) guanine: a selective inhibitor of herpes-group virus replication. Proc Natl Acad Sci USA 80: 4139–4143

Field JK, Spandidos DA, Malliri A, Gosney JR, Yiagnisis M, Stell PM (1991) Elevated p53 expression correlates with a history of heavy smoking in squamous cell carcinoma of the head and neck. Br J Cancer 64: 573–577

Field JK, Spandidos DA, Stell PM (1992) Overexpression of p53 gene in head and neck cancer, linked with heavy smoking and drinking. Lancet 339: 502–503

Flescher E, Talal N (1991) Do viruses contribute to the development of Sjogren's syndrome? Am J Med 90: 283–285

Fluckiger R, Laifer G, Itin P, Meyer B, Lang C (1994) Oral hairy leukoplakia in a patient with ulcerative colitis. Gastroenterol 106: 506–508

Forbes BA (1989) Acquisition of cytomegalovirus infection: an update. Clin Microbiol Rev 2: 204–216

Fox JD, Briggs M, Ward P, Tedder RS (1990) Human herpesvirus 6 in salivary glands. Lancet ii: 590–593

Fox RI (1989) Viral genomes in lymphomas of patients with Sjogren's syndrome. In: Talal N (ed) Sjogren's syndrome: a model for understanding autoimmunity. Academic, London, pp 141–147

Fox RI, Pearson G, Vaughan JH (1986) Detection of Epstein-Barr virus-associated antigens and DNA in salivary gland biopsies from patients with Sjogren's syndrome. J Immunol 137: 3162–3168

Fox RI, Luppi M, Kang HI, Pisa P (1991) Reactivation of Epstein-Barr virus in Sjogren's syndrome. Springer Semin Immunopathol 13: 217–231

Fox SF, Meiller TF, Lohr JT, Sydiskis RJ (1987) Evaluation of a monoclonal antibody typing system for herpes simplex virus. Oral Surg Oral Med Oral Pathol 64: 165–170

Fraga-Fernandez J, Vicandi-Plaza B (1992) Diagnosis of hairy leukokplakia by exfoliative cytologic methods. Am J Clin Pathol 97: 262–266

Frazer IH, Leonard JH, Schonrock J, Wright RG, Kearsley JH (1993) HPV DNA in oropharyngeal squamous cell cancers: comparison of results from four DNA detection methods. Pathology 25: 138–143

Freeman JL, McIvor NP, Feinmesser R, Cheung RK, Dosch HM (1994) Epstein-Barr virus and nasopharyngeal carcinoma: bringing molecular genetics strategies to head and neck oncology. J Otolaryngol 23: 130–134

Frenkel N, Schirmer EC, Wyatt LS, Katsafanas G, Roffman E, Danovich RM, June CH (1990) Isolation of a new herpesvirus from human CD4+ T cells. Proc Natl Acad Sci USA 87: 748–752

Friedman-Kien AE (1986) Viral origin of hairy leukoplakia. Lancet ii: 694

Friedman-Kien AE, Saltzman BR, Cao YZ et al (1990) Kaposi's sarcoma in HIV-negative homosexual men. Lancet 335: 168–169

Gail MH, Pluda JM, Rabkin CS et al (1991) Projections of the incidence of non-Hodgkin's lymphoma related to acquired immunodeficiency syndrome. J Natl Cancer Inst 83: 695–701

Gallina G, Cumbo V, Messina P et al (1985) HLA-A, B and C antigens in Sicilian patients with recurrent herpes labialis. IRCS Med Sci 13: 374–373

Garlick JA, Calderon S, Buchner A, Mitrani-Rosenbaum S (1989) Detection of human papillomavirus (HPV) DNA in focal epithelial hyperplasia. J Oral Pathol Med 18: 172–177

Garry RF, Fermin CD, Hart DJ, Alexander SS, Donehower LA, Luo-Zhang H (1990) Detection of a human intracisternal A-type retroviral particle antigenically related to HIV. Science 250: 1127–1129

Gaston JS, Rowe M, Bacon P (1991) Sjogren's syndrome after infection by Epstein-Barr Virus. J Rheumatol 17: 558–561

Gentry LO, Zeluff B (1988) Infection in the cardiac transplant patient. In: Rubin RH, Young LS (eds) Clinical approach to infection in the compromised host, 2nd edn. Plenum Medical, New York, pp 623–648

Gershon AA, National Institute of Allergy and Infectious Diseases Varicella Vaccine Collaborative Study Group (1990) Live attenuated varicella vaccine: protection in healthy adults compared with leukaemic children. J Infect Dis 161: 661–666

Gibson JR, Klaber MR, Harvey SG, Tosti A, Jones D, Yeo JM (1986) Prophylaxis against herpes labialis with acyclovir cream – a placebo-controlled study. Dermatologica 172: 104–107

Gilligan K, Rajadurai P, Resnick L, Raab-Traub N (1990) Epstein-Barr virus small nuclear RNAs are not expressed in permissively infected cells in AIDS-associated leukoplakia. Proc Natl Acad Sci USA 87: 8790–8794

Glaser R, Kiecolt-Glaser JK, Speicher CE, Holliday JE (1985) Stress, loneliness, and changes in herpesvirus latency. J Behav Med 8: 249–260

Glaser R, Rice J, Sheridan et al (1987) Stress-related immune suppression: health implications. Brain Behav Immun 1: 7–20

Glick M, Cleveland DB, Salkin LM, Alfaro-Miranda A, Fielding AF (1991) Intraoral cytomegalovirus lesion and HIV-associated periodontitis in a patient with acquired immunodeficiency syndrome. Oral Surg Oral Med Oral Pathol 72: 716–720

Gluckman E, Lotsberg J, Devergie A et al (1983a) Oral acyclovir prophylactic treatment of herpes simplex infection after bone marrow transplantation. J Antimicrob Chemother 12 [Suppl B]: 161–167

Cluckman E, Lotsberg J, Devergie A et al (1983b) Prophylaxis of herpes infections after bone-marrow transplantation by oral acyclovir. Lancet 2: 706–708

Gonik B, Seibel M, Berkowitz A, Woodin MB, Mills K (1991) Comparison of two enzyme-linked immunosorbent assays for detection of herpes simplex virus antigen. In Clin Microbiol 29: 436–438

Gopal MR, Thomson BJ, Fox J, Tedder RS, Honess RW (1990) Detection by PCR of HHV-6 and EBV DNA in blood and oropharynx of healthy adults and HIV-seropositives. Lancet 335: 1598–1599

Gottlieb MS, Schroff R, Schanker HM et al (1981) Pneumocystis carinii pneumonia and mucosal candidiasis in previously healthy homosexual men: evidence of a new acquired cellular immunodeficiency. N Engl J Med 305: 1425–1431

Grattan CEH, Small D, Kennedy CTC, Scully C (1986) Oral herpes simplex infection in bullous pemphigoid. Oral Surg Oral Med Oral Pathol 61: 40–43

Green JA, Spruance SL, Wenerstrom G, Pipkorn MW (1985) Post-herpetic erythema multiforme prevented with prophylactic oral acyclovir. Ann Intern Med 102: 632–633

Green TL, Eversole LR (1989) Oral lymphomas in HIV-infected patients: associated with Epstein-Barr virus DNA. Oral Surg Oral Med Oral Pathol 67: 437–442

Green TL, Greenspan JS, Greenspan D, DeSouza YG (1989) Oral lesions mimicking hairy leukoplakia: a diagnostic dilemma. Oral Surg Oral Med Oral Pathol 67: 422–426

Greenberg MS, Cohen SG, Boosz B, Friedman H (1987a) Oral herpes simplex infections in patients with leukemia. JADA 114: 483–486

Greenberg MS, Friedman H, Cohen SG, Ol SH, Laster L, Starr S (1987b) A comparative study of herpes simplex infections in renal transplant and leukemic patients. J Infect Dis 156: 280–287

Greenberg MS, Dubin G, Stewart JCB, Cumming CG, MacGregor RR, Freidman HM (1995) Relationship of oral disease to the presence of cytomegalovirus DNA in the saliva of AIDS patients. Oral Surg Oral Med Oral Pathol 79: 175–179

Greenspan D, Greenspan JS, Conant M, Petersen V, Silverman S, DeSouza Y (1984) Oral "hairy" leukoplakia in male homosexuals: evidence of association with both papillomavirus and a herpes-group virus. Lancet ii: 831–834

Greenspan D, de Villiers EM, Greenspan JS et al (1988) Unusual HPV types in oral warts in association with HIV infection. J Oral Pathol 17: 482–487

Greenspan D, Greenspan JS, DeSouza YG, Levy JA, Ungar AM (1989) Oral hairy leukoplakia in an HIV-negative renal transplant recipient. J Oral Pathol Med 18: 32–34

Greenspan D, Greenspan JS, Pindborg JJ, Schiodt M (1990) AIDS and the dental team, 2nd edn. Munksgaard, Copenhagen

Greenspan JS, Green D (1989) Oral hairy leukoplakia: diagnosis and management. Oral Surg Oral Med Oral Pathol 67: 396–403

Greenspan JS, Greenspan D, Lennette ET, Abrams B, Conant M, Petersen V, Freese H (1985) Replication of Epstein-Barr virus within the epithelial cells of "hairy" leukoplakia, an AIDS-associated lesion. N Engl J Med 313: 1564–1571

Greer RO, Eversole LR, Poulson TC, Boone ME, Lindenmuth JE, Crosby L (1987) Identification of human papillomavirus DNA in smokeless tobacco-associated keratoses from juveniles, adults and older adults using immunocytochemical and in situ DNA hybridization techniques. Gerodontics 3: 201–208

Greer RO Jr, Eversole LR, Crosby LK (1990) Detection of human papillomavirus-genomic DNA in oral epithelial dysplasias, oral smokeless tobacco-association leukoplakias, and epithelial malignancies. J Oral Maxillofac Surg 48: 1201–1205

Griffiths PD, Grundy JE (1988) The status of CMV as a human pathogen. Epidemiol Infect 100: 1–15

Grimwood R, Major M, Huff J, Weston W (1983) Complement deposition in the skin of patients with herpes-associated erythema multiforme. J Am Acad Dermatol 9: 199

Groot RH, van Merekesteyn JPR, Bras J (1990) Oral manifestations of non-Hodgkin's lymphoma in HIV infected patients. Int J Oral Maxillofac Surg 19: 194–196

Grose C, Litwin V (1988) Immunology of the varicella-zoster virus glycoproteins. J Infect Dis 157: 877–881

Gross G,Wiegand H, Zentgraf H (1988) Epstein-Barr virus detection in oral hairy leukoplakia in AIDS patients, in leukoplakias and on normal tongue epithelia in HIV-negative patients. Z Hantks 63: 44–48

Grossman ME, Stevens AW, Cohen PR (1993) Brief report: herpetic geometric glossitis. N Engl J Med 329: 1859–1860

Guinan ME, Wolinsky SM, Reichman RC (1985) Epidemiology of genital herpes simplex virus infection. Epidemiol Rev 7: 127–146

Gusterson BA, Anbazhagan R, Warren W, Midgely C, Lane DP, O'Hare M, Stamps A, Carter R, Jayatilake H (1991) Expression of p53 in premalignant and malignant squamous epithelium. Oncogene 6: 1785–1789

Haddad J, Deny P, Munz-Gother C et al (1992) Lymphocytic sialadenitis of Sjogren's syndrome associated with chronic hepatitis C virus liver disease. lancet 339: 321–323

Hamzaoui K, Ayed K, Slim A, Hamza M, Touraine J (1990) Natural killer cell activity, interferon gamma and antibodies to herpes viruses in patients with Behcet's disease. Clin Exp Immunol 79: 28–34

Hann IM, Prentice HG, Blacklock HA et al (1983) Acyclovir prophylaxis against herpes virus infections in severely immunocompromised patients: randomized double blind trial. Br Med J 287: 384–388

Harabuchi Y, Yamanaka N, Kataura A et al (1990) Epstein-Barr virus in nasal T-cell lymphomas in patients with lethal midline granuloma. Lancet i: 128

Harbour DA, Hill TJ, Blyth WA (1983) Recurrent herpes simplex in the mouse: inflammation in the skin and activation of virus in ganglia following peripheral stimulation. J Gen Virol 64: 1491–1498

Harnett GB, Farr TJ, Pietroboni GR, Bucens MR (1990) Frequent shedding of human herpesvirus 6 in saliva. J Med Virol 32: 139–142

Haverkos HW, Friedman-Kien AE, Doetman DP, Morgan WM (1990) The changing incidence of Kaposi's sarcoma among patients with AIDS. J Am Acad Dermatol 22: 1250–1253

Henderson S, Rowe M, Gregory C et al (1991) Induction of bcl-2 expression by Epstein-Barr virus latent membrane protein 1 protects infected B cells from programmed cell death. Cell 65: 1107

Henke PR, Guerin-Reverchon I, Milde-Langosch K, Stromme-Koppang H, Loning T (1989) In situ detection of human papillomavirus types 13 and 32 in focal epithelial hyperplasia of the oral mucosa. J Oral Pathol Med 18: 419–421

Herndier GB, Werner A, Arnstein P et al (1994) Characterisation of a human Kaposi's sarcoma cell line that induces angiogenic tumors in animals. AIDS 8: 575–581

Hersman J, Meyers JD, Thomas ED, Buckner CD, Clift R (1982) The effect of granulocyte transfusions upon the incidence of cytomegalovirus infection after allogeneic marrow transplantation. Ann Intern Med 96: 149–52

Hidaka Y, Liu Y, Yamamoto M, Mori R, Miyazaki C, Kusuhara K, Okada K, Ueda K (1993) Frequent isolation of human herpes virus 7 from saliva samples. J Med Virol 40: 343–346

Hill TJ (1985) Herpes simplex virus latency. In: Roizman B (ed) The herpes viruses, vol 3. Plenum, New York, pp 175–240

Hill PA, Lamey PJ (1986) Oral herpes zoster with contralateral skin involvement. Br Dent J 161: 217–218

Hirsch JM, Johannson SL, Vahlne A (1984a) Effect of snuff and herpes simplex virus-1 on oral mucosa. Possible association with the development of squamous cell carcinoma. J Oral Pathol 13: 52–62

Hirsch JM, Svennerholm B, Vahlne A (1984b) Inhibition of herpes simplex virus replication by tobacco extracts. Cancer Res 44: 1991–1997

Ho M (1990) Epidemiology of cytomegalovirus infections. Rev Infect Dis 19: 5701–5710

Hommel DJ, Brown ML, Kinzie JJ (1987) Response to radiotherapy of head and neck tumours in AIDS patients. Am J Surg 154: 443–446

Honig JF, Becker MJ, Brinck Y, Korabiowska M (1995) Detection of human papillomavirus DNA sequences in leucocytes: a new approach to identify hematological markers of HPV infection in patients with oral SCC. Bull Group Int Rech Sci Stomatol Odontol 38: 25–31

Hopp JR, Collins FJV, Ross A, Myall RWT (1982) A review of Burkitt's lymphoma: importance of radiographic diagnosis. J Maxillfac Surg 10: 240–245

Hording U, Nielsen HW, Dangaard S, Albeck H (1994) Human papillomavirus types 11 and 16 detected in nasopharyngeal carcinomas by the polymerase chain reaction. Laryngoscope 104: 99–102

Horiuchi H, Mishima K, Ichijima K, Sugimura M Ishida T, Kirita T (1995) Epstein-Barr virus in the proliferative diseases of squamous epithelium in the oral cavity. Oral Surg Oral Med Oral Pathol 79: 57–63

Hsu MM, Chang YL, Ko JY, Chen CL, Kao YF (1994) Epstein-Barr virus harboring in the parotid gland without tumor association. J Formos Med Assoc 93: 104–109

Huang YQ, Li JJ, Kaplan MH et al (1995) Human herpesvirus-like nucleic acid in various forms of Kaposi's sarcoma. Lancet 345: 759–761

Huff JW, Weston WL (1989) Recurrent erythema multiforme. Medicine (Baltimore) 68: 133

Hyman RW (ed) (1987) Natural history of varicella-zoster virus. CRC Press, Gainsville, Florida

Isaacs D, Menser M (1990) Modern vaccines: measles mumps, rubella and varicella. Lancet 335: 1384–1387

Itin P, Rufli I, Rudlinser R, Lathomas G, Hurer H, Podrinec M, Gurdat A (1988) Oral hairy leukoplakia in a HIV-negative renal transplant patient: a marker for immunosuppression. Dermatologica 17: 126–128

Iwasaka T, Yokoyama M, Hayashi Y, Sugimori H (1988) Combined herpes simplex virus type 2 and human papillomavirus type 16 or 18 deoxyribonucleic acid leads to oncogenic transformation. Am J Obstet Gynecol 159: 1251–1255

Jabbar AAR, Al-Samarou Am, Al-Amar NS (1991) HLA antigens associated with susceptibility to herpes simplex virus infection. Dis Markers 9: 281–287

Jacobsen MA, Mills J (1988) Serious cytomegalovirus disease in the acquired immunodeficiency syndrome (AIDS). Ann Intern Med 108: 585–594

Jalal H, Sanders CM, Prime SS, Scully C, Maitland NJ (1992) Detection of human papillomavirus type 16 DNA in oral squames from normal young adults. J Oral Pathol Med 28: 465–470

Jalal H, Scully C, Maitland NJ, Porter S, Luker J Detection of Epstein-Barr virus DNA in oral squames from HIV seropositive persons by polymerase chain reaction. J Oral Path Med (in press)

Jarrett RF, Clark DA, Josephs SF, Onions DE (1990) Detection of human herpesvirus-6 DNA in peripheral blood and saliva. J Med Virol 32: 73–76

Johnson FB (1982) Chemical interactions with herpes simplex type 2 virus: enhancement of transformation by selected chemical carcinogens and procarcinogens. Carcinogenesis 3: 1235–1240

Johnson TL, Plieth DA, Crissman JD, Sarkar FH (1991) HPV detection by polymerase chain reaction (PCR) in verrucous lesions of the upper aerodigestive tract. Mod Pathol 4: 461

Jones AC, Migliorati CA, Baughman RA (1992) The simultaneous occurrence of oral herpes simplex virus, cytomegalovirus, and histoplasmosis in an HIV-infected patient. Oral Surg Oral Med Oral Pathol 74: 334–339

Jones AC, Freedman PD, Phelan JA, Baughman RA, Kerpel SM (1993) Cytomegalovirus infections of the oral cavity. Oral Surg Oral Med Oral Pathol 73: 76–85

Kameyama T, Sujaku C, Yamamot S, Hwang C, Shillitoe E (1988a) Shedding of herpes simplex virus type 1 into saliva in a Japanese population. J Oral Pathol 17: 478–481

Kameyama T, Sujaku C, Yamamoto S et al (1988b) Shedding of herpex simplex virus type 1 into saliva. J Oral Pathol 17: 478–481

Kameyama T, Futami M, Nakayoshi N, Sujaku C, Yamamoto S (1989) Shedding of herpes simplex virus type 1 into saliva in aptients with orofacial fracture. J Med Virol 28: 78–80

Kampgen E, Burg G, Wank R (1988) Association of herpes simplex virus-induced erythema multiforme with human leukocyte antigen DQw3. Arch Dermatol 124: 1372

Kanas RJ, Jensen JL, Abrams AM (1987) Cytomegalovirus as a manifestation of the acquired immune deficiency syndrome. Oral Surg Oral Med Oral Pathol 64: 183–189

Kanas RJ, Abrams AM, Jensen JL, Wuerker RB, Handlers JP (1988a) Oral hairy leukoplakia: ultrastructural observations. Oral Surg Oral Med Oral Pathol 65: 333–338

Kanas RJ, Abrams AM, Recher L, Jansen JL, Handlers JP, Wuerker RB (1988b) Oral hairy leukoplakia: a light microscopic and immunohistochemical study. Oral Surg Oral Med Oral Pathol 66: 334–340

Kaner RJ, Baird A, Mansukhani A et al (1990) Fibroblast growth factor receptor is a portal of cellular entry for herpes simplex virus type 1. Science 248: 1410–1413

Kanitakis J, Euvrard S, LeFrancois N, Hermier C, Thivolet J (1991) Oral hairy leukoplakia in a HIV-negative renal graft recipient. Br J Dermatol 124: 483–486

Karameris A, Gorgoulis V, Iliopoulos A (1992) Detection of the Epstein Barr viral genome by an in situ hybridization method in salivary gland biopsies from patients with secondary Sjogren's syndrome. Clin Exp Rheumatol 10: 327–332

Karja J, Syrjanen S, Usenius T, Vornanen M, Collan Y (1988) Oral cancer in children under 15 years of age. A clinicopatholgocial and virological study. Acta Otolaryngol (Stockh) 449: 145–149

Karp JE, Broder S (1991) Acquired immunodeficiency syndrome and non-Hodgkin's lymphomas. Cancer Res 51: 4743-4756

Kashima KH, Kutcher M, Kessis T, Levin LS, de Villiers E-M, Shah K (1990) Human papillomavirus in squamous cell carcinoma, leukoplakia, lichen planus, and clinically normal epithelium of the oral cavity. Ann Otol Rhinol Laryngol 99: 55-61

Kaugars GE, Burns JC (1989) Non-Hodgkin's lymphoma of the oral cavity associated with AIDS. Oral Surg Oral Med Oral Pathol 67: 433-436

Kazmierowski JA, Peizner DS, Wuepper KD (1982) Herpes simplex antigen in immune complexes of patients with erythema multiforme. J Am Med Assoc 247: 2547

Kellowski J, Syrjanen S, Syrjanen K, Yliskoski M (1990) Oral mucosal changes in women with genital HPV infection. J Oral Pathol Med 19: 12-148

Kellowski JK, Syrjanen SM, Chang F, Yliskoski M, Syrjanen KJ (1992a) Southern blot hybridization and PCR in detection of oral human papillomavirus (HPV) infections in women with genital HPV infections. J Oral Pathol Med 21: 459-464

Kellowski JK, Syrjanen S, Yliskoski M, Syrjanen K (1992b) Dot blot hybridization in detection of human papillomavirus (HPV) infections in oral cavity in women with genital HPV infections. J Oral Microbiol Immum 7: 19-23

Kessler HH, Benson CH, Urbanski P (1988) Regression of oral hairy leukoplakia during zidovudine therapy. Arch Intern Med 148: 2490-2497

Kido S, Kondon K, Kondon T, Morishima T, Takashashi M, Yamanishi K (1990) Detection of human herpesvirus 6 DNA in throat swabs by polymerase chain reaction, J Med Virol 32: 139-142

Kiecolt-Glaser JK, Kennedy S, Malkoff S et al (1988) Marital discord and immunity in males. Psychom Med 50: 213-229

Kitasato H, Delius H, Zur Hausen H, Sorger K, Rosl F, de Villiers EM (1994) Sequence rearrangements in the upstream regulation region of human papillomavirus type 6: are these involved in malignant transition? J Gen Virol 75: 1157-1162

Kiyabu MT, Shibata D, Arnheim N, Martin WJ, Fitzgibbons (1989) Detection of human papillomavirus in formalin-fixed, invasive squamous carcinomas using the polymerase chain reaction. Am J Surg 13: 221

Kohl S (1985) Herpes simplex virus immunology: problems, progress and promises. J Infect Dis 152: 435-440

Krueger GRF, Wassermann K, de Clerk LS et al (1990) Latent herpesvirus-6 in salivary and bronchial glands. Lancet 336: 590-593

Kucera LS, Daniel LW, Waite M (1983) 2-O-Tetradecanoyl-phorbol-13-acetate enhancement of the tumorigenic potential of herpes simplex virus type 2 transformed cells. Oncology 40: 357-362

Kuhn JE, Dunkler G, Munk K, Braun RW (1987) Analysis of the IgM and IgG antibody response against herpes simplex virus type 1 (HSV 1) structural and non-structural proteins. J Med Virol 23: 135-150

Kumari TV, Thankamani H, Prabha B, Sasidharan VK, Vasudevan DM (1985) Detection of antibodies against HSV in patients with oral cancers. Indian J Cancer 21: 137-140

Lafferty WE, Coombs RW, Benedetti J, Critchlow MS, Corey L (1987) Recurrences after oral and genital herpes simplex virus infection. Influence of site of infection and viral type. N Engl J Med 316: 1444-1449

Lalwani AK, Snyderman NL (1991) Pharyngeal ulceration in AIDS patients secondary to cytomegalovirus infection. Ann Otol Rhinol Laryngol 100: 484-487

Lamey P-J, Waterhouse JP, Ferguson MM (1982) Pleomorphic salivary adenoma: virally-induced pleomorphic salivary adenoma in the CFLP mouse. Am J Pathol 109: 129-132

Langford A, Kunze R, Timm H, Ruf B, Reichart P (1990) Cytomegalovirus associated oral ulcerations in HIV-infected patients. J Oral Pathol Med 19: 71-76

Langford A, Dienemann D, Schuman D et al (1990) Oral manifestations of AIDS-associated non-Hodgkin's lymphomas. Int J Oral Maxillofac Surg 20: 136-141

Larsen ET, Duggan MA, Inoue M (1994) Absence of human papilloma virus DNA in oropharyngeal spindle cell squamous carcinomas. Am J Clin Pathol 101: 514-518

Larsson PA, Johansson SL, Vahlne A, Hirsch JM (1989) Snuff tumorigenesis: effects of long-term snuff administration after initiation with 4-nitroquinoline N-oxide and herpes simplex virus type-2. J Oral Pathol Med 18: 187–192

Larsson PA, Edstron S, Westin T, Nordkrist A, Hirsch HM, Vahlne A (1991) Reactivity against herpes simplex virus in patients with head and neck cancer. Int J Cancer 49: 14–18

Laskin OL (1985) Acyclovir and suppression of frequently recurring herpetic whitlow. Ann Intern Med 102: 494–495

Laskin OL, Cederberg DM, Mills J, Eson LJ, Mildvan D, Spector SA (1987) Ganciclovir for the treatment and suppression of serious infections caused by cytomegalovirus. J Infect Dis 155: 323–327

Lawton GM, Thomas SJ, Schonrock J, Monsour FM, Frazer IH (1992) Prevalence of genital human papillomaviruses in normal oral mucosa: a comparison of methods for sample collection. J Oral Pathol Med 21: 265–269

Leading Article (1985) EBV and persistent malaise. Lancet i: 1017–1018

Leading Article (1989) Recurrent erythema multiforme and herpes simplex virus. Lancet ii: 1311

Leading Article (1990) Postherpetic neuralgia. Lancet 336: 537–538

Leess FR, Kessler DJ, Mickel RA (1987) Non-Hodgkin's lymphoma of the head and neck in patients with AIDS. Arch Otolaryngol Head Neck Surg 113: 1104–1106

Legendre C, Russell AS, Jeannet M (1982) HLA antigens in patients with recrudescent herpes simplex infections. Tissue Antigens 19: 85–89

Leight I, Mowbray J, Levene G, Sutherland S (1985) Recurrent and continuous erythema multiforme: a clinical and immunological study. Clin Exp Dermatol 10: 58

Leimola-Virtanen RE, Happonen PR, Syrjanen SM (1995) Cytomegalovirus (CMV) and Helicobacter pylori (HP) found in oral mucosal ulcers. J Oral Pathol Med 24: 14–17

Lemak MA, Davis M, Bean SF (1986) Oral acyclovir for the prevention of herpes-associated erythema multiforme. J Am Acad Dermatol 15: 50

Lenoir GM, Delecluse HJ (1989) Lymphoma and immunocompromised host. In: Revilland JP, Wierzbicki N (eds) Immune disorders and opportunistic infections. Suresness Foundation Franco-Allemande, pp 173–183

Leport C, Harzic M, Pignon JM et al (1987) Benign cytomegalovirus mononucleosis in non-AIDS, HIV-infected patients. Lancet ii: 214

Lerner CW, Tapper ML (1984) Opportunistic infection complicating acquired immune deficiency syndrome: clinical features of 25 cases. Medicine (Baltimore) 63: 155–164

Lerner M, Andrews N, Miller J et al (1981) Two small RNAs encoded by Epstein-Barr virus and complexed with protein are precipitated by antibodies from patients with systemic lupus. Proc Natl Acad Sci USA 78: 805–809

Levy JA, Ferro F, Greenspan D, Lennette ET (1990) Frequent isolation of HHV-6 from saliva and high seroprevalence of the virus in the population. Lancet i: 1047–1050

Ley C, Bauer HM, Reingold A (1991) Determinants of genital human papillomavirus infection in young women. JNCI 83: 991–1003

Leyvraz S, Heule W, Chahinian AP et al (1985) Association of Epstein-Barr virus with thymic carcinoma. N Engl J Med 312: 1296–1299

Liebowitz D (1994) Nasopharyngeal carcinoma: the Epstein-Barr virus association. Semin Oncol 21: 376–381

Lin-Greenberg A, Villacin A, Moussa G (1990) Lymphomatoid granulomatosis presenting as ulcerodestructive gastrointestinal tract lesions in patients with human immunodeficiency virus infection. Arch Intern Med 150: 2581–2583

Lipson SM, Salo RJ, Leonardi GP (1991) Evaluation of five monoclonal antibody-based kits or reagents for the identification and culture confirmation of herpes simplex virus. J Clin Microbiol 29: 466–469

Lo SC, Shih JW, Newton PB III et al (1989) Virus-like infectious agent (VLIA) is a novel pathogenic mycoplasma: mycoplasma incognitus. Am J Trop Med Hyg 41: 586–600

Loeser JD (1986) Herpes zoster and postherpetic neuralgia. Pain 25: 1172–1181

Loning T, Ikenberg H, Becker J, Gissmann L, Hoepfer I, zur Hausen H (1985) Analysis of oral papillomas, leukoplakias, and invasive carcinomas for human papillomavirus type related DNA. J Invest Dermatol 84: 417–420

Loning T, Henke RP, Reichart P, Becker J (1987a) In situ hybridisation to detect Epstein-Barr virus DNA in oral tissues of HIV-infected patients. Virchows Arch [A] 412: 127–133

Loning T, Meichsner M, Milde-Langosch K et al (1987b) HPV DNA detection in tumours of the head and neck: a comparative light microscopy and DNA hybridization study. Otorhinology 49: 259–269

Lowhagen GB, Janesn E, Nordenfelt E, Lycke E (1990) Epidemiology of genital herpes infections in Sweden. Acta Derm Venereol (Stockh) 70: 330–334

Lozada-Nur F, Shillitoe EJ (1985) Erythema multiforme and herpes simplex virus. J Dent Res 64: 930

Lozada-Nur F, Silverman S Jr, Migliorati C et al (1984) The diagnosis of AIDS and AIDS-related complex in the dental office: findings in 171 homosexual males. CDA J 12: 21–25

Lozada-Nur F, Cram D, Gorsky M (1992) Clinical response to levamisole in thirty-nine patients with erythema multiforme. Oral Surg Oral Med Oral Pathol 74: 294–298

Lucht E, Albert J, Linde A (1993) Human immunodeficiency type 1 and cytomegalovirus in saliva. J Med Virol 39: 156–162

Lucin P, Pavic I, Polic B, Jonjic S, Koszinowski UH (1992) Gamma interferon-dependent clearance of cytomegalovirus infection in salivary glands. J Virol 66: 1977–1984

Lumerman H, Freedman P, Kerpel S, Cale A (1990) Screening for oral hairy leukoplakia by cytologic examination. Diagn Cytopathol 6: 225

Lynn WA, Davidson RN, Wansbrough-Jones MH (1987) Successful use of oral acyclovir to prevent herpes simplex-associated erythema multiforme. J Infect 15: 192–193

Mabruk MJEMF, Flint S, Toner M et al (1994) In situ hybridization and the polymerase chain reaction in analysis of biopsies and exfoliative cytology specimens for definitive diagnosis of oral hairy leukoplakia (OHL). J Oral Pathol Med 24: 302–308

Mabruk MJEMF, Flint SR, Toner M, Leonard N, Sheils O, Coleman DC, Atkins GJ (1995) Detection of Epstein-Barr virus DNA in tongue tissues from AIDS autopsies without clinical evidence of oral hairy leukoplakia. J Oral Pathol Med 24: 109–112

Macher AM, Richert CM, Straus SE et al (1983) Death in the AIDS patient: role of cytomegalovirus. N Engl J Med 309: 1454

Macleod RI, Long LQ, Soames JV (1990) Oral hairy leukoplakia in an HIV-negative renal transplant patient. Br Dent J 169: 208–209

MacPhail LA, Greenspan D, Schiodt M, Drennan DP, Mills J (1989) Acyclovir-resistant, foscarnet-sensitive oral herpes simplex type II lesion in a patient with AIDS. Oral Surg Oral Med Oral Pathol 67: 427–432

MacPhail LA, Hilton JF, Heinic GS, Greenspan D (1995) Direct immunofluorescence vs culture for detecting HSV in oral ulcers: a comparison. JADA 126: 74–78

Madden C, Beckmann AM, Thomas DB, McKnight B, Sherman KJ, Ahley RL, Corey L, Daling JR (1992) Human papillomaviruses, herpes simplex viruses and the risk of oral cancer in men. Am J Epidemiol 135: 1093

Madinier I, Doglio A, Cagnon L, Lefebvre JC, Monteil RA (1992) Epstein-Barr virus DNA detection in gingival tissues of patients undergoing surgical extractions. Br J Oral Maxillofac Surg 30: 237–243

Mai M, Sutker NW, Husberg B, Klintmaim G, Gonwa T (1989) DHPG (ganciclovir) improves survival in CMV pneumonia. Transplant Proc 21: 2263–2265

Maitland NJ, Scully C (1994) Frequency of EBV-DNA detection in Sjogren's syndrome. Am J Med 96: 97–98

Maitland NJ, Cox MF, Prime SS, Scully C, Meanwell CA (1987) Detection of human DNA virus-like sequences in human oral tissues. Br J Cancer 56: 245–250

Maitland NJ, Bromidge T, Cox MF, Prime SS, Meanwell CA, Scully C (1989) Detection of human papillomavirus genes in human oral tissue biopsies and cultures by polymerase chain reaction. Br J Cancer 59: 698–703

Maitland NJ, Lynas C, Bromidge T, Crane I, Flint SR, Cox MF, Prime SS, Scully C (1991) Presence and expression of latent viruses in oral tissues. In: Johnson NW (ed) Oral cancer: detection of patients and lesions at risk. Cambridge University Press, Cambridge, pp 317–339

Maitland N, Flint S, Scully C, Crean S (1995) Detection of cytomegalovirus and Epstein-Barr virus in labial salivary glands in Sjogren's syndrome and non-specific sialadenitis. J Oral Pathol Med 24: 293–298

Malmstrom M et al (1990) Herpes simplex antigens and inflammatory cells in oral lesions in recurrent erythema multiforme. Acta Derm Venereol 70: 405

Mandal BK (1987) Herpes zoster and the immunocompromised. J Infect 14: 1–15

Mangano MF, Hodinka RL, Spivak JG (1992) Detection of human cytomegalovirus by polymerase chain reaction. In: Becker Y, Darai G (eds) Diagnosis of human viruses by polymerase chain reaction technology. Springer, Berlin Heidelberg New York, pp 147–156

Manzella JP, McConville JH, Valenti W, Menegus MA, Swierkosz EM, Arens M (1984) An outbreak of herpes simplex virus 1 gingivostomatitis in a dental hygiene practice. JAMA 252: 2019–2022

Mao EJ, Smith CJ (1993) Detection of Epstein-Barr virus (EBV) DNA by the polymerase chain reaction (PCR) in oral smears from healthy individuals and patients with oral squamous cell carcinoma. J Oral Pathol Med 22: 12–17

Marder MZ, Barr CE, Mandel ID (1985) Cytomegalovirus presence and salivary composition in acquired immune deficiency syndrome. Oral Surg Oral Med Oral Pathol 60: 372–376

Mariette X, Gozlan J, Clerc D, Bisson M, Morinet F (1991) Detection of Epstein-Barr virus DNA by in situ hybridization and polymerase chain reaction in salivary gland biopsy specimens from patients with Sjogren's syndrome. Am J Med 90: 286–294

Marquart KH, Oehlschlaegel G (1985) Mycoplasma-like structures in a Kaposi's sarcoma not associated with AIDS. Eur J Clin Microbiol 4: 73–74

Marquart KH, Engst R, Oehlschlaegel G (1991) An 8 year history of Kaposi's sarcoma in an HIV-negative bisexual man. AIDS 5: 346–348

Martin P, Vass WC, Schiller JT, Lowy DR, Vehu TJ (1989) The bovine papillomavirus E5 transforming protein can stimulate the transforming activity of EGF and CSF receptors. Cell 59: 21–32

Mathew A, Cheng HM, Sam CK, Joab I, Prasad U, Cochet C (1994) A high incidence of serum IgG antibodies to the Epstein-Barr virus replication activator protein in nasopharyngeal carcinoma. Cancer Immunol Immunother 38: 68–70

Matthews JB, Scully C, Jovanovic A, Van der Waal I, Yeudall WA, Prime SS (1993) Relationship of tobacco-alcohol use to p53 expression in patients with lingual squamous carcinomas. Oral Oncol Eur J Cancer 29B: 285–290

Matz B, Schlehofer JR, zur Hausen H (1984) Identification of a gene function of herpes simplex virus type 1 essential for amplification of simian virus 40 DNA sequences in transformed hamster cells. Virology 134: 328–337

Matz B, Schlehofer JR, zur Hausen H, Huber B, Fanning E (1985) HSV- and chemical carcinogen-induced amplification of SV40 DNA sequences in tranformed cells in cell-line-dependent. Int J Cancer 35: 521–525

McKinnon WW, Weisse C, Reynolds C et al (1989) Chronic stress, leucocyte subpopulations and humoral response to latent viruses. Health Psych 8: 389–402

McMillan JA, Weiner LB, Higgins AM, Lamparella VJ (1993) Pharyngitis associated with herpes simplex virus in college students. Pediatr Infect Dis J 12: 280–284

Melbye M, Grossman RJ, Goedert JJ et al (1987) Risk of AIDS after herpes zoster. Lancet i: 728–731

Merigan T (1981) Immunosuppression and herpesviruses. In: Nahmias AJ, Dowdle WR, Schinazi RF (eds) The human herpesviruses. Elsevier, New York, pp 308–316

Meyers JD (1989) Chemoprophylaxis of viral infection in immunocompromised patients. Eur J Cancer Clin Oncol 25: 1369–1374

Meyers JD, Thomas ED (1988) Infection complicating bone marrow transplantation. In: Rubin RH, Young LS (eds) Clinical approach to infection in the compromised host, 2nd edn. Plenum Medical, New York, pp 525–556

Meyers JD, Reed EC, Shepp DH et al (1988) Acyclovir for prevention of cytomegalovirus infection and disease after allogeneic marrow transplantation. N Engl J Med 318: 70–75

Migliorati C, Jones A, Baughman P (1993) Use of exfoliative cytology in the diagnosis of oral hairy leukoplakia. Oral Surg Oral Med Oral Pathol 76: 704–710

Milde K, Loning T (1986) Detection of papillomavirus DNA in oral papillomas and carcinomas: application of in situ hybridization with biotinylated HPV 16 probes. J Oral Pathol 15: 292–296

Millar EP, Traulis MJ (1994) Herpes zoster of the trigeminal nerve: the dentists role in diagnosis and management. J Can Dent Assoc 60: 450–453

Miller CS, Redding SW (1992) Diagnosis and management of orofacial herpes simplex virus infections. Dent Clin North Am 36: 879-895

Miller CS, Zeuss MS, White DK (1994) Detection of HPV DNA in oral carcinoma using polymerase chain reaction together with in situ hybridization. Oral Surg Oral Med Oral Pathol 77: 480-486

Miller WE, Edwards RH, Walling DM, Raab-Traub N (1994) Sequence variation in the Epstein-Barr virus latent membrane protein 1. J Gen Virol 75: 2729-2740

Mindel A (1991) Is it meaningful to treat patients with recurrent herpetic infections. Scand J Infect [Suppl] 78: 27-32

Mitchell M, Rubin DMD, Carmen A, Gatta DMD, Gerard M, Cozzi DDS (1989) Non-Hodgkin's lymphoma of the buccal gingiva as the initial manifestation of AIDS. J Oral Maxillofac Surg 47: 1311-1313

Mitrani-Rosenbaum S, Tsvieli R, Tur-Kaspa R (1989) Oestrogen stimulates differential transcription of human papillomavirus type 16 in SiHa cervical carcinoma cells. J Gen Virol 70: 2227-2232

Mittal K, Neri A, Feiner H, Schinella R, Alfonso F (1990) Lymphomatoid granulomatosis in the acquired immunodeficiency syndrome. Cancer 63: 1345-1349

Miura S, Smith CC, Burnett JW, Aurelian L (1992) Detection of viral DNA within skin of healed recurrent herpes simplex infection and erythema multiforme lesions. J Invest Dermatol 98: 68

Miyasaka N, Saito I, Haruta J (1994) Possible involvement of Epstein-Barr virus in the pathogenesis of Sjogren's syndrome. Clin Immunol Immunopathol 72: 166-170

Molin L (1987) Oral acyclovir prevents herpes simplex virus-associated erythema multiforme. Br J Dermatol 116: 109

Montgomery MT, Redding SW, Le Maistre CF (1986) The incidence of oral herpes simplex virus infection in patients undergoing cancer chemotherapy. Oral Surg Oral Med Oral Pathol 61: 238-242

Montilla P, Dronda F, Moreno S, Expeleta C, Bellas C, Buzon L (1987) Lymphomatoid granulomatosis and the acquired immunodeficiency syndrome. Ann Intern Med 106: 166-167

Moore PS, Chang Y (1995) Detection of herpesvirus like DNA sequences in Kaposi's sarcoma lesions from persons with and without HIV infection. N Engl J Med 332: 1181-1185

Moore RD, Kessler H, Richman DD, Flexner C, Chaisson RE (1991) Non-Hodgkin's lymphoma in patients with advanced HIV infection treated with zidovudine. JAMA 267: 2208-2211

Mosadomi A (1984) Burkitt's lymphoma of the mouth and jaws. In: Shklar G (ed) Oral cancer: the diagnosis, therapy, management and rehabilitation of the oral cancer patient. Saunders, Philadelphia, pp 283-292

Munger K, Werness Ba, Dyson N, Phelps WC, Harlow E, Howley PM (1989) Complex formation of human papillomavirus E7 proteins with the retinoblastoma tumor supressor gene product. EMBO J 8: 4099-4105

Muretto P, Ferenczy A (1992) Association of human papillomavirus type 16 with intraepithelial neoplasia of the vulva and oral cavity. Cervix 10: 55-56

Myerson D, Hackman RC, Nelson JA, WardDC, McDougall JK (1984) Widespread evidence of histologically occult cytomegalovirus. Hum Pathol 15: 430-439

Myskowski PL, Straus DJ, Safai B (1990) Lymphoma and other HIV-associated malignancies. J Am Acad Dermatol 22: 1253-1260

Nagao Y, Sata M, Tanikawa K, Itoh K, Kameyama T (1995) High prevalence of hepatitis C virus antibody and RNA in patients with oral cancer. J Oral Pathol Med 24: 354-360

Naghashfar Z, Sawda E, Kutcher MA et al (1985) Identification of genital tract papillomaviruses JHPV-6 and HPV-16 in warts of the oral cavity. J Med Virol 17: 313-324

Nahass GT, Goldstein BA, Zhu WY, Serfling U, Penneys NS, Leonardi CL (1992) Comparison of Tzanck smear, viral culture and DNA diagnostic methods in detection of herpes simplex and varicella-zoster infection. JAMA 268: 2541-2544

Naher H, Gissmann L, von Knebel Doebertiz C et al (1991) Detection of Epstein-Barr virus DNA in tongue epithelium of human immunodeficiency virus-infected patients. J Invest Dermatol 97: 421-424

Nassrin N, Taiba K, Hanman N, Hannan M, al-Sedairy S (1994) A molecular study of EBV DNA and p53 mutations in nasopharyngeal carcinoma of Saudi Arab patients. Cancer Lett 29: 189–198

Newman C, Polk BF (1987) Resolution of hairy leukoplakia during therapy with 9-(1-3,dihydroxy-2-propoxymethyl) guanine (DHPG). Ann Intern Med 107: 348–350

Nideobitek G, Young LS, Lau R et al (1991) Epstein-Barr virus infection in oral hairy leukoplakia: virus replication in the absence of detectable latent phase. J Gen Virol 72: 3035–3046

Noble-Topham SE, Fliss DM, Hartwick WJ, McLachlin CM, Freeman JL, Moyek AM, Andrulis IL (1993) Detection and typing of human papillomavirus in verrucous carcinoma of the oral cavity using the polymerase chain reaction. Arch Otol Head and Neck Surg 119: 1299–1304

Norris SA, Kessler HA, Fife KH (1987) Severe, progressive herpetic whitlow caused by an acyclovir-resistant virus in a patient with AIDS. J Infect Dis 157: 209–210

Ogawa H, Kazuyama Y, Hashiguchi K (1990) Detection of herpes simplex virus, varicella zoster virus and cytomegalovirus in aphthous stomatitis. Nippon Jibiinkoka Gakkaikaiho 93: 920

Ogden GR, Kiddie RA, Lunny DP, Lane DP (1992) Assessment of p53 protein expression in normal, benign and malignant oral mucosa. J Pathol 166: 389–394

Oh JS, Paik DI, Christensen R, Akoto-Amanfu E, Kim K, Park NH (1989) Herpes simplex virus enhances the 7,12-dimethylbenz-(a)anthracene (DMBA)-induced carcinogenesis and amplification and over expression of c-erb-B-1 protooncogene in hamster buccal pouch epithelium. Oral Surg Oral Med Oral Pathol 68: 428–435

O'Hare P, Hayward GS (1985) Three transacting regulatory proteins of herpes simplex virus modulate immediate – early gene expression in a pathway involving positive and negative feedback regulation. J Virol 56: 723–733

Okabe M, Chiba S, Tamina T, Chiba Y, Nakao T (1983) Longitudinal studies of cytomegalovirus-specific cell-mediated immunity in congenitally infected infants. Infect Immun 41: 128–131

Orton PW, Huff JC, Tonnesen MG, Weston WL (1984) Detection of a herpes simplex viral antigen in skin lesions of erythema multiforme. Ann Intern Med 101: 48

Ostwald C, Muller P, Basten M, Rutsatz K, Sonnenburg M, Milde-Langosch K, Loning T (1994) Human papillomavirus DNA in oral squamous cell carcinomas and normal mucosa. J Oral Pathol Med 23: 220–225

Overall JC (1984) Dermatologic viral disease. In: Gallasso GJ, Merigan TC, Buchanan RA (eds) Antiviral agents and viral disease of man, 2nd edn. Raven, New York, pp 247–312

Padayachee A (1994) Human papillomavirus (HPV) types 2 and 57 in oral verrucae demonstrated by in situ hybridization. J Oral Pathol Med 23: 413–417

Palefsky JM, Silverman S, Abdel-Salaam M, Daniels TE, Greenspan JS (1995) Association between proliferative verrucous leukoplakia and infection with human papillomavirus type 16. J Oral Pathol Med 24: 193–197

Pao CC, Tsai PL, Chang YL, Hsieh TT (1992) Non-sexual papillomavirus transmission routes. Lancet 339: 1479–1480

Papadopoulos GK, Moutsopoulos HM (1992) Slow viruses and the immune system in the pathogenesis of local tissue damage in Sjogren's syndrome. Ann Rheum Dis 51: 136–138

Park NH, Herbosa EG, Sapp JP, Li KK (1986) Herpes simplex virus (HSV) infection with simulated snuff-dipping induces oral cancer in hamsters. J Dent Res 65: 276

Park K, Cherrick H, Min G-M, Park NH (1990) Active HSV-1 immunization prevents the co-carcinogenic activity of HSV-1 in the oral cavity of hamsters. J Oral Pathol Med 70: 186–190

Park NH, Dokko H, Li SL, Cherrick HM (1991) Synergism of herpes simplex virus and tobacco-specific N'-nitrosamines in cell transformation. J Oral Maxillofac Surg 49: 276–281

Park NH, Li SL, Xie JF, Cherrick HM (1992) In vitro and animal studies of the role of viruses in oral carcinogenesis. Oral Oncol Eur J Cancer 28B: 145–152

Pass RF, Stagno S, Britt WJ, Alford CA (1983) Specific cell-mediated immunity and the natural history of congenital infection with cytomegalovirus. J Infect Dis 148: 953–961

Pater A, Bayatpour M, Pater MM (1990) Oncogenic transformation by human papillomavirus type 16 deoxyribonucleic acid in the presence of progesterone or progestin from oral contraceptives. Am J Obstet Gynecol 162: 1099–1103

Patton DF, Shirley P, Raab-Traub N et al (1990) Defective viral DNA in Epstein-Barr virus associated oral hairy leukoplakia. J Virol 64: 397

Patton L, McMillan CW, Webster WP (1990) American Burkitt's lymphoma: a 10 year review and case study. Oral Surg Oral Med Oral Pathol 69: 307–316

Peckham CS (1991) Cytomegalovirus infection: congenital and neonatal disease. Scand J Infect [Suppl] 78: 82–87

Pedersen A (1989) Varicella zoster virus and recurrent aphthous ulceration. Lancet i: 1203

Pedersen A, Hornsleth A (1993) Recurrent aphthous ulceration: a possible clinical manifestation of reactivation of varicella zoster or cytomegalovirus infection. J Oral Pathol Med 22: 64–68

Pedersen A, Madsen HO, Vestergaard BP, Ryder LP (1993) Varicella-zoster virus DNA in recurrent aphthous ulcers. Scand J Dent Res 101: 311–313

Peitroboni GR, Harnett GB, Bucens MR, Honess RW (1988) Isolation of human herpesvirus 6 from saliva. Lancet I: 1235

Perl TM, Haugen TH, Pfaller MA, Hollis R, Laeman AD, Whitley RJ, Nicholson D, Hunter GA, Wenzel RP (1992) Transmission of herpes simplex virus type 1 infection in an intensive care unit. Ann Intern Med 117: 584–586

Pfugfelder SC, Roussel TJ, Culbertson WW (1987) Primary Sjogren's syndrome after infectious mononucleosis. JAMA 257: 1049–1050

Phelan JA, Klein RN (1988) Resolution of oral hairy leukoplakia during treatment with azidothymidine. Oral Surg Oral Med Oral Pathol 65: 717–720

Pialoux G, Ravisse P, Trotot P, Dupont B (1991) Cytomegalovirus infection of the submandibular gland in a patient with AIDS. Rev Infect Dis 13: 338

Polk BF, Fox R, Brookmeyer R et al (1987) Predictors of the acquired immunodeficiency syndrome developing in a cohort of seropositive homosexual men. N Engl J Med 316: 61–66

Preblud SR (1986) Varicella: complications and costs. Pediatrics 78: 728–735

Preblud SR, Orenstein WA, Bart KJ (1984) Varicella: clinical manifestations, epidemiology, and health impact in children. Pediatr Infect Dis 3: 505–509

Preiksaitis JK, Diaz-Mitoma F, Mirzayans F, Roberts S, Tyrrell DLJ (1992) Quantitative oropharyngeal Epstein-Barr virus shedding in renal and cardiac transplant recipients: relationship to immunosuppressive therapy, serologic responses and the risk of post transplant lymphoproliferative disorder. J Infect Dis 166: 986–994

Purtilo DT (1980) Immunopathology of infectious mononucleosis and other complications of Epstein-Barr virus infections. Sommers SC, Rosen PP (eds) Pathology annual, part 1, vol 15. Appleton-Century Crofts, New York, pp 253–299

Purtilo DT, Sakamoto K (1981) Epstein-Barr virus and human disease: immune responses determine the clinical and pathological expression. Hum Pathol 12: 677–679

Purtilo DT, Sakamoto K, Barnabei V et al (1982) Epstein-Barr virus-induced diseases in boys with the x-linked lymphoproliferative syndrome (XLP). Am J Med 73: 49–56

Raab-Traub N, Rajadurai P, Flynn K, Lanier A (1991) Epstein-Barr virus infection in carcinoma of the salivary gland. J Virol 65: 7032–7036

Rabeneck L, Popovic M, Gartner S (1990) Acute HIV infection presenting with painful swallowing and oesophageal ulcers. JAMA 263: 2318–2322

Raborn G, McCaw WT, Grace M, Percy J (1988) Treatment of herpes labialis with acyclovir: review of three clinical trials. Am J Med 85 [Suppl 2A]: 39–42

Raborn GW, McGow WT, Grace M, Tyrell LD, Samuels SM (1987) Oral acyclovir and herpes labialis: a randomised double-blind placebo-controlled study. JADA 115: 38–42

Rady PL, Yen A, Rollefson JL et al (1995) Herpesvirus-like DNA sequences in non-Kaposi's sarcoma sin lesions of transplant patients. Lancet 345: 1339–1340

Rager-Zisman B, Quan PC, Rosner M et al (1987) Role of NK cells in protection of mice against herpes simplex virus-1 infection. J Immunol 138: 884–888

Rapp F (1981) Transformation by herpes simplex viruses. In: Essex M, Todaro G, zur Hausen H (eds) Viruses in naturally occurring cancers. Cold Spring Harbor Conf Cell Prolif 7: 63–80

Redding SW (1990) Role of herpes simplex virus reactivation in chemotherapy-induced oral mucositis. NCI Mongr 9: 103–105

Reed EC, Wolford JL, Kopecky KJ et al (1990) Ganciclovir for the treatment of cytomegalovirus gastroenteritis in bone marrow transplant patients. A randomized placebo-controlled trial. Ann Intern Med 112: 505–510

Reichart PA, Langford A, Gelderblom HR, Phle HD, Becker J, Wolf H (1989) Oral hairy leukoplakia: observations in 95 cases and review of the literature. J Oral Pathol Med 18: 410–415

Resnick L, Herbst JS, Ablashi DV, Atherton S, Frank B, Rosen L, Horowitz N (1988) Regression of oral hairy leukoplakia after orally administered acyclovir therapy. JAMA 259: 384–388

Ringden O, Lonnqvist B, Paulin T et al (1986) Pharmacokinetics, safety, and preliminary clinical experiences using foscarnet in the treatment of cytomegalovirus infections in bone marrow and renal transplant recipients. J Antimicrob Chemother 17: 373–387

Roizman B, Sears AE (1987) An inquiry into the mechanaism of herpes simplex virus latency. Annu Rev Microbiol 41: 543–571

Rook AH (1988) Interactions of cytomegalovirus with the human immune system. Infect Dis 10: 460–467

Rooney CM, Rowe M, Wallace LE, Rickinson AB (1985) Epstein-Barr virus positive Burkitt's lymphoma cells not recognised by virus-specific T-cell surveillance. Nature 317: 629–631

Rouse BT (1985) Immunopathology of herpesvirus infections. In: Roizman B, Lopez C (eds) The herpesviruses: immunobiology and prophylaxis of human herpesvirus infections, vol 4. Plenum, New York, pp 103–119

Rowe M, Rowe DT, Gregory DM, Young LS, Farrell PJ, Rupani H, Rickinson AB (1987) Differences in B cell growth phenotype reflect novel patterns of Epstein-Barr virus latent gene expresssion in Burkitts lymphoma cells. EMBO J 6: 2743–2751

Rowe M, Young LS, Cadwallader K et al (1989) Distinction between Epstein-Barr virus type A (EBNA 2A) and type B (EBNA 2B) isolates extends to the EBNA 3 family of nuclear proteins. J Virol 63: 1031

Rowe NH, Heine CS, Kowalski CJ (1982) Herpetic whitlow: an occupational disease of practising dentists. JADA 105: 471–473

Rubin MM, Gatta CA, Cozzi GM (1989) Non-Hodgkin's lymphoma of the buccal gingiva as the initial manifestation of AIDS. J Oral Maxillofac Surg 47: 1311–1313

Rubin RH (1988) Infection in the renal and liver transplant patient. In: Rubin RH, Young LS (eds) Clinical approach to infection in the compromised host, 2nd edn. Plenum Medical, New York, pp 557–621

Rubin RH, Tolkoff-Rubin NE (1984) The problem of cytomegalovirus infection in transplantation. In: Morris PJ, Tilney NL (eds) Progress in transplantation. Churchill Livingstone, Edinburgh, pp 89–114

Rush JD, Ng VL, Hopewell PC, Hadley WK, Mills J (1989) Comparative recovery of cytomegalovirus from saliva, mucolysed induced sputum and bronchoalveolar lavage fluid from patients at risk for or with acquired immunodeficiency syndrome. J Clin Microbiol 27: 2864–2865

Ryder JW, Croen K, Kleinschmidt-DeMasters BK et al (1986) Progressive encephalitis three months after resolution of cutaneous zoster in a patient with AIDS. Ann Neurol 19: 182–188

Sacks SL (1984) Frequency and duration of patient observed recurrent genital herpes simplex virus infection: characterisation of the nonlesional prodrome. J Infect Dis 150: 873–877

Saemundsen AK, Purtilo DT, Sakamoto K et al (1981) Documentation of EBV infection in immunodeficient patients with lymphoproliferative diseases by EBV complimentary RNA/DNA and viral DNA/DNA hybridisation. Cancer Res 41: 4237–4242

Saito I, Servenius B, Compton T, Fox RI (1989) Detection of Epstein-Barr virus DNA by polymerase chain reaction in blood and tissue biopsies from patients with Sjogren's syndrome. J Exp Med 169: 2191–2198

Sakai E, Tsuchida N (1992) Most human squamous cell carcinomas in the oral cavity contain mutated p53 tumor-suppressor genes. Oncogene 7: 927–933

Sakaoka H, Sait H, Sekine K et al (1987) Genomic comparison of herpes simplex virus type 1 isolates from Japan, Sweden and Kenya. J Gen Virol 68: 749–764

Salahuddin SZ, Abalashi DV, Markham PD, Josephs SF, Sturzeneger S, Kaplan M, Halligan G, Biberfeld P, Wong-Staal F, Kramarsky B, Gallow RC (1986) Isolation of a new virus, HBLV, in patients with lymphoproliferative disorders. Science 234: 596–601

Sample J, Young L, Martin B et al (1990) Epstein-Barr virus types 1 and 2 differ in their EBNA-3A, EBNA-3B and EBNA-3C genes. J Virol 64: 4084

Sandvej K, Krenacs L, Hamilton-Dutoit SJ, Rindum JL, Pindborg JJ, Pallesen G (1992) Epstein-Barr virus latent and replicative gene expression in oral hairy leukoplakia. Histopathology 20: 387–395

Saral R, Burns WH, Laskin OL, Santos GW, Lietman PS (1981) Acyclovir prophylaxis of herpes simplex virus infections: a randomized, double-blind, controlled trial in bone-marrow transplant recipients. N Engl J Med 305: 63–67

Schalling M, Ekman M, Kaaya EE, Linde A, Biberfeld P (1995) A role for a new herpes virus (KSHV) in different forms of Kaposi's sarcoma. Nature Med 1: 707–708

Schantz SP, Shillitoe EJ, Brown B, Campbell B (1986) Natural killer cell activity and head and neck cancer: a clinical assessment. J Natl Cancer Inst 77: 869–875

Scheffner M, Werness BA, Huibregtse JM, Levine AJ, Howley PM (1990) The E6 oncoprotein encoded by human papillomavirus types 16 and 18 promotes the degradation of p53. Cell 63: 1129–1136

Schiffman MH (1994) Epidermiology of cervical human papillomavirus infections. In: Compans RW, Cooper M, Koprowski H et al (eds) Current topics in microbiology and immunology, vol 86. Springer, Berlin Heidelberg New York, pp 56–81

Schinazi FR, delBene V, Scott RT, Dudley-Thorpe JB (1986) Characterization of acyclovir-resistant and -sensitive herpes simplex viruses isolated from patients with an acquired immune deficiency. J Antimicrob Chemother 18 [Suppl B]: 127–134

Schiodt M, Greenspan D, Daniels TE et al (1989) Parotid gland enlargement associated with labial sialadenitis in HIV infected patients. J Autoimmun 2: 415–426

Schiodt M, Norgard T, Greenspan JS (1995) Oral hairy leukoplakia in an HIV-negative woman with Behcet's syndrome. Oral Surg Oral Med Oral Pathol 79: 53–56

Schlefhofer JR, Gissmann L, Matz B, zur Hausen H (1983) Herpes simplex virus-induced amplification of SV40 sequences in transformed Chinese hamster embryo cells. Int J Cancer 32: 99–103

Schmidt-Westhausen A, Gelderblom HR, Reichart PA (1990) Oral hairy leukoplakia in an HIV seronegative heart transplant patient. J Oral Pathol Med 19: 192

Schmidt-Westhausen A, Gelderblom HR, Hetzer R, Reichart PA (1991) Demonstration of Epstein-Barr virus in scrape material of lateral border of tongue in heart transplant patients by negative staining electron microscopy. J Oral Pathol Med 20: 215–217

Schmidt-Westhausen A, Gelderblom HR, Neuhaus P, Reichart PA (1993) Epstein-Barr virus in lingual epithelium of liver transplant patients. J Oral Pathol Med 22: 274–276

Schubert MM, Epstein JB, Lloyd ME, Cooney E (1993) Oral infections due to cytomegalovirus in immunocompromised patients. J Oral Pathol Med 22: 268–273

Sciubba J, Brandsma J, Schwartz M, Barrezueta N (1989) Hairy leukoplakia: an AIDS-associated opportunistic infection. Oral Surg Oral Med Oral Pathol 67: 404–410

Sciubba JJ, Schwartz MH (1987) Hairy leukoplakia and Epstein-Barr virus. Oral Surg Oral Med Oral Pathol 65: 563–584

Sculley TB, Apolloni A, Hurren L, Moss DJ, Cooper DA (1990) Coinfection with A- and B-type Epstein-Barr virus in human immunodeficiency virus-positive subjects. J Infect Dis 162: 643

Scully C (1983) Viruses and cancer: herpes viruses and tumors in the head and neck. Oral Surg Oral Med Oral Pathol 56: 285–292

Scully C (1985) Ulcerative stomatitis, gingivitis and rash: a diagnostic dilemma. Oral Surg Oral Med Oral Pathol 59: 261–263

Scully C (1989a) Orofacial herpes simplex virus infections. Oral Surg Oral Med Oral Pathol 68: 701–710

Scully C (1989b) Sjogren's syndrome: no demonstrable association by serology of secondary Sjogren's syndrome with cytomegalovirus. J Oral Pathol Med 19: 43–44

Scully C (1989c) Orofacial herpes simplex virus infections: current concepts on the epidemiology, pathogenesis and treatment and disorders in which the virus may be implicated. Oral Surg Oral Med Oral Pathol 68: 701–710

Scully C (1992) Viruses and oral squamous carcinoma. Oral Oncol Eur J Cancer 28B: 57–60

Scully C (1993) Are viruses associated with aphthae and oral vesiculoerosive disorders? Br J Oral Maxillofac Surg 31: 173–177

Scully C (1995) Infectious disease. In: Millard HD, Mason DK (eds) 1993 world workshop on oral medicine. University of Michigan, Michigan

Scully C, Bagg J (1992) Viral infections in dentistry. Curr Opin Dent 9: 8–11

Scully C, Cawson RA, Griffiths M (eds) (1990) Occupational hazards to dental staff. Br Dent J

Scully C, Samaranayake LP (1992) Clinical virology in dentistry and oral medicine. Cambridge University Press, Cambridge

Scully C, Eglin RP, Ward-Booth P, McGregor IA, Boyle P (1982) Human oral squamous cell carcinoma: evidence for RNA complementary to herpes simplex DNA. IRCS Med Sci 10: 531

Scully C, Prime SS, Maitland NJ (1985) Papillomaviruses: their possible role in oral disease. Oral Surg Oral Med Oral Pathol 60: 166–174

Scully C, Maitland NJ, Cox MF, Prime SS (1987) Human papillomavirus DNA and oral mucosa. Lancet I: 336

Scully C, Cox MF, Prime SS, Maitland NJ (1988) Papillomaviruses: the current status in relation to oral disease. Oral Surg Oral Med Oral Pathol 65: 526–532

Scully C, Epstein JB, Porter SR (1989) Oral hairy leukoplakia (leading article). Lancet ii: 1194

Scully C, Epstein JB, Porter SR, Cox MF (1991a) Viruses and chronic diseases of the oral mucosa. Oral Surg Oral Pathol Oral Med 72: 537–544

Scully C, Prime SS, Cox M, Maitland NJ (1991b) Infectious agents in the aetiology of oral cancer. In: Johnson NW (ed) "Oral cancer: detecction of patients and lesions at risk". Cambridge University Press, Cambridge, pp 96–113

Seal LA, Toyama PS, Fleet KM et al (1991) Comparison of standard culture methods, a shell vial assay, and a DNA probe for the detection of herpes simplex virus. J Clin Microbiol 29: 650–652

Sedlacek TV, Lindheim S, Eder C (1989) Mechanisms for human papillomavirus transmission at birth. Am J Obstet Gynecol 161: 55–59

Selby PJ, Powles RL, Easton D et al (1989) The prophylactic role of intravenous and long-term oral acyclovir after allogeneic bone marrow transplantation. Br J Cancer 59: 434–438

Shattles WG, Brooker SM, Venables PJW, Clark DA, Maini RN (1992) Expression of antigen reactive with a monoclonal antibody to HTLV-1 P19 in salivary glands in Sjogren's syndrome. Clin Exp Immunol 89: 46–51

Shepp DH, Newton BA, Dandliker PS (1985) Oral acyclovir therapy for mucocutaneous herpes simplex virus infections in immunocompromised marrow transplant recipients. Ann Intern Med 102: 783–785

Shillitoe EJ (1991) Relationship of viral infection to malignancies. Curr Opin Dent 1: 398–403

Shillitoe EJ, Alspaugh MA (1985) Antibody to cytomegalovirus in various connective tissue disorders. J Rheumatol 12: 642–643

Shillitoe EJ, Greenspan D, Greenspan JS, Hansen LS, Silverman S (1982) Neutralising antibody to herpes simplex virus type 1 in patients with oral cancer. Cancer 49: 2315–2320

Shillitoe EJ, Greenspan D, Greenspan JS, Silverman S (1983) Immunoglobulin class of antibody to herpes simplex virus in patients with oral cancer. Cancer 51: 65–71

Shin KH, Min BM, Cherrick HM, Park NH (1994) Combined effects of human papillomaviurs-18 and N-methyl-N-nitrosoguanidine on the transformation of normal human oral keratinocytes. Mol Carcinog 9: 76–86

Shindoh M, Sawada Y, Kogho T, Amemiya A, Fujinaga K (1992) Detection of human papillomavirus DNA sequence in tongue squamous cell carcinoma utilizing the polymerase chain reaction method. Int J Cancer 50: 167–171

Shroyer KR, Greer RO (1991) Detection of human papillomavirus DNA by in situ hybridization and polymerase chain reaction in premalignant and malignant oral lesions. Oral Surg Oral Med Oral Pathol 71: 708

Shroyer KR, Greer RO, Fankhouser CA, McGuirt WF, Marshall R (1993) Detection of human papillomavirus DNA in oral verrucous carcinoma by polymerase chain reaction. Mod Pathol 6: 669–672

Shuster EA, Beneke JS (1985) Monoclonal antibody for rapid laboratory detection of cytomegalovirus infections: characterisation and diagnostic application. Mayo Clin Proc 60: 577–585

Sixbey JW, Nedrud JG, Raab-Traub N, Hanes RA, Pagano JS (1984) Epstein-Barr virus replication in oropharyngeal epithelial cells. N Engl J Med 310: 1225–1230

Sixbey JW, Shirley P, Chesney PJ, Buntin DM, Resnick L (1989) Detection of a second widespread strain of Epstein-Barr virus. Lancet ii: 761

Smith S, Ross JR, Scully C (1984) An unusual oral complication of herpes zoster infection. Oral Surg Oral Med Oral Pathol 57: 388–389

Snijders P, Schulten E, Mullink H et al (1990) Detection of human papillomavirus and Epstein-Barr virus DNA sequences in oral mucosa HIV infected patients by the polymerase chain reaction. Am J Pathol 137: 659

Snijders PJF, Meijer DJLM, Van den Brule AJC, Schrijnemakers HFJ, Snow GB, Walboomers JMM (1992) Human papillomavirus (HPV) type 16 and 33 E6/E7 region transcripts in tonsillar carcinomas can originate from integrated and episomal HPV DNA. J Gen Virol 73: 2059–2066

Soderholm AL, Lindquiet C, Heikinheimo K, Rosell K, Happonen RP (1990) Non-Hodgkin's lymphomas presenting through oral symptoms. Int J Oral Maxillofac Surg 19: 131–134

Somers KD, Merrick MA, Kopez ME, Incognito LS, Schechter GL, Casey G (1992) Frequent p53 mutations in head and neck cancer. Cancer Res 52: 5997–6000

Spector SA, Hirata KK, Neuman TR (1984) Identification of multiple cytomegalovirus strains in homosexual men with acquired immunodeficiency syndrome. J Infect Dis 150: 953–956

Spruance SL (1984) Pathogenesis of herpes simplex labialis: excretion of virus in the oral cavity. J Clin Micro 19: 675–679

Spruance SL (1985) Pathogenesis of herpes simplex labialis: experimental induction of lesions with U-V light. J Clin Microbiol 22: 366–368

St Onge G, Bezahler GH (1982) Giant esophageal ulcer associated with cytomegalovirus. Gastroenterology 83: 127–130

Stagno S, Whitley RJ (1985) Herpes virus infections of pregnancy. N Engl J Med 313: 1270–4

Stagno S, Reynolds DW, Pass RF, Alford CA (1980) Breast milk and the risk of CMV infection. N Engl J Med 302: 1073–1076

Stanberry LR (1986) Herpesvirus latency and recurrence. Prog Med Virol 33: 61–77

Stow PJ, Glynn CJ, Minor B (1989) EMLA cream in the treatment of postherpetic neuralgia: efficacy and phamacokinetic profile. Pain 39: 301–305

Strand A, Vahlne A, Svennerholm B, Wallin J, Lycke E (1986) Asymptomatic virus shedding in men with genital herpes infection. Scand J Infect Dis 18: 195–197

Straus SE, Rooney JF, Sever JL et al (1985) Herpes simplex virus infection: biology, treatment and prevention. Ann Intern Med 103: 404–410

Straus SE, Ostrove JM, Inchauspe G et al (1988) Varicella-zoster virus infection. Ann Intern Med 108: 221–237

Su IJ, Hsu YS, Chang YC, Wang IW (1995) Herpesvirus-like DNA sequence in Kaposi's sarcoma from AIDS and non-AIDS patients in Taiwan. Lancet 345: 722–723

Sugihara K, Reupke H, Schmidt-Westhausen A, Phle HD, Gelderblom HR, Reichart PA (1990) Negative staining EM for the detection of Epstein-Barr virus in oral hairy leukoplakia. J Oral Pathol Med 19: 367–370

Sumida T, Yonaha F, Maeda T et al (1994) Expression of sequences homologous to HTLV-1 tax gene in the labial salivary glands of Japanese patients with Sjogren's syndrome. Arthritis Rheum 37: 545–550

Suttmann U, Willers H, Gurdelmann R, Hopken I, Schededl H, Deicher H (1988) Cytomegalovirus infection in HIV-infected individuals. Infection 16: 111–114

Syrjanen KJ (1989) Epidemiology of human papillomavirus (HPV) infections and their associations with genital squamous cell cancer. APMIS 97: 957–970

Syrjanen S (1992) Viral infections in oral mucosa. Scand J Dent Res 100: 17–31

Syrjanen S, Laine P, Valle SL (1988) Demonstration of Epstein-Barr virus (EBV) DNA in oral hairy leukoplakia using in situ hybridisation with biotinylated probe. Proc Finn Dent Assoc 84: 127–132

Syrjanen S, Laine P, Happonen RP, Niemela M (1989) Oral hairy leukoplakia is not a specific sign of HIV-infection but related to immunosuppression in general. J Oral Pathol Med 18: 28–31

Syrjanen S, Karja V, Change F, Johansson B, Syrjanen K (1990) Epstein-Barr virus involvement in salivary gland lesions associated with Sjogren's syndrome. ORL 52: 254–259

Syrjanen S, Scully C. Human papillomaviruses (HPV) and oral health and disease. J Oral Pathol Med (in press)

Syrjanen SM (1990) Basic concepts and practical applications of recombinant DNA techniques in detection of human papillomavirus infections. APMIS 98: 95–110

Syrjanen SM, Syrjanen KJ, Lamberg MA (1986) Detection of human papillomavirus DNA in oral mucosal lesions using in situ DNA-hybridization applied on paraffin sections. Oral Surg Oral Med Oral Pathol 62: 660–667

Syrjanen SM, Syrjanen KJ, Happonen RP et al (1987) In situ DNA hybridization analysis of human papillomavirus (HPV) sequences in benign oral mucosal lesions. Arch Dermatol Res 279: 543–549

Syrjanen SM, Syrjanen KJ, Happonen RP (1988) Human papillomavirus (HPV) DNA sequences in oral precanerous lesions and squamous cell carcinoma demonstrated by in situ hybridization. J Oral Pathol Med 17: 273–278

Szaki T, Miwata H, Matsui Y et al (1990) Varicella zoster virus DNA in throat swabs. Arch Dis Child 65: 333–334

Taieb A, Fontan I, Maleville J (1985) Acyclovir therapy for eczema herpeticum in infants. Arch Dermatol 121: 1380

Takashashi K, Sonoda S, Kawakami K, Miyata K, Oki T, Nagata T, Okuno T, Yamanishi K (1988) Human herpesvirus 6 and exanthem subitum. Lancet i: 1463

Talacko AA, Teo CG, Griffin BE, Johnson NW (1991) Epstein Barr virus receptors but not viral DNA are present in normal and malignant oral epithelium. J Oral Pathol Med 20: 20–25

Talal N, Dauphinee MJ, Dang H, Alexander SS, Hart DJ, Garry RF (1990) Detection of serum antibodies to retroviral proteins in patients with primary Sjogren's syndrome (autoimmune exocrinopathy). Arthritis Rheum 33: 774–781

Terada K, Katamine S, Eguchi K et al (1994) Prevalence of HTLV-1 in Sjogren's syndrome. Lancet 344: 1116–1119

Thom JJ, Oxholm P, Andersen KH (1988) High levels of complement fixing antibodies against cytomegalovirus in patients with primary Sjogren's syndrome. Clin Exp Rheumatol 6: 71–74

Thomas JA, Felix DH, Wray D, Southam JC, Cubie HA, Crawford DH (1991) Epstein-Barr virus gene expression and epithelial cell differentiation in oral hairy leukoplakia. Am J Pathol 139: 1369–1380

Toghill PJ, McGaughey M (1972) Cytomegalovirus esophagitis. Br Med J 2: 294

Tovi F, Hadar T, Sidi J et al (1985) The significance of specific IgA antibodies in the serum in the early diagnosis of zoster. J Infect Dis 152: 230

Tseng CJ, Lin CY, Wang RL (1992) Possible transplacental transmission of human papillomavirus. Am J Obstet Gynecol 166: 35–40

Tsuchiya H, Tomita Y, Shirasawa H, Tanzawa H, Sato K, Simizu B (1991) Detection of human papillomavirus in head and neck tumors with DNA hybridization and immunohistochemical analysis. Oral Surg Oral Med Oral Pathol 71: 721–725

Tyan Y-S, Liu S-T, Ong W-R, Chen M-L, Shu C-H, Chang Y-S (1993) Detection of Epstein-Barr virus and human papillomavirus in head and neck tumours. J Clin Microbiol 31: 53–56

Ueda K, Kusuhara K, Hirose M, Okada K, Miyazaki C, Tokugawa K, Nakayama M, Yamanishi K (1989) Exanthem subitum and antibody to human herpesvirus-6. J Infect Dis 159: 750–752

Uschendorf PR, Schofer H, Rumme U, Nilbradt R (1988) Therapy of oral hairy leukoplakia with acyclovir. Hautarzt 39: 36–38

Vasudevan DM, Raghunath PN, Shanavas KR, Vijayakumar T, Antony A (1991a) Detection of HSV1 DNA segments in human oral cancer biopsies by dot-blot and in situ DNA hybridisation techniques. J Exp Clin Cancer Res 10: 291–294

Vasudevan DM, Shanavas KR, Kala V, Vijayakumar T, Kumari TV (1991b) Association of herpes group of viruses with oral cancer. In: Varma AK (ed) Oral oncology. Macmillan, New York, pp 113–116

Verano L, Michalski FJ (1990) Herpes simplex virus antigen direct detection in standard virus transport medium by Du Pont Herpchek enzyme-linked immunosorbent assay. J Clin Microbiol 28: 2555–2558

Vestey JP, Norval M (1992) Mucocutaneous infections with herpes simplex virus and their management. Clin Exp Dermatol 17: 221–237

Vilde JL, Perronne C, Huchon A et al (1985) Association of Epstein-Barr virus with lethal midline granuloma. N Engl J Med 313: 1161

Villar LA, Massanari RM, Mitros FA (1984) Cytomegalovirus infection with acute erosive esophagitis. Am J Med 76: 924–928

Walling DM, Raab-Traub N (1994) Epstein-Barr virus intrastrain recombination in oral hairy leukoplakia. J Virol 68: 7909–7917

Walling DM, Edmiston SN, Sixbey JW, Abdel-Hamid M, Resnick L, Raab-Traub N (1992) Coinfection with multiple strains of the Epstein-Barr virus in human immunodeficiency virus-associated hairy leukoplakia. Proc Natl Acad Sci USA 89: 6560–6564

Walling DM, Perkins AG, Webster-Cyriaque J, Resnick L, Raab-Traub N (1994) The Epstein-Barr virus EBNA-2 gene in oral hairy leukoplakia: strain variation genetic deletion, and transcriptional expression. J Virol 68: 7918–7926

Walling DM, Clark M, Markovitz DM, Frank TS, Braun DK, Eisenberg E, Krutchkoff DJ, Felix DH, Raab-Traub N (1995) Epstein-Barr virus coinfection and recombination in nonhuman immunodeficiency virus-associated oral hairy leukoplakia. J Infect Dis 171: 1122–1130

Warnakulasuriya KAAS, Johnson NW (1992) Expression of p53 mutant nuclear phosphoprotein in oral carcinoma and potentially malignant oral lesions. J Oral Pathol Med 21: 404–408

Warren WP, Balcarek K, Smith R, Pass RF (1992) Comparison of rapid methods of detection of cytomegalovirus in saliva with virus isolation in tissue culture. J Clin Microbiol 30: 786–789

Watts SL, Brewer EE, Fry TL (1991) Human papillomavirus DNA types in squamous cell carcinomas of the head and neck. Oral Surg Oral Med Oral Pathol 71: 701–707

Werness BA, Levine AJ, Howley PM (1990) Association of human papillomavirus types 16 and 18 E6 proteins with p53. Science 248: 76–79

Westheim AI, Tenser RB, Marks JG (1987) Acyclovir resistance in a patient with chronic mucocutaneous herpes simplex infection. J Am Acad Dermatol 17: 785–880

Weston WL, Brice SL, Jester JD, Lane AT, Stockert S, Huff JC (1992) Herpes simplex virus in childhood erythema multiforme. Pediatrics 89: 32–34

Whitley RJ, Gnann JW (1992) Acyclovir: a decade later. N Engl J Med 327: 782–789

Whitley RJ, Alford CA, Hirsch MS, Schooley RT, Luby JP, Aoki FY, Hanley D, Nahmias AJ, Soong SJ (1986) Vidarabine versus acyclovir therapy in herpes simplex encephalitis. N Engl J Med 314: 144–149

Whittingham S, McNeilage J, Mackay IR (1985) Primary Sjogren's syndrome after infectious mononucleosis. Ann Intern Med 102: 490–493

Wildy P (1985) Herpes viruses: a background. Br Med Bull 41: 339–344

Wildy P (1986) Herpesvirus. Intervirology 25: 117–140

Wildy P, Gell PGH (1985) The host response to herpes simplex virus. Br Med Bull 41: 86–91

Wiley D (1988) MHC gene in cytomegalovirus. Nature 331: 209–210

Wilkes M, Fortin AH, Felix JC et al (1988) Value of necropsy in acquired immunodeficiency syndrome. Lancet 2: 85–88

Winston DJ, Pollard RB, Ho WG et al (1982) Cytomegalovirus immune plasma in bone marrow transplant recipients. Ann Intern Med 97: 11–18

Wolf BC, Martin AW, Neiman RS et al (1990) The detection of Epstein-Barr virus in hairy cell leukemia cells by in situ hybridization. Am J Pathol 136: 717–723

Wolf H, Bogedain C, Schwarzmann F (1993) Epstein-Barr virus and its interaction with the host. Intervirology 35: 26–39

Wood MJ (1991) Herpes zoster and pain. Scand J Infect [Suppl] 78: 53–61

Woods KV, Shillitoe EJ, Spitz MR, Schantz SP, Adler-Storthz K (1993) Analysis of human papillomavirus DNA in oral squamous cell carcinomas. J Oral Pathol Med 22: 101–108

Woodworth CD, Doniger J, DiPaolo JA (1989) Immortalization of human foreskin keratinocytes by various human papillomavirus DNAs corresponds to their association with cervical carcinoma. J Virol 63: 159–164

WuDunn D, Spear P (1989) Initial interaction of herpes simplex virus with cells is binding to heparan sulfate. J Virol 63: 52–58

Wyatt LS, Rodriguez WJ, Balachandran N, Frenkel N (1991) Human herpesvirus 7: antigenic properties and prevalence in children and adults. J Virol 65: 6260–6265

Yamanishi K, Okuno T, Shiraki K, Takashashi M, Kondo T, Asano Y, Kurata T (1988) Identification of human herpesvirus-6 as a causal agent for exanthem subitum. Lancet i: 1065–1067

Yao QY, Ogan P, Rowe M, Wood M, Rickinson AB (1989) Epstein-Barr virus-infected B cells persist in the circulation of acyclovir-treated virus carriers. Int J Cancer 43: 67–71

Yao QY, Rowe M, Young LS, Rickinson AB (1991) The Epstein-Barr virus: dominance of a single growth transforming isolate in the blood and in the oropharynx of healthy virus carriers. J Gen Virol 72: 1579

Yeudall WA (1992) Human papillomaviruses and oral neoplasia. Oral Oncol Eur J Cancer 28B: 61–66

Yeudall WA, Campo MS (1991) Human papillomavirus DNA in biopsies of oral tissues. J Gen Virol 72: 173

Yin XY, Donovan-Peluso M, Whiteside TL et al (1991) Gene amplification and gene dosage in cell lines derived from squamous cell carcinoma of the head and neck. Genes Chromosomes Cancer 3: 443–454

Yoshikawa T, Suga S, Asano Y (1991) Human herpesvirus infection in bone marrow transplant. Blood 78: 1381–1384

Youle PW, Hawkins DA, Collins P et al (1988) Acyclovir-resistant herpes in AIDS treated with foscarnet. Lancet 2: 341–342

Young LS, Dawson CW, Clark D et al (1988) Epstein-Barr virus gene expression in nasopharyn-geal carcinoma. J Gen Virol 69: 1051–1065

Young LS, Alfieri C, Hennessy K et al (1989a) Expression of Epstein-Barr virus transformation-associated genes in tissues of patients with EBV lymphoproliferative disease. N Engl J Med 321: 1080–1085

Young LS, Bevan LS, Johnson MA, Blomfield PI, Bromidge T, Maitland NJ (1989b) The poly-merase chain reaction: a new epidemiological tool for investigating cervical human papillomavirus infection. Br Med J 298: 14–18

Young LS, Lau R, Rowe M et al (1991) Differentiation associated expression of the Epstein Barr virus BZLF1 transactivator protein in oral hairy leukoplakia. J Virol 65: 2868

Young SK, Min KW (1991) In situ DNA hybridization analysis of oral papillomas, leukoplakias, and carcinomas for human papillomavirus. Oral Surg Oral Med Oral Pathol 71: 726–729

Zeuss MS, Miller CS, Whilte DK (1991) In situ hybridization analysis of human papillomavirus DNA in oral mucosal lesions. Oral Surg Oral Med Oral Pathol 71: 714–720

Zhang X, Langford A, Becker J, Rabamus JP, Pohle HD, Reichart P, Gelderblom H (1988) Ultra-structural and immunohistochemical findings in oral hairy leukoplakia. Virchows Arch [A] 412: 533–542

Ziegler JL, Beckstead JA, Volberding PA et al (1984) Non-Hodgkin's lymphoma in 90 homosexual men. Relation to generalised lymphadenopathy and the acquired immunodeficiency syn-drome. N Engl J Med 311: 565–570

Zimmerman SJ, Moses E, Sofat N et al (1991) Evaluation of a virual, rapid, membrane enzyme immunosassay for the detection of herpes simplex virus antigen. J Clin Microbiol 29: 842–845

Zur Hausen H, de Villiers EM (1994) Human papillomaviruses. Annu Rev Microbiol 48: 427–447

Oral Pathology of Acquired Immunodeficiency Syndrome and Oro-facial Kaposi's Sarcoma*

P.A. REICHART

---

*This work is dedicated to the late Professor Jens J. Pindborg, Copenhagen.

Current Topics in Pathology
Volume 90, G. Seifert (Ed.)
© Springer-Verlag Berlin Heidelberg 1996

1 Introduction

The present volume on oral pathology focuses on diagnostic and prognostic aspects of oral diseases. The acquired immunodeficiency syndrome (AIDS) was first described in 1981, and diagnostic criteria for both the clinical and histopathological aspects of the disease were considered to be of particular importance. Early adequate diagnosis of oral lesions, which in many cases are indicators of the human immunodeficiency virus (HIV) disease, is relevant for early treatment and thus to a certain extent prognosis.

1.1 Factors Relevant to Diagnosis

Clinical and histopathological diagnosis of oral lesions associated with HIV infection and AIDS may be influenced by several parameters. Whether or not the HIV serostatus is known may play a certain role in the diagnosis. In cases in which the HIV-positive serostatus is known, diagnoses such as hairy leukoplakia (HL) and Kaposi's sarcoma (KS) may be biased by this knowledge. In addition, the stage of the disease – according to the Centers for Disease Control (CDC) classification – may also influence diagnostic decision processes. A number of pitfalls have been described both for clinical and histopathological diagnoses. Exact knowledge of the history and serostatus of a patient will enable the oral pathologist to arrive at an adequate diagnosis. Close cooperation between the clinician and the oral pathologist is warranted.

1.2 Prognosis

Some oral manifestations have been recognised as markers and indicators of HIV infection and AIDS. Oral candidiasis, HL and KS, in particular, need to be mentioned as markers. The prognostic value of HL for the development and course of the disease has been clearly shown. Some other opportunistic infections such as herpes zoster and cytomegalovirus (CMV) infection have some prognostic significance for the development and course of HIV disease. The prognosis for patients with HIV infection has been improved mainly through improved control of opportunistic infections such as candidiasis, toxoplasmosis, *Pneumocystis carinii* pneumonia infection (PcP) and viral diseases.

2 Classification

Several classifications of oral manifestations in HIV infection have been published and revised. The EC Clearinghouse on Oral Problems Related to HIV Infection and WHO Collaborating Centre on Oral Manifestations of the Immunodeficiency

Virus published a classification and diagnostic criteria for oral lesions in HIV infection in 1993 (EC 1993). The classification was based on presumptive and definitive criteria.

2.1 Presumptive and Definite Criteria for the Diagnosis of Oral Lesions in Human Immunodeficiency Virus Infection

Presumptive criteria predominantly relate to the initial clinical appearance of a lesion. These diagnostic criteria were not considered to be perfect because of the fact that patients with other diseases may present with similar appearances. A working knowledge of oral mucosal diseases is mandatory, and the spectrum of differential diagnoses must always be considered. The definite criteria are those necessary to establish a reliable diagnosis requiring further clinical or laboratory tests. These include histopathological procedures and the application of refined techniques such as electron microscopy, in situ hybridisation, polymerase chain reaction (PCR) and other molecular biological techniques.

2.2 Classification Groups

Oral lesions in HIV infection were classified into three groups:

- *Group I*: Lesions strongly associated with HIV infection, including candidiasis, HL, several types of periodontal disease, KS and non-Hodgkin's lymphoma.
- *Group II*: Lesions less commonly associated with HIV infection, including some bacterial infections, salivary gland disease, ulcerations not otherwise specified (NOS) and a number of viral infections both of the herpes virus group and the human papillomavirus group.
- *GroupIII*: Lesions seen in HIV infection, some of which are rare and therefore may only have been recorded anecdotally. Bacterial, fungal and viral infections as well as drug reactions or neurological disturbances have been recorded.

Since HIV infection has become a pandemic, geographical differences of manifestations may still be noticed in the future. Tropical diseases such as mycotic infections or leprosy and numerous other diseases may make further revisions of the present classification necessary.

3 Lesions Strongly Associated with Human Immunodeficiency Virus Infection (Group I)

3.1 Candidiasis

Oral candidiasis, the "disease of the diseased", is probably one of the most frequent opportunistic infections in the course of IIIV infection. During IIIV infection, all patients develop oral candidiasis at some time of the disease process. It has been considered as a forerunner of AIDS, and an average of one in three patients are affected by some type of oral candidiasis (SAMARANAYAKE 1992; SAMARANAYAKE and HOLMSTRUP 1989). Of particular importance is the fact that oral candidiasis is not usually observed in individuals 25–54 years of age, an age-group typically affected by HIV infection. Occurrence of signs of oral candidiasis in this group of patients suggests an underlying immuno-incompetence, probably related to an HIV infection. From the clinical point of view, the appearance of the variants of oral candidiasis is similar in the immunocompetent and immunocompromised subjects. Some variations, however, exist in the clinical pattern of oral candidiasis associated with HIV infection, and these are related to factors such as inadequate dosage of antifungals, poor compliance, shift of species or resistance to drugs. All areas of the oral cavity may be affected by oral candidiasis, however, the buccal mucosa, the tongue, the palate and the floor of the mouth are involved most frequently. Different types of oral candidiasis may be seen in one patient.

3.1.1 Erythematous Candidiasis

Erythematous candidiasis may be easily overlooked, particularly in patients whose HIV serostatus is unknown. Diagnostic presumptive criteria are red areas usually located on the palate and dorsum of the tongue, but occasionally on the buccal mucosa. White spots and plaques may be seen, but these are not usually conspicuous. Figure 1a shows a characteristic erythematous candidiasis of the dorsum of tongue characterised by loss of papillae with a glossy red appearance. Clinical symptoms are minimal. Due to contact of the tongue with the palate, a palatal erythematous candidiasis is usually observed at the same time. The undefined nature of erythematous candidiasis is exemplified by the relatively poor definitive criteria. The detection of *Candida albicans* and/or response to antifungal therapy may help to establish the diagnosis.

3.1.1.1 Laboratory Findings. As mentioned above, the detection of *Candida albicans* by microbiological culture may help to establish the diagnosis. It must, however, be remembered that *Candida albicans* is a saprophyte of the oral cavity and as such may be found in up to 20%–50% of normal individuals. Quantification of *Candida albicans* may be helpful, and it has been shown that the number of colony-forming units of *Candida albicans* may be considered as an indicator for the presence of clinical disease. Smears to demonstrate blastospores or candidal hyphae may be helpful, although the latter are not usually found in erythematous candidiasis. The fact that *Candida albicans* is a dimorphic agent causing different types of oral candidiasis further complicates the situation.

3.1.1.2 Histopathology. No systematic studies of the histopathology of erythematous candidiasis associated with HIV infection exist.

Histopathologically, erythematous candidiasis is characterised by an epithelial atrophy with loss of rete ridges, subepithelial inflammatory infiltration, hyperaemia and occasional microabscesses. Penetration of the epithelium with hyphae is the exception. Preliminary studies have been conducted to show the significance of calprotectin, an antibacterial and antimycotic protein located in keratinocytes of normal mucosa and that of erythematous and other types of candidiasis (EVERSOLE et al. 1993). It was demonstrated that calprotectin production in oral epithelium of erythematous and pseudomembranous candidiasis is up-regulated (Fig. 1b).

3.1.2 Pseudomembranous Candidiasis

Presumptive criteria of pseudomembranous candidiasis are white or yellow spots or plaques that may be located in any part of the oral cavity and can be wiped off to reveal an erythematous surface which may bleed. The definite criteria for the demonstration of pseudomembranous candidiasis are response of the lesions to antifungal therapy and tests for the presence of *Candida albicans*. These are not essential for diagnosis, but they may enhance it, particularly in cases resistant to antifungal therapy. Smears and/or cultures may be performed (EC 1993). Cytological smears, however, stained by periodic acid – Schiff (PAS) are revealing when the presence of candidal hyphae is shown.

3.1.2.1 Histopathology. As with erythematous candidiasis, no systematic studies on the histopathology of pseudomembranous candidiasis in HIV infection have been published. The indicative finding is the demonstration of hyphae in the surface epithelium down to the spinous cell layer. Parakeratosis, acanthosis and spongiosis may be seen. Intra-epithelial microabscesses are characteristic. Subepithelially, some inflammatory changes may be observed, although these may be minimal due to the immunodeficiency and lack of response. Figure 1c shows the hyphae in a biopsy of pseudomembranous candidiasis. Occasionally, deeper penetration of hyphae beyond the basal membrane into the subepithelial connective tissue has been observed (REICHART et al. 1995). In an ultrastructural study of pseudomembranous candidiasis, the principle of thigmotropism of *Candida albicans* was shown (REICHART et al. 1995). In addition, ability of the hyphae to detach desmosomes has been demonstrated (Fig. 1d,e).

Fig. 1. a Erythematous candidiasis of the dorsum of tongue in a human immunodeficiency virus (HIV)-positive patient. The red, glossy appearance is characteristic. **b** Section of pseudomembranous candidiasis stained with antibodies against calprotectin showing marked staining of the superficial epithelial cells. Moderate inflammatory infiltration is seen subepithelially. APAAP, ×250. **c** Same patient as in Fig. 1b, revealing the characteristic hyphae in the superficial layer of the epithelium. PAS, ×250. **d** Transmission electron microscopy of pseudomembranous candidiasis. Two cross-sections of hyphae, one in the intercellular space, the other through an epithelial cell, are seen. In addition, multiple bacteria are also found. ×30000. **e** Scanning electron microscopical view of epithelial surface of a pseudomembranous candidiasis. Hyphae are seen penetrating the surface in several locations. The penetration in between epithelial gaps is called "thigmotropism". ×3000

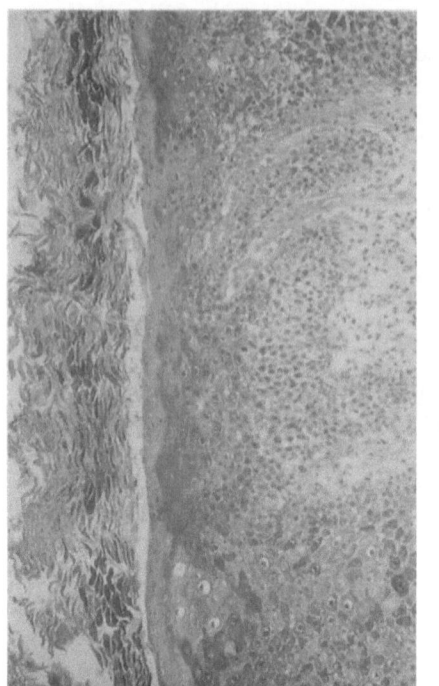

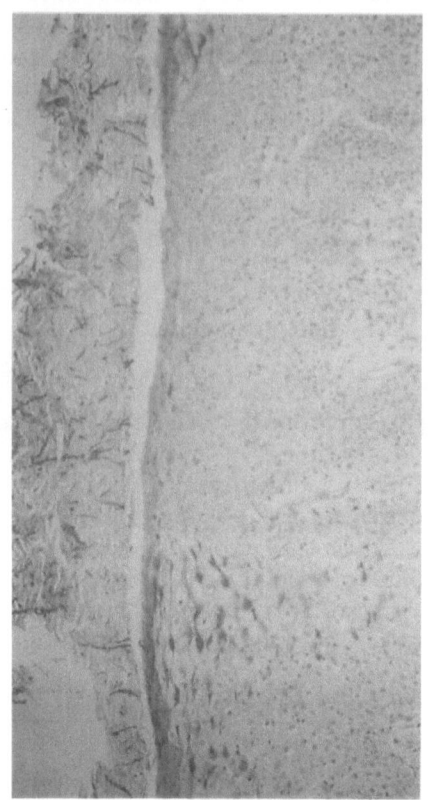

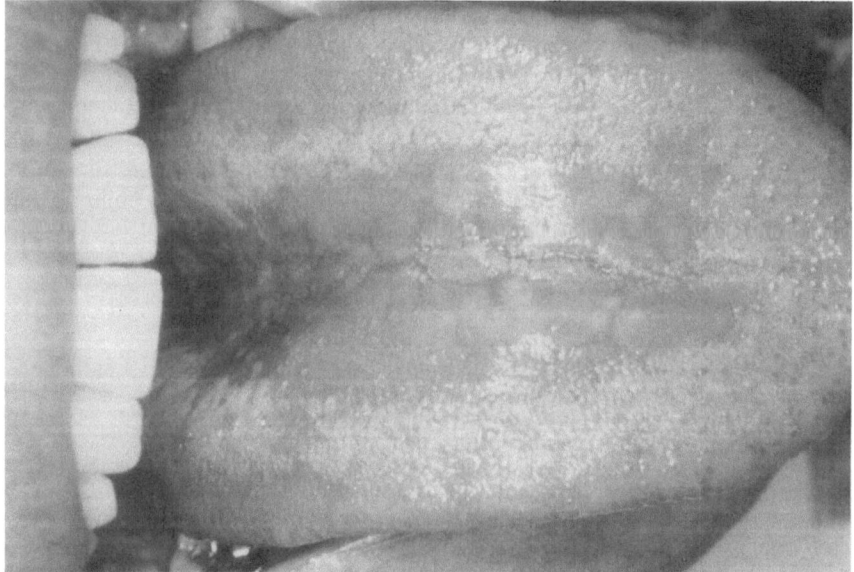

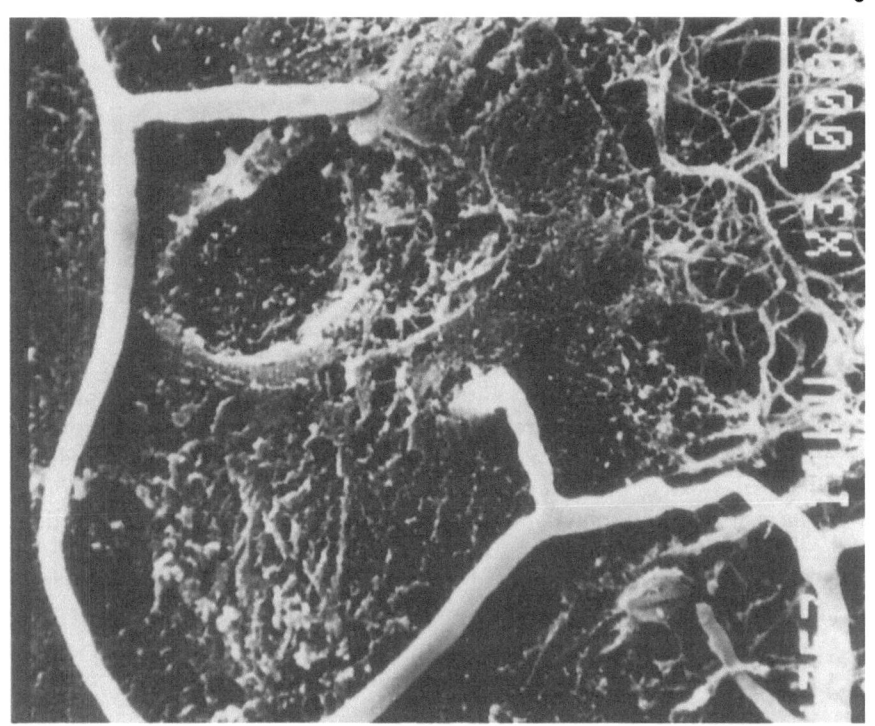

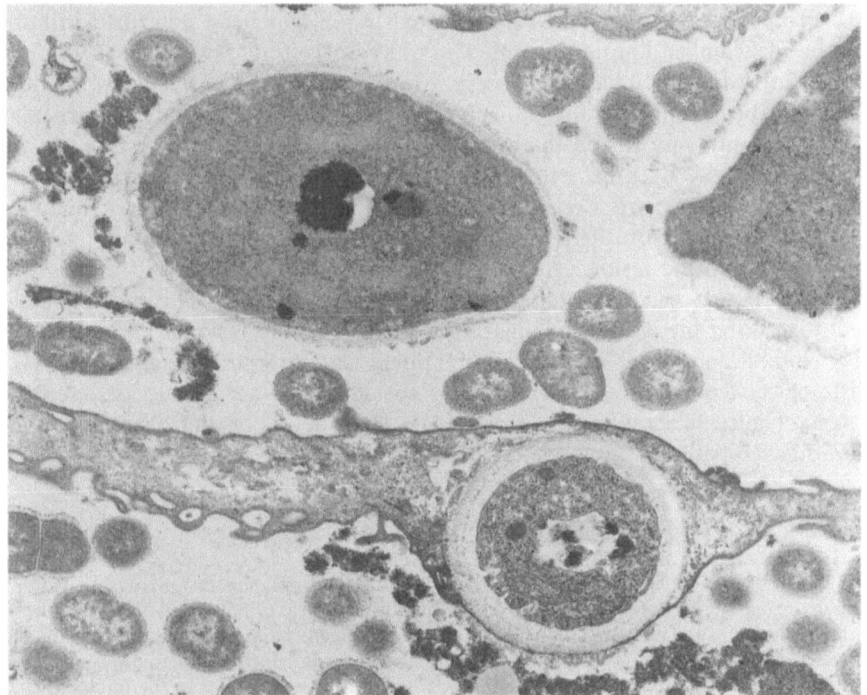

3.1.3 Other Types of Oral Candidiasis

Angular cheilitis and denture-induced stomatitis may be observed in patients with HIV infection. Both variants of oral candidiasis can be diagnosed clinically. Recently, a papillary variant of oral candidiasis in HIV-infected patients has been described (REICHART et al. 1994).

3.1.4 Prognosis

The prognosis of oral candidiasis in HIV infection is determined by the fact that eradication of *Candida albicans* by antifungal treatment is not possible. Antifungal medication results in disappearance of clinical signs and symptoms; however, recolonisation occurs as soon as treatment is interrupted or dosage is reduced. Dentinal caries has recently been described as a reservoir for *Candida albicans* (ROEDER et al. 1995). In some centres, prophylaxis has been introduced in patients whose CD4$^+$ cell count is below 200/mm^3. Azoles, particularly fluconazole and itraconazole, are the drugs of choice, but a number of patients in the final stage of AIDS develop resistance to azole therapy.

3.2 Hairy Leukoplakia

HL, an Epstein-Barr virus (EBV)-associated lesion, has been described in both immunodeficient and immunocompetent individuals (for a review, see PINDBORG and REICHART 1995). It has been observed in all risk groups and occurs worldwide. It has not been found in any other mucosal lining except the lateral border of the tongue and, very rarely, the buccal mucosa. There is no explanation of why HL preferentially occurs in this site. For correct diagnosis, both clinical and laboratory findings are necessary. Clinical presumptive criteria are bilateral whitish/grey lesions on the lateral margins of the tongue. Vertical corrugations are typical, and the lesion can not be removed. HL may extend to the ventral and dorsal surfaces of the tongue, where it is usually flat. The most reliable definitive criterion is the demonstration of EBV in the lesions. Persistence of the white lesions after antifungal treatment supports the diagnosis of HL. Histological features are not sufficiently specific to be acceptable as definitive criteria. Figure 2a shows an example of HL at the lateral border of tongue in an HIV-infected patient.

Fig. 2. a Hairy leukoplakia at the lateral border of tongue revealing the corrugated pattern partially extending to the lower surface of the tongue. **b** Biopsy of hairy leukoplakia showing surface epithelium and intense staining for virus capsid antigen of numerous nuclei, revealing the presence of Epstein-Barr virus. APAAP, ×200. **c** Transmission electron micrograph of a thin section of hairy leukoplakia, revealing multiple herpesvirus-like particles in the interepithelial space. ×25 000

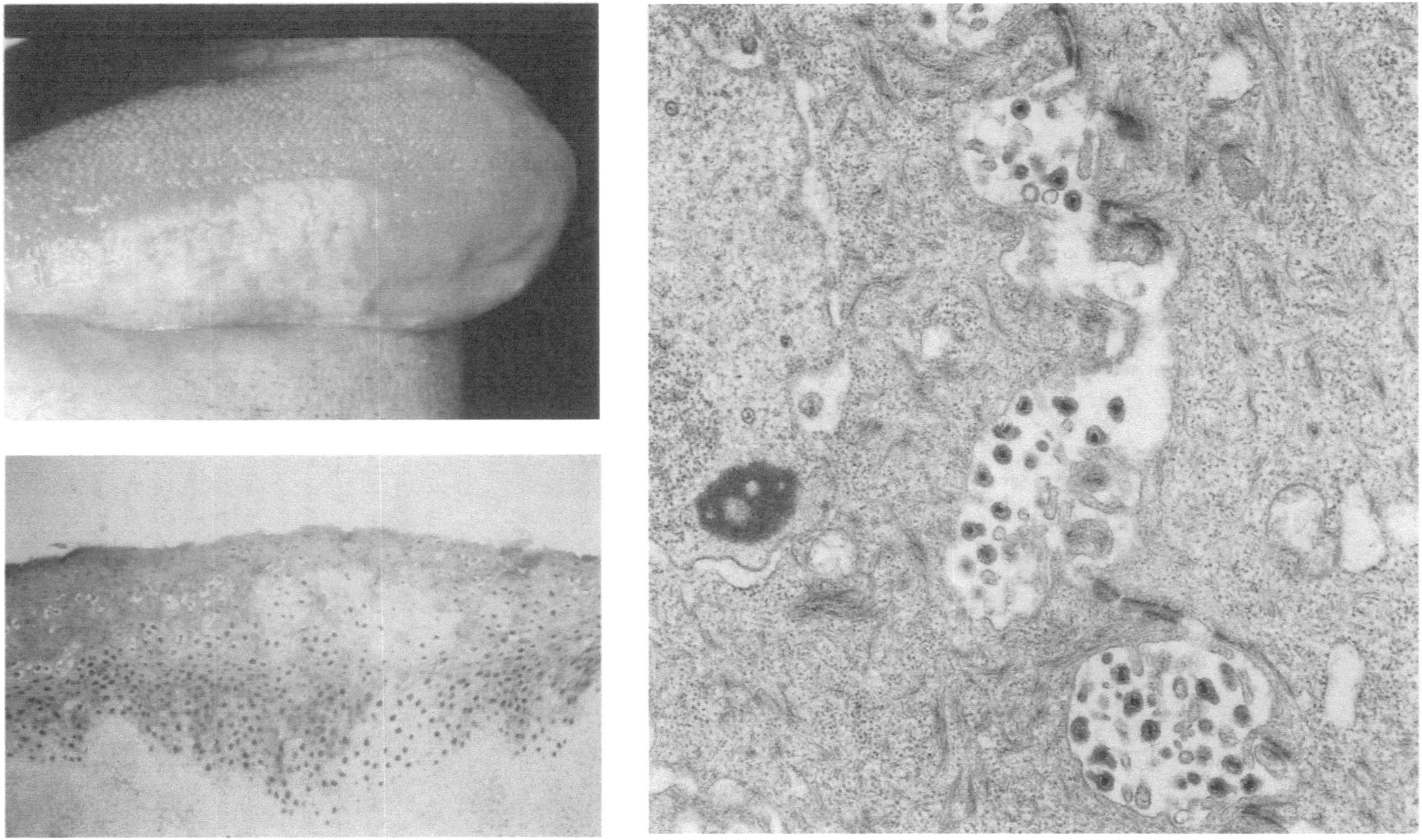

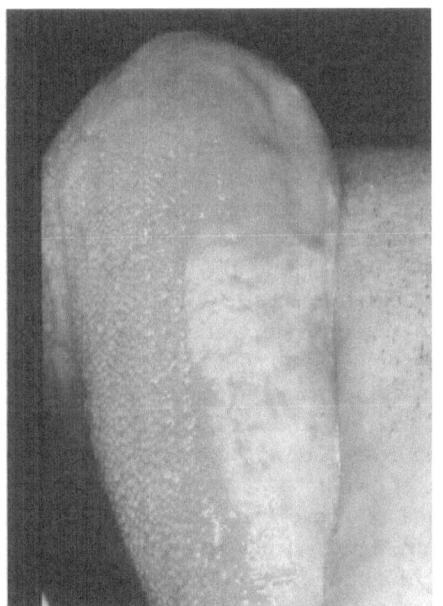

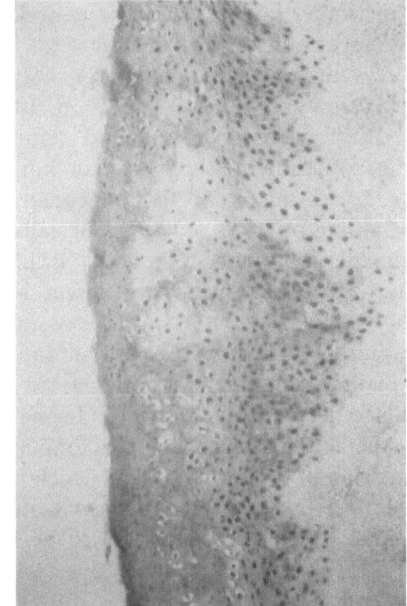

3.2.1 Histopathology

When HL was first described in 1984, it was compared to the histopathology of the flat wart of the skin. Histological features characterising HL are keratin projections, parakeratosis and acanthosis, ballooning of cells in the prickle cell layer, little or no inflammation and mild epithelial atypia in some cases. Basophilic nuclear inclusion bodies of epithelial cells in the prickle cell layer are an indication of viral infection. In 43%–100% of cases of HL, candidal infection may be demonstrated in PAS sections. An absence of Langerhans cells in HL has been described (DANIELS et al. 1987). Due to the unspecified histological appearance of HL, but also due to problems related to sectioning (ANDERSEN et al. 1990) and bias caused by lack of information about the HIV serostatus of the patient, HL may become a pitfall from the morphological point of view (SCHULTEN et al. 1991). To avoid misinterpretations, demonstration of EBV is mandatory. Numerous techniques have been suggested to demonstrate EBV, including immunohistochemistry (Fig. 2b), in situ hybridisation, negative-staining electron microscopy and electron microscopy (EPSTEIN et al. 1995). The disadvantage of electron microscopy is that this method allows for the demonstration of herpesvirus-type particles but not for the identification of EBV. Demonstration of viral capsid antigen in either biopsies or cytological smears allows for the unequivocal demonstration of EBV. A number of electron microscopy studies on the fine structure of HL have been published (ZHANG et al. 1988; GREENSPAN et al. 1989; EL-LABBAN et al. 1990). The presence of *Candida albicans* hyphae was revealed electron microscopically in a number of cases. Characteristic koilocyte-like cells showed pycnotic nuclei and condensed chromatin. Virus particles of the herpesvirus group may be observed in and around koilocytotic cells as well as in intercellular spaces. Isometric viral nucleocapsids have a diameter of 100nm. Budding processes may also be observed. Fully assembled herpes-virus-type particles have an identical diameter of 150nm (Fig. 2c). In addition, tubulo-reticular structures with a diameter of 35nm were observed, and remnants of membrane were found in close approximation to the nuclei of koilocytotic cells. One study has shown that the expression of proteins encoded by EBV-transactivated genes depends on the differentiation of epithelial cells in HL (BECKER et al. 1991a). The EBV immediate early gene product BZLF1 was localised to the cytoplasm of the basal epithelial layer by indirect immunofluorescence. To date, this is the only study in which it was possible to demonstrate that, in immunocompromised and probably also in immunocompetent patients, EBV may move with increasing differentiation from the cytoplasm to the nucleus of epithelial cells, where it is co-activated during the terminal differentiation of epithelium at the lateral border of the tongue. Figure 2c shows herpesvirus-type viral particles in a biopsy of HL which were shown to be EBV by immunohisto-chemical methods. Non-invasive methods to prove the presence of EBV in lesions which clinically seem to be HL are easier to perform, because it may be difficult to take a biopsy due to lack of compliance of many HIV-infected patients.

3.2.2 Prognosis

Although HL is associated with EBV, this lesion has not been demonstrated to be pre-cancerous. Single cases of oral carcinoma, however, have been described. The presence of HL is considered as a predictor for the development of AIDS, and three quarters of patients with HL develop AIDS in 2–3 years (MONIACI et al. 1990). Treatment of HL is unnecessary in most cases, but regression of the lesion has been observed concurrent with antiviral treatment for other viral infections. HL lesions seem to recur after discontinuation of treatment.

3.3 Kaposi's Sarcoma

In 1872, M. Kaposi first described a lesion which he termed idiopathic multiple pigmented sarcoma of skin. This type of classical KS was rare and mainly occurred in elderly men of southern and eastern European descent. Oral manifestations of Kaposi's classical type were extremely rare. Four different subtypes of KS are currently differentiated:

1. The classical European or Mediterranean KS
2. The endemic African KS
3. KS occurring in transplant patients under immunosuppressive therapy
4. Epidemic KS associated to AIDS (eKS)

The fourth subtype, eKS, was first described in 1981 in young homosexual or bisexual men from New York. KS in HIV infection is an AIDS-defining lesion. Oral eKS was shown to predominantly occur in male homosexual patients (REICHART et al. 1993); it is rare in heterosexuals, intravenous drug users (IDU), women and children. Patients are affected at an average age of 38 years. Presumptive criteria describing and defining eKS are one or more erythematous, slightly bluish or violaceous macules or swellings with or without ulceration, predominantly seen on the palate, gingiva or tongue. (Fig. 3a). The characteristic histological appearance on biopsy allows a definitive diagnosis to be made. Most eKS lesions are 1–3 cm in diameter. Oral eKS lesions may be non-pigmented (REICHART and SCHIÖT 1989) and may also involve the jaw bones (LANGFORD et al. 1991a). Whenever the HIV serostatus is known, diagnosis of eKS is not to difficult. This is particularly so in those cases in which skin lesions precede those of the oral mucosa. Clinical

Fig. 3. a Oral Kaposi's sarcoma on dorsum of tongue, a characteristic site after palatal and gingival location. b Biopsy of Kaposi's sarcoma showing spindle-shaped cells and early formation of vessel-like structures. Numerous extravasated erythrocytes are also seen. H&E, ×200. c Semi-thin section of oral Kaposi's sarcoma. Large vascular spaces with protruding endothelial cells are seen. Toludine blue, ×350. d Transmission electron micrograph (TEM) of a thin section of oral Kaposi's sarcoma showing protruding endothelial cells in an newly formed vascular structure. Nuclei are irregular and large. ×5000. e TEM of tumour cells of Kaposi's sarcoma, which are often spindle-shaped with large oval nuclei with small rims of condensed chromatin. ×5000

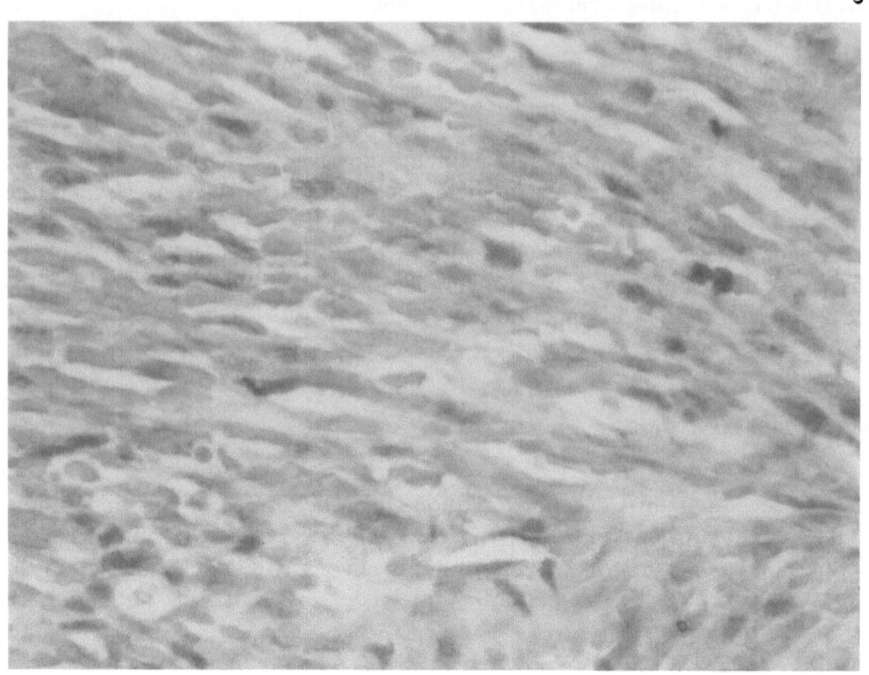

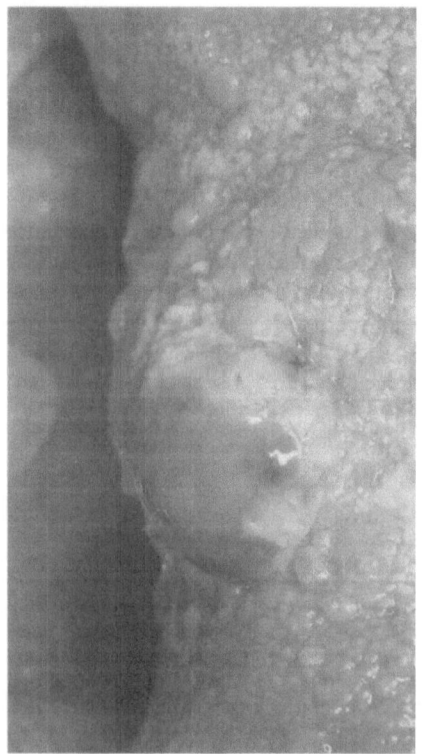

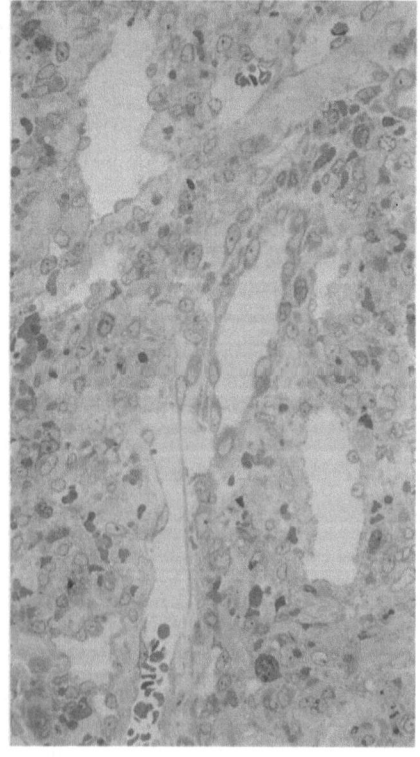

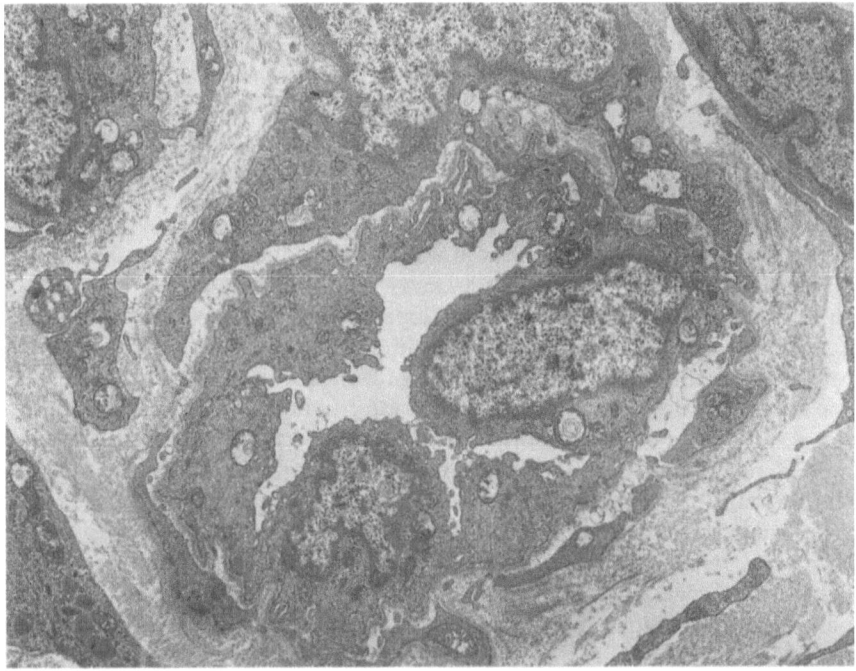

e

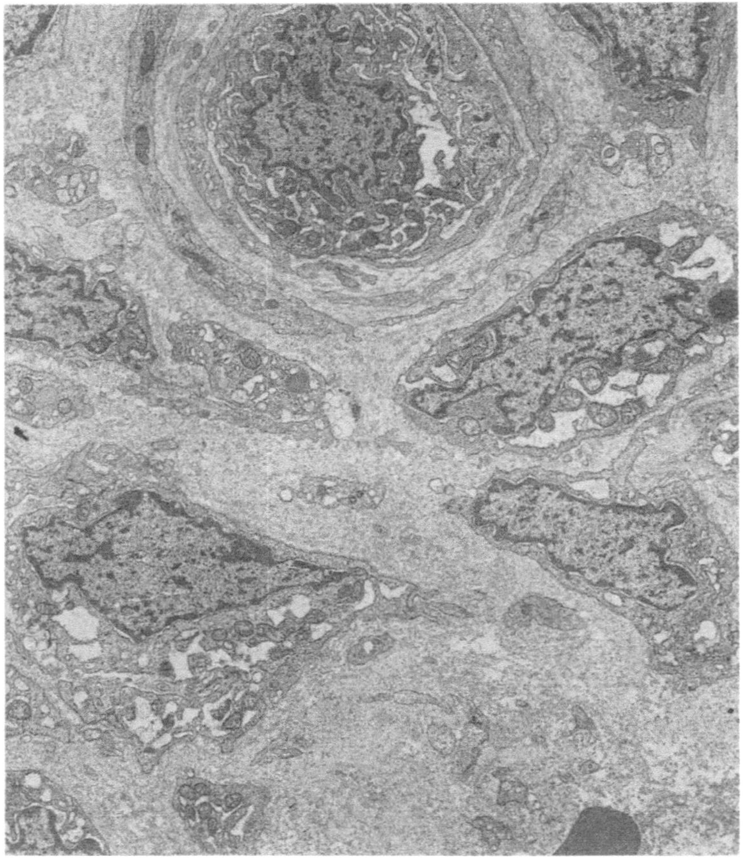

d

differential diagnosis includes other pigmented lesions such as haematoma, haemangioma, tattoos and other neoplasms of vascular origin.

3.3.1 Histopathology

Light and electron microscopic features of the classical and African subtypes of KS and eKS are identical (GREEN et al. 1984). Since oral KS was extremely rare in the pre-AIDS era, this histopathological diagnosis was not routine. It has now become much more frequent, and oral pathologists must be aware of the fact that, histologically, eKS tissue may mimic granulation tissue with numerous vessels, as seen in peri-apical granuloma. Other lesions derived from vascular structures may also show similarities. Early eKS lesions show dilated, thin-walled vascular spaces with polymorphous endothelial cells. These protrude into the vascular lumen. Endothelial cells appear to be enlarged and show small amounts of cytoplasm containing polymorphic electron-lucent nuclei. Late stages of eKS characterised by tumour growth show a decrease in atypical vessels. The interstitial, spindle-shaped cells with enlarged oval nuclei prevail. Vessel-like spaces are filled with erythrocytes, and extravascular erythrocytes are common. Macrophages that phagocytose erythrocytes are seen, as are deposits of haemosiderin, and inflammatory cells may be seen around vessel-like spaces. Mitoses of tumour cells are rare (Fig. 3b,c). A 10-year retrospective, histopathological study of oral KS (REGEZI et al. 1993) has recently confirmed these findings. In addition, it was stated that eKS expresses the CD34 antigen, which may be useful in the diagnosis of small, well-delineated oral lesions lacking the classic KS features. Antigen CD34 may also be helpful to differentiate eKS from bacillary angiomatosis, pyogenic granuloma, epithelioid haemangioma or other spindle cell proliferations.

The ultrastructure of eKS shows a number of specific features. Endothelial cells are characterised by enlarged nuclei showing a marked lobulated surface and little marginal chromatin (Fig. 3d,e). Basal membranes are interrupted and connected by tight, intermediate or gap junctions or desmosomes. Weibel-Palade bodies are characteristic organelles of endothelial cells and are found in oral eKS lesions. In addition, intracytoplasmic aggregates of tubular structures with an average diameter of 24–35 μm are characteristic. Extravasated erythrocytes are seen on electron microscopy and in histopathology (KUNTZ et al. 1987). It was interesting to see similar ultrastructural findings in vessels of uninvolved oral mucosa of patients with HIV infection. Features as seen in eKS such as swollen endothelial cells, loss of cellular junctions, interruptions of the basal membrane, presence of Weibel-Palade bodies and tubular structures were also observed. These findings were interpreted as features of a disregulated vascular neogenesis (ZHANG et al. 1989). Studies of the extracellular matrix in eKS showed that stains for basement membrane components revealed distinct patterns of distribution. A delicate and partly fragmented lining of basement membrane around the sinusoid-like vascular spaces was seen, as well as an occasional diffuse interstitial fluorescence in the tumour stroma. From these findings, a vascular cell origin of the endothelial and spindle cell components of eKS was likely (BECKER et al. 1991b). Intense fluorescence was noted for procollagens type I and III and collagen type VI. It was concluded that procollagens type I and III and collagen type VI are synthesized de novo by cells of the tumour stroma. In another study, immunoelectron microscopy showed an atypical pattern and a quantitive shift of collagens type I, III and VI in eKS. Collagen fibrils in eKS consisted of collagen type I. However, there was a marked loss of thick fibre bundles of collagens types I and III in eKS compared to normal oral mucosa. Collagen type VI was increased. This abundance of collagen type VI in a pattern comparable to early stages of wound healing suggested that the eKS stroma resembles an early organisational stage of the interstitial and vascular extracellular matrix. It appeared that the eKS stroma resulted from a continous autocrine and paracrine stimulation of cell growth and collagen synthesis (BECKER et al. 1991c).

Other studies have focused on immunocompetent cells in eKS. Of interest was the fact that both eKS lesions and uninvolved oral mucosa of HIV-infected patients show infiltration with CD4+ cells. In early eKS lesions, a marked increase of CD8+ cells was found compared to later tumour stages. In addition, the number of HLA DR+ cells was increased. Findings were interpreted as indicating the influence of eKS growth factors on the inflammatory reaction during the course of systemic immunosuppression characteristic of HIV infection (TABATA et al. 1993).

3.3.2 Aetiology and Pathogenesis

Both the aetiology and the pathogenesis of eKS are still unclear. However, as early as 1983 (LOZADA et al. 1983) a number of possible factors which may be associated with eKS and probably other neoplasms were pinpointed, including higher than normal incidence of antibodies titers to CMV, multiple opportunistic infections (e.g. venereal diseases, herpetic infections, PcP, oral candidiasis), heavy drug usage and marked sexual activity. While some of these factors are still considered valid, the aetiologic relationship of HIV and eKS has also been discussed. There are several possible mechanisms by which oncogenic RNA viruses such as retroviruses may cause malignancy (REICHART 1991). In particular, the role of the HIV *tat* gene has been considered of importance (CREMER et al. 1990). Human papillomavirus type 16-related DNA sequences were found in eKS, and it was suggested that this may have a role in the pathogenesis of eKS (HUANG et al. 1992). A transmissible agent was suspected, and eKS was considered a sexually transmitted infection (BERAL et al. 1990). As such, eKS occurred in 1% of men with haemophilia and 21% of homosexual or bisexual men. While agents such as CMV, hepatitis B virus, human herpesvirus-6 (HHV-6), HIV and *Mycoplasma penetrans* have been suspected to be associated with eKS, in December 1994 herpesvirus-like DNA sequences in AIDS-associated KS were identified (CHANG et al. 1994). These sequences were termed KS-associated herpesvirus-like sequences (KSHV), defining a possible new human herpesvirus. Of interest is the fact that these KSHV sequences are also found in HIV-negative patients with KS. In addition, KSHV DNA sequences are also found in AIDS-related body cavity-based lymphomas. The possible aetio-pathogenic role of KSHV is underlined by the observation that remissions of eKS were observed in patients who received foscarnet. Foscarnet is an antiviral drug used for treatment of infections with herpesviruses. Generally, numerous growth factors have been identified which promote the growth of eKS cells. Autocrine and paracrine mechanisms are involved. A major growth factor for eKS has been identified as oncostatin M (NAIR et al. 1992).

Figure 4 shows a model for the pathogenesis of eKS. In principal, HIV-infected cells release viral and other cellular factors probably capable of stimulating activation and proliferation of cells of mesenchymal origin which may be endothelial cells. These acquire the spindle-shaped morphology characteristic of eKS cells. KS cells then start to produce cytokines, which maintain and amplify the cellular response via autocrine and paracrine pathways. Paracrine activation of normal cells leads to fibroblast proliferation, neoangiogenesis and inflammatory cell infiltration. If the initial stimulus persists, a vicious cycle may be established, resulting in tumour transformation.

It must be remembered that eKS is, by definition, a multicentric, hyperplastic proliferation and not a true neoplastic and metastatic expansion. As such, it is not a true sarcoma, at least at the beginning of the disease, but is considered as a type of multicentric hyperplasia.

3.3.3 Prognosis

The prognosis of oral eKS is poor. In one study (REICHART et al. 1993), average survival time of 124 patients was 1 year and 9 months (range, 3 months to 4 years and 6 months). A total of 57.3% of patients evaluated in that study died. Treatment is palliative, consisting of local or systemic administration of cytostatic drugs (bleomycin, vinblastine, vincristine, actinomycin D, doxorubicin, etoposide and others and combinations thereof). In addition, interferon-α_2 has been used as an immunomodulatory treatment, and radiation (dosage, 20 Gy) has also been used. Treatment modalities and results for oral eKS are still not satisfactory, and it should be made clear that "many patients require infinite treatment for control of lesions."

3.4 Non-Hodgkin's Lymphoma

Non-Hodgkin's lymphoma (NHL) is observed in 77% of AIDS patients and Hodgkin's lymphoma in 23%. After eKS, HIV-related malignant lymphomas are the most common malignancies observed in AIDS patients. Presumptive criteria of NHL include firm, elastic, often reddish or purplish swellings with or without ulceration. The gingiva, palatal mucosa and fauces are the most common sites. Definite criteria are based on characteristic histological appearance on biopsy, supported by appropriate immunocytochemical or molecular biological investigations. Malignant lymphomas grow rapidly, and ulceration is therefore a common finding (LANGFORD et al. 1991b). When situated on gingival tissue, NHL lesions cannot be differentiated from necrotising stomatitis or infection. The histological spectrum of NHL is wide, including lymphoblastic, centroblastic, immunoblastic, highly malignant and unclassifiable types. Furthermore, the histological pattern of

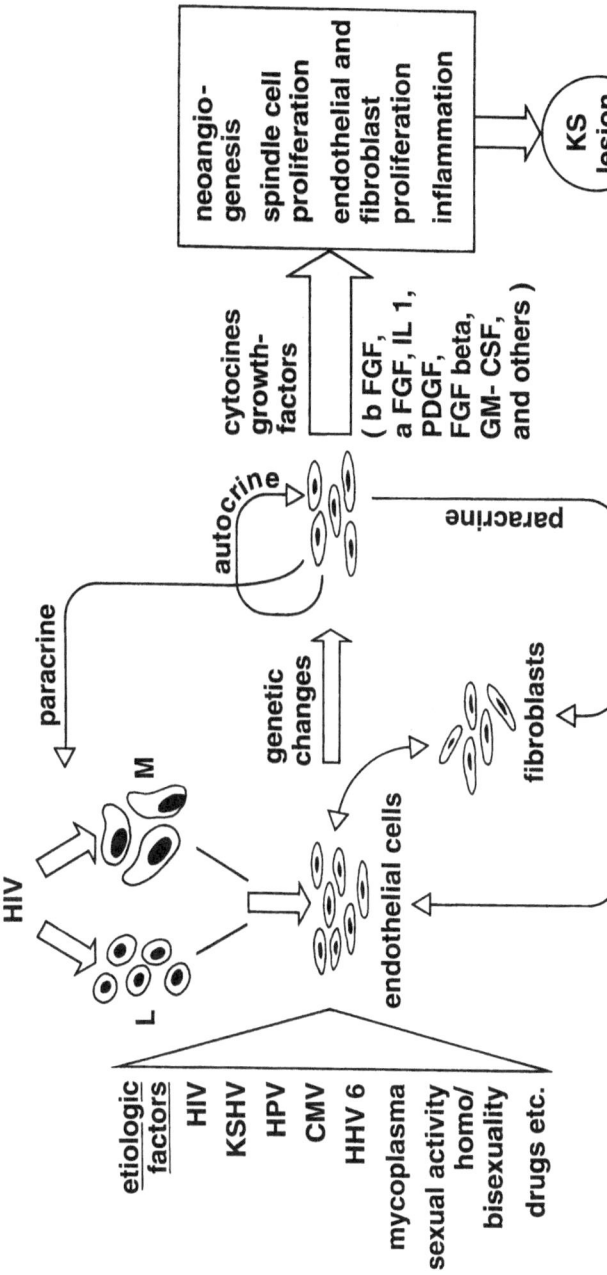

Fig. 4. Causative factors and pathogenesis of Kaposi's sarcoma (*KS*). Mainly autocrine and paracrine stimuli account for the formation of the KS tumour cell. *M*, macrophages; *L*, lymphocytes; *HIV*, human immunodeficiency virus; *KSHV*, KS herpesvirus; *HPV*, human papillomavirus; *CMV*, cytomegalovirus; *HHV*, human herpesvirus; *FGF*, fibroblast growth factor; *bFGF*, basic FGF; *aFGF*, acidic FGF; *PDGF*, platelet-derived growth factor; *GM-CSF*, granulocyte-macrophage colony-stimulating factor

non-Hodgkin's lymphoma ranges from large pleomorphic lymphoblasts to small, non-cleaved cells. A relation to EBV has been documented for both NHL and Hodgkin's lymphoma; however, not all B cell lymphomas show EBV DNA.

3.4.1 Prognosis

The prognosis of NHL in AIDS patients is very poor, and survival of patients is counted in months. Treatment involves chemotherapy with various cytotoxic drugs.

3.5 Periodontal Diseases

Periodontal diseases associated with HIV infection and AIDS are still the subject of controversy. In the classification system drawn up by the European Community (EC 1993), it was stated that, in addition to the specific forms of periodontal disease, it should be appreciated that chronic marginal gingivitis and adult periodontitis can occur in patients with HIV infection. The clinical appearances of these conditions may, however, be altered or exaggerated as a result of immuno-suppression. Periodontal diseases are considered by some as the same periodontal diseases seen in normal patients with some exaggerated features and by others as specific diseases particular to HIV infection or AIDS.

3.5.1 Linear Gingival Erythema

Linear gingival erythema (LGE) is described as a distinct, firey-red band along the margin of the gingiva (Fig. 5a). The amount of erythema is disproportionally intense for the amount of plaque seen. No ulceration is present, and there is no evidence of pocket or attachment loss. There are currently no definite criteria, and LGE is diagnosed clinically. It has been suggested that a feature of LGE is that it does not respond well to oral hygiene measures and to the removal of dental plaque and calculus. The microbiology of this lesion is controversial; however, *Candida albicans* seems to be involved in the aetiology (GRBRIC et al. 1995). The specificity of LGE and its association to HIV infection and AIDS has been questioned by several clinicians; similar, if not identical changes have been observed in debilitated patients.

Biopsy is not recommended for making the definite diagnosis.

3.5.2 Necrotising (Ulcerative) Gingivitis

Destruction of one or more interdental papillae is a presumptive criterion of necrotising gingivitis. In the acute stage of the process, ulceration, necrosis and sloughing is seen with ready haemorrhage and a characteristic odour. As in all the

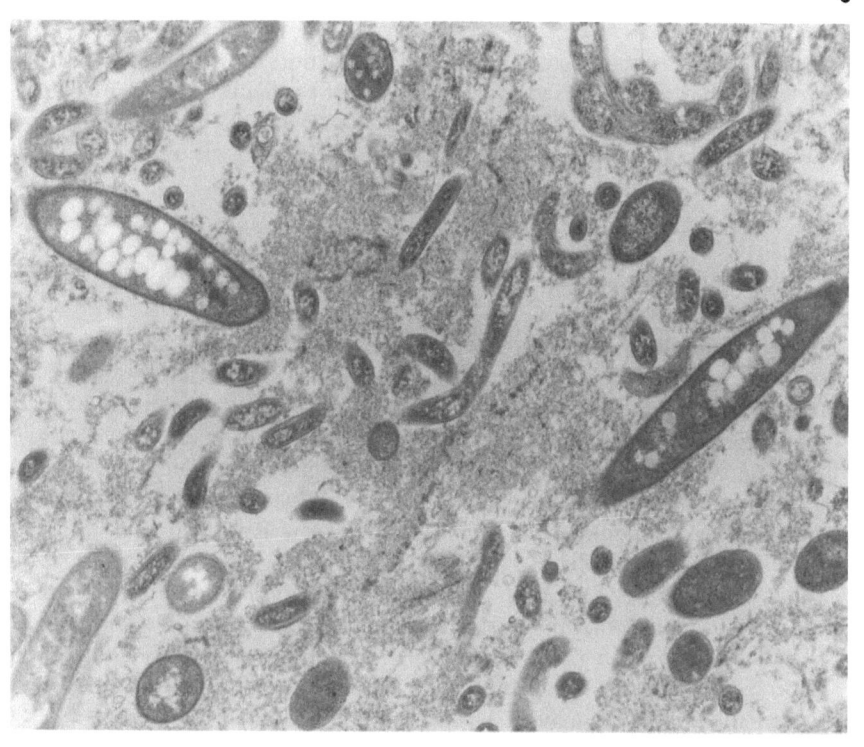

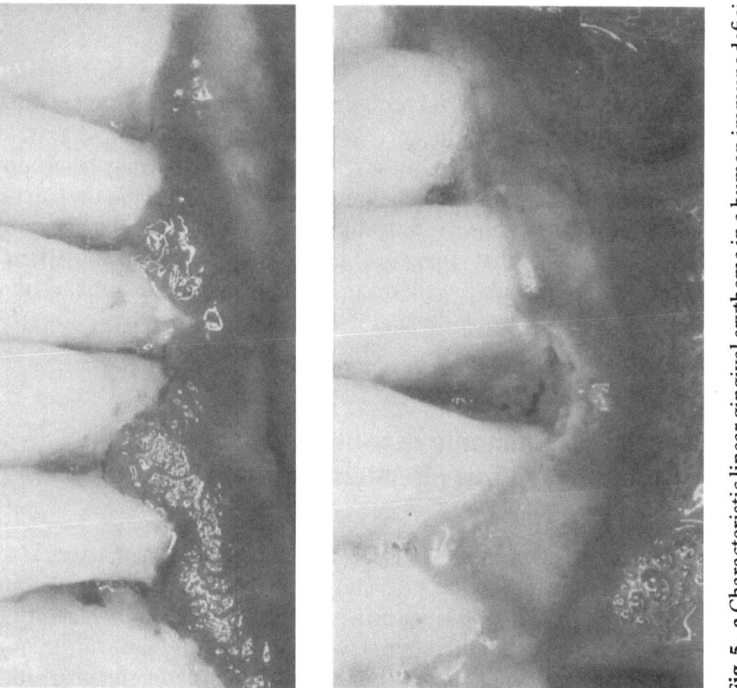

Fig. 5. a Characteristic linear gingival erythema in a human immunodeficiency virus (HIV)-positive patient. b Necrotising gingivitis with characteristic loss of papilla in an HIV-positive patient. c Transmission electron micrograph of numerous spirilliform bacteria and cocci in a biopsy of necrotising gingivitis.

other periodontal diseases associated with HIV infection or AIDS, no definite criteria are available. Figure 5b shows a typical loss of papilla in an HIV-infected patients. Necrotising gingivitis has been reported in 5%–11% of HIV-infected individuals (HOLMSTRUP and WESTERGAARD 1994). Most patients only show necrotic tops of the interdental papilla.

3.5.3 Necrotising (Ulcerative) Periodontitis

Necrotising periodontitis is characterised by presumptive criteria such as soft tissue loss as a result of ulceration or necrosis. Exposure, destruction or segregation of bone is seen, and teeth may become loose. There may be severe pain. As in LGE and necrotising gingivitis, no definite criteria are known for necrotising periodontitis. A study carried out by the U.S. National Institute of Dental Research of 200 HIV-seropositive patients found that the type of periodontitis seen in these patients did not have unique or pathognomonic characteristics that could set it apart from the periodontal disease in HIV-seronegative patients (RILEY et al. 1992). The microbiology of both necrotising gingivitis and necrotising periodontitis show micro-organisms such as *Borrelia*, gram-positive cocci, β-haemolytic streptococci and *Candida albicans* (ZAMBON et al. 1990). Figure 5c shows a thin section of a biopsy of necrotising periodontitis with numerous organisms invading the marginal gingival tissue.

3.5.4 Prognosis

Periodontal diseases in HIV infection and AIDS have been overestimated as to their prevalence and significance. As with periodontal diseases in non-immunocompromised patients, these lesions and diseases may be prophylactically avoided by appropriate oral hygiene measures, although rapid destruction of periodontal tissue has been observed. It must be stressed that the periodontal lesions are interrelated and that they are not individual characteristic entities. A necrotising stomatitis may well occur as a result of necrotising gingivitis or periodontitis. More severe lesions, however, seem to be rare.

4 Lesions Less Commonly Associated with Human Immunodeficiency Virus Infection (Group II)

Group II comprises some bacterial infections of mycobacterial origin and viral infections including herpes simplex virus, human papillomavirus and varicella zoster virus. In addition, other diseases such as NOS ulceration, salivary gland disease and melanotic hyperpigmentation are part of this group. Of particular interest are NOS ulcerations and human papillomavirus-induced oral lesions.

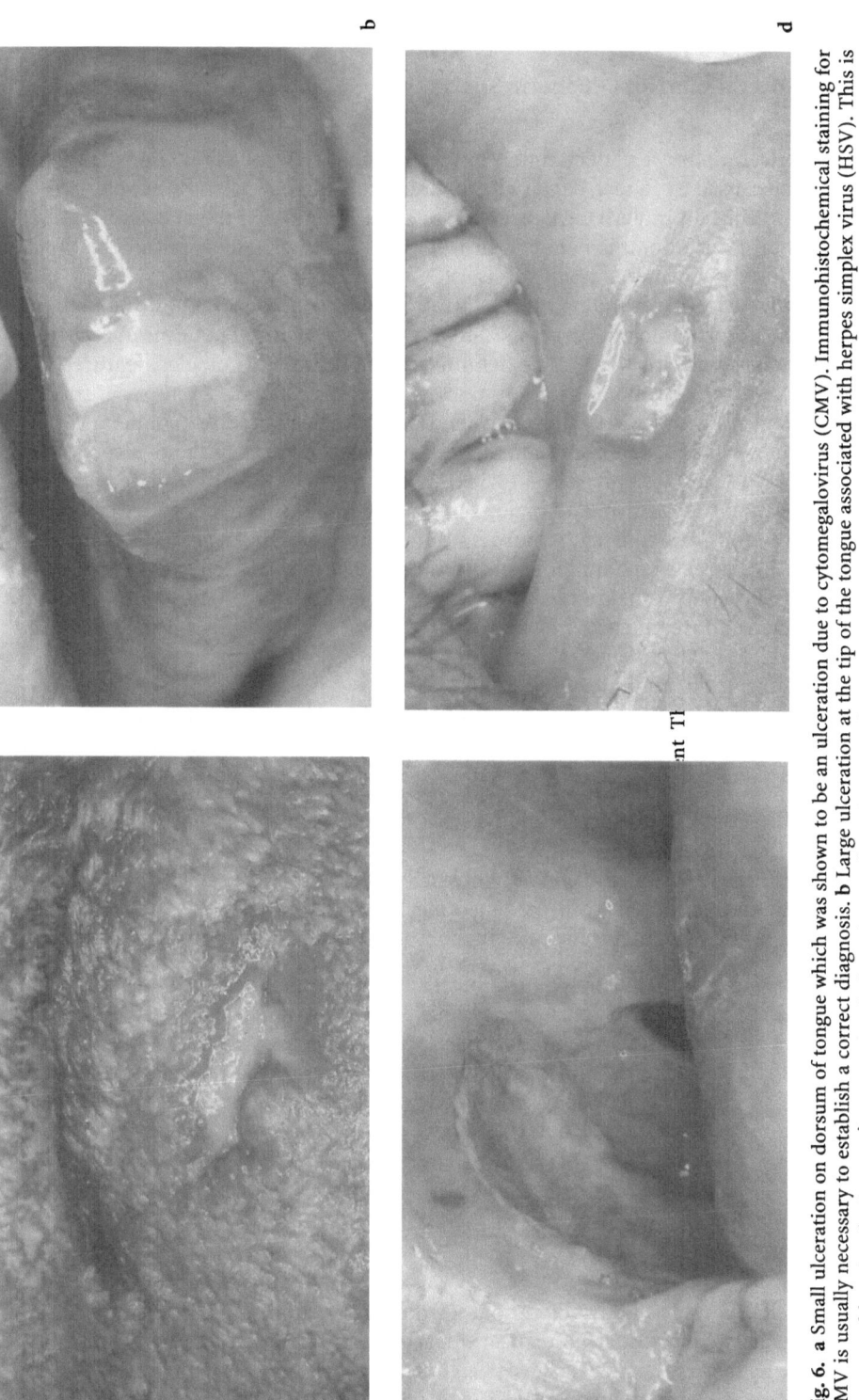

Fig. 6. a Small ulceration on dorsum of tongue which was shown to be an ulceration due to cytomegalovirus (CMV). Immunohistochemical staining for CMV is usually necessary to establish a correct diagnosis. **b** Large ulceration at the tip of the tongue associated with herpes simplex virus (HSV). This is an unusual location for herpesvirus-associated ulceration. **c** Ulceration not otherwise specified on the fauces and palate of an AIDS patient. Histology is nonconclusive Chronic recurrent ulcer on lipmucosa of an AIDS patient. The characteristic clinical morphology of this type of aphthae is seen.

4.1 Ulcerations Not Otherwise Specified

Oral ulcerations are very common in the course of HIV infection and AIDS. They may be caused by fungal, bacterial and viral infections as well as by neoplasia (Fig. 6a–d). While an underlying cause may be found in most of the above-mentioned types of ulceration, this is not so in NOS ulcerations. These were called atypical ulceration in former classifications. NOS ulcerations are characterised by presumptive criteria, including those ulcerations with a predilection for the pharynx and palate which do not correspond to any of the recognised patterns of recurrent aphthous stomatitis (RAS). The definite criteria include histological features of a non-specific ulceration. Viral or bacterial cultures fail to identify a specific aetiological agent (EC 1993). NOS ulcerations have been described under a variety of names such as major aphthous-like ulcers or recurrent aphthous ulcers of the major type. In one study, 66% of 75 HIV-seropositive patients presented with the uncommon herpetiform and major types of ulcerations. Patients with this type of ulceration were significantly more immunosuppressed than those with minor or herpetiform recurrent aphthous ulcerations in that they had fewer CD4$^+$ and CD8$^+$ lymphocytes (MACPHAIL et al. 1991). NOS ulcerations are often painful and not responsive to treatment. They may persist for weeks. Treatment usually involves topical tetracyclines and steroids; however, resistant ulceration has also been treated with thalidomide.

The aetiology and pathogenesis of NOS ulcerations is still not clear. Several mechanisms may be operative in the aetio-pathogenesis of such ulcers (REICHART 1992):

1. A directly or indirectly antibody-mediated mechanism
2. A T cell-mediated mechanism
3. Antibody-dependent cellular cytotoxicity
4. A natural killer (NK) cell-mediated mechanism
5. A specific or non-specific immunocomplex-mediated mechanism

The diagnosis is mainly based on clinical appearance and history of the ulceration. No reliable histopathological criteria have yet been found to characterise NOS ulceration. To a certain extent diagnosis is also made by exclusion of other causes, such as fungal, bacterial and viral agents. The prognosis is fair because the disease process may be considerably shortened with local or systemic steroids and/or thalidomide. Recurrences, however, may occur.

4.2 Human Papillomavirus Infections

Epithelial verruca-like proliferations of the oral mucosa have been reported in HIV-positive individuals. Verruca vulgaris, condyloma acuminatum and focal epithelial hyperplasia (FEH) have been described. Lesions may either occur as tiny proliferations or may involve large areas of the oral mucosa (Fig. 7a). Lesions are associated with human papillomavirus, especially type 7 or other types including

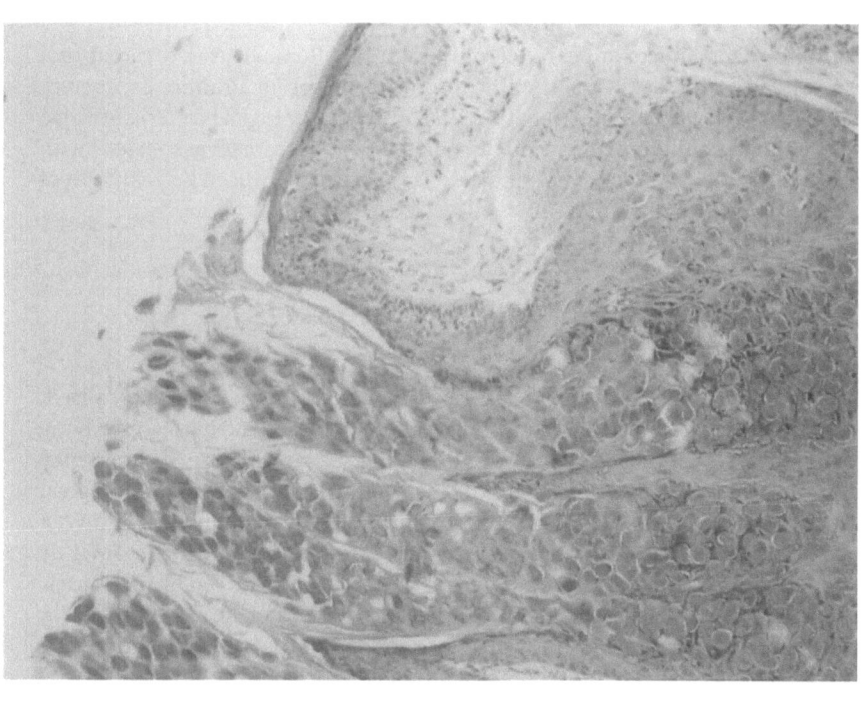

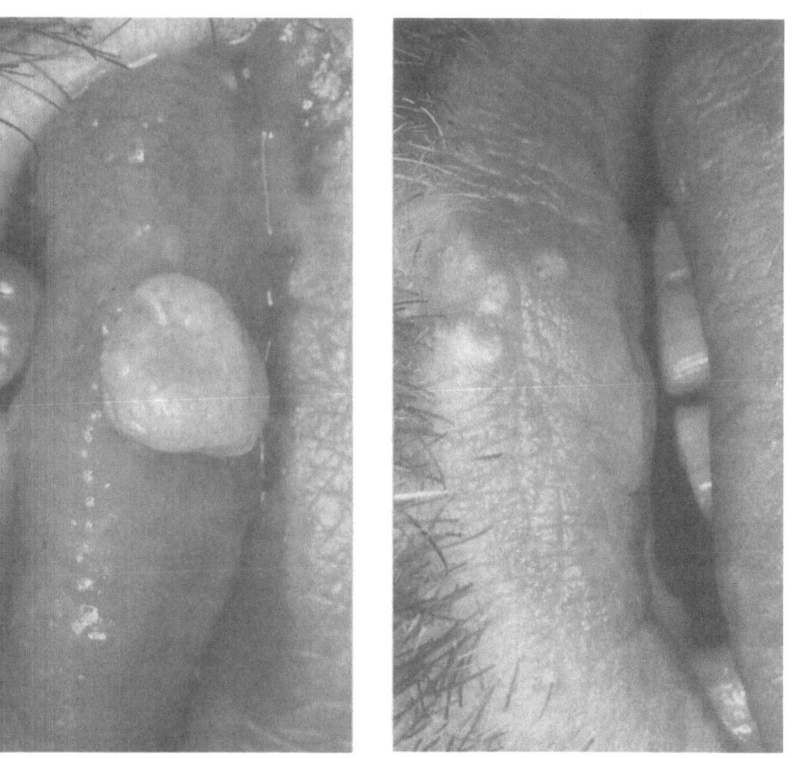

Fig. 7. a Human papillomavirus (HPV)-associated proliferation at the lateral border of tongue of a human immunodeficiency virus (HIV)-positive patient. In this case the lesion had a more papilloma-like appearance. **b** On the upper lip of this HIV-positive patient, the characteristic lesions caused by molluscum contagiosum are seen. **c** Histological section of molluscum contagiosum-associated lesion, showing characteristic eosinophilic intracytoplasmic inclusion bodies These cells show hyperplastic growth and form large continuous lobules H&E ×200

13, 18 and 42. The clinical appearance of human papillomavirus-associated oral mucosa lesions is the same in immunocompromised as in immunocompetent subjects (for a review, see SYRJÄNEN 1995). The histopathological criteria are also identical. Human papillomavirus is not associated (as was initially suspected) with HL. Cryosurgery, laser therapy or surgical excision are usually used in treatment of oral papillomatous lesions.

4.3 Necrotising Stomatitis

Necrotising stomatitis is characterised by presumptive criteria such as localised, acute, painful ulcerative necrotic lesions of the oral mucosa that expose underlying bone or penetrate or extend into neighbouring tissues. These lesions may extend from areas of necrotising periodontitis. Definite criteria show histological features of non-specific ulceration. Microbiological studies fail to identify a specific aetiologic agent. Extensive noma-like cases of necrotising stomatitis have been described, and perforation of facial skin may be observed in such cases. As has already been discussed, necrotising stomatitis is not an entity in itself, but is usually determined by gingival or periodontal necrosis. The prognosis in such extensive cases of necrotising stomatitis is poor, and the disease may be life-threatening.

4.4 Human Immunodeficiency Virus Associated Salivary Gland Disease

HIV-associated salivary gland disease (HIV-SGD) encompasses non-neoplastic changes of the salivary glands with enlargement of one or more of the major salivary glands with or without xerostomia. Diseases such as benign lympho-epithelial lesion, cystic lymphoid hyperplasia of the parotid gland, lymphadenopathy of the parotid gland, parotid swelling or enlargement, sicca complex syndrome and Sjögren's syndrome are considered to belong to HIV-SGD (SCHIÖDT 1992). HIV-SGD appears to be rather uncommon in adult HIV patients (0%–0.8%), but it has been observed in 0%–58% of HIV-infected children (SCHIÖDT 1992). The age distribution of patients with HIV-SGD is characterized by two groups: children born of HIV-infected mothers and adults between 20 and 60 years of age. Men are affected in over 90% of cases. Intravenous drug users are affected in 61% and homosexual men in 39% of cases. The main symptom is swelling of one or more of the major salivary glands, most often the parotid. A total of 91% of patients with HIV-SGD or Sjögren's syndrome-like conditions complained of a dry mouth. The parotid gland is affected in more than 90% of patients, while the submandibular gland is only affected in 2%. Diagnostic procedures involve measurement of salivary flow rates, labial salivary gland biopsy, eye examinations and serological examination for antinuclear antibodies, rheumatoid factor and Sjögren's syndrome antibodies A and B. HIV-SGD has a characteristic appearance on computed tomography (CT) and magnetic resonance imaging (MRT).

Multicentric cysts within salivary glands are characteristic. Histopathology uniformly reveals lympho-epithelial lesions or cysts. The lesion is composed of hyperplastic intraparotid lymph nodes or a lymphocytic infiltrate within the salivary gland tissue or both. Epimyoepithelial islands are seen within the lymphoid tissue, and a cystic lumen is seen centrally. The inflammatory infiltrate is dominated by CD8+ cells. Labial salivary gland biopsy shows focal sialadenitis comparable to Sjögren's syndrome, with a predominance of CD8+ cells. The prognosis of HIV-SGD is favourable, although no definitive treatment has so far been described. The pathogenesis of HIV-SGD is unknown.

5 Lesions Seen in Human Immunodeficiency Virus Infection (Group III)

Group III of the classification (EC 1993) comprises rare diseases and lesions. Bacterial infections caused by *Enterobacteriaceae* and other agents have been described. Fungal infections comprise those of rare diseases such as cryptococcosis, geotrichosis, histoplasmosis, mucormycosis and others. Viral infections include CMV and molluscum contagiosum (Fig. 7b,c). Lesions in group III include drug reactions, epithelioid angiomatosis and neurological disturbances of facial nerves.

All of these lesions are anecdotal and have only been described in rare instances. Their occurrence may not necessarily be associated with HIV infection. Due to geographical differences, other types of rare infections may be included in group III in the future. One example is penicilliosis, which is rare in Europe and North America, but rather prevalent as an oral lesion in South-East Asia, particularly in Thailand.

References

Andersen L, Philipsen HP, Reichart PA (1990) Macro- and microanatomy of the lateral border of the tongue with special reference to oral hairy leukoplakia. J Oral Pathol Med 19: 77–80

Becker J, Leser U, Marschall M, Langford A, Jilg W, Gelderblom H, Reichart P, Wolf H (1991a) Expression of proteins encoded by Epstein-Barr virus trans-activator genes depends on the differentation of epithelial cells in oral hairy leukoplakia. Proc Natl Acad Sci USA 88: 8332–8336

Becker J, Schuppan D, Reichart P (1991b) The extracellular matrix in oral Kaposi's sarcoma (AIDS): the immunohistochemical distribution of collagens type IV, V, VI, of procollagens type I and II of laminin and of undulin. Virchows Arch [A] Pathol Anat Histopathol 412: 161–168

Becker J, Schuppan D, Rabanus JP, Gelderblom HR, Reichart P (1991c) Immunoelectron microscopy shows an atypical pattern and a quantitative shift of collagens type I, III and VI in oral Kaposi's sarcoma of AIDS. Virchows Arch [A] Pathol Anat Histopathol 419: 237–244

Beral V, Petermann TA, Berkelman RL, Jaffe HW (1990) Kaposi's sarcoma among persons with AIDS - a sexually transmitted infection? Lancet 335: 123–128

Chang Y, Cesarman E, Pessin M, Lee F, Culpepper J, Knowles D, Moore P (1994) Identification of herpesvirus-like DNA sequences in AIDS-associated Kaposi's sarcoma. Science 226: 1865–1869

Cremer KJ, Spring SB, Gruber J (1990) Role of human immunodeficiency virus type I and other viruses in malignancies associated with aquired immunodeficiency disease syndrome. J Natl Cancer Inst 82: 1016–1024

Daniels TE, Greenspan D, Greenspan JS, Lennette E, Schiödt M, Petersen V, de Souza Y (1987) Absence of Langerhans cells in oral hairy leukoplakia, an AIDS-associated lesion. J Invest Dermatol 89: 178–182

EC Clearinghouse on Oral Problems Related to HIV Infection and WHO Collaborating Centre on Oral Manifestations of the Immunodeficiency Virus (1993) Classification and diagnostic criteria for oral lesions in HIV infection. J Oral Pathol Med 22: 289–291

El-Labban N, Pindborg JJ, Rindum J, Nielsen (1990) Further ultrastructural findings in epithelial cells of hairy leukoplakia. J Oral Pathol Med 19: 24–34

Epstein JB, Fatahzadeh M, Matisic J, Anderson G (1995) Exfoliative cytology and electron microscopy in the diagnosis of hairy leukoplakia. Oral Surg Oral Med Oral Pathol Oral Radiol Endod 79: 564–569

Eversole L, Miyasaki KT, Christensen RE (1993) Keratinocyste expression of calprotectin in oral inflammatory mucosal diseases. J Oral Pathol Med 22: 303–307

Grbric JT, Mitchell-Lewis DA, Fine JB, Phelan JA, Bucklan RS, Zambon JL, Lamster IB (1995) The relationship of candidiasis to linear gingival erythema in HIV-infected homosexual men and parenteral drug users. J Periodontol 66: 30–37

Green TL, Beckstead JH, Lozada-Nur F, Silverman S, Hansen LS (1984) Histopathologic spectrum of oral Kaposi's sarcoma. Oral Surg 58: 306–314

Greenspan JS, Rabanus J-P, Petersen V, Greenspan D (1989) Fine structure of EBV-infected keratinocytes in oral hairy leukoplakia. J Oral Pathol Med 18: 565–572

Holmstrup P, Westergaard J (1994) Periodontal diseases in HIV-infected patients. J Clin Periodontol 21: 270–280

Huang YQ, Li JJ, Rush MG, Poiesz BJ, Nicolaides A, Jacobson M, Zhang WG, Coutavas E, Abbott MA, Friedman-Kien AE (1992) HPV-16-related DNA sequences in Kaposi's sarcoma. Lancet 339: 515–518

Kuntz AA, Gelderblom HR, Winkel T, Reichart PA (1987) Ultrastructural findings in oral Kaposi's sarcoma (AIDS). J Oral Pathol 16: 372–379

Langford A, Pohle HD, Reichart P (1991a) Primary intraosseous AIDS-associated Kaposi's sarcoma: report of two cases with initial jaw involvement. Int J Oral Maxillofac Surg 20: 366–368

Langford A, Pohle H-D, Reichart P (1991b) Oral manifestations of AIDS-associated non-Hodgkin's lymphomas. J Oral Maxillofac Surg 20: 136–141

Lozada F, Silverman S, Migliorati CA, Conant MA, Volberding PA (1983) Oral Manifestations of tumour and opportunistic infections in the acquired immunodeficiency syndrome (AIDS): findings in 55 homosexual men with Kaposi's sarcoma. Oral Surg Oral Med Oral Pathol 56: 491–494

MacPhail L, Greenspan D, Feigal DW, Lennette ET, Greenspan JS (1991) Recurrent aphthous ulcers in association with HIV infection. Oral Surg Oral Med Oral Pathol 71: 678–683

Moniaci D, Greco D, Flecchia G, Raiteri R, Sinicco A (1990) Epidemiology, clinical features and prognostic value of HIV-1 related oral lesions. J Oral Pathol Med 19: 477–481

Nair BC, De Vico AL, Nakamura S, Copeland TD, Chen Y, Patel A, O'Neil T, Oroszlan S, Gallo RC, Sarngadharan MG (1992) Identification of major growth factor for AIDS-Kaposi's sarcoma cells as oncostatin M. Science 255: 1430–1432

Pindborg JJ, Reichart PA (1995) Atlas of diseases of the oral cavity in HIV infection, 1st edn. Munksgaard, Copenhagen

Regezi JA, Mac Phail LA, Daniels TE, Greenspan JS, Greenspan D, Dodd CL, Lozada-Nur F, Heinic GS, Chinn H, Silverman S Jr, Hansen LS (1993) Oral Kaposi's sarcoma: a 10-year retrospective histopathologic study. J Oral Pathol Med 22: 292–297

Reichart PA (1991) Oral manifestations of recently described viral infections, including AIDS. Curr Opin Dent 1: 377–383

Reichart PA (1992) Oral ulceration and iatrogenic disease in HIV infection. Oral Surg Oral Med Oral Pathol 73: 212–214

Reichart PA, Schiödt M (1989) Non-pigmented oral Kaposi's sarcoma (AIDS): report of two cases. Int J Oral Maxillofac Surg 18: 197–199

Reichart PA, Langford A, Pohle HD (1993) Epidemic oro-facial Kaposi's sarcoma (eKS) – report on 124 cases. Oral Oncol Eur J Cancer 29B: 187–189

Reichart PA, Schmidt-Westhausen A, Samaranayake LP, Philipsen HP (1994) Candida associated palatal papillary hyperplasia in HIV infection. J Oral Pathol Med 23: 403–405

Reichart PA, Philipsen HP, Schmidt-Westhausen A, Samaranayake LP (1995) Pseudo-membranous oral candidiasis in HIV infection: ultrastructural findings. J Oral Pathol Med 24: 276–281

Riley C, London JP, Burmeister JA (1992) Periodontal health in 200 HIV seropositive patiens. J Oral Pathol Med 21: 124–127

Roeder L, Flaitz C, Jacob L, Nichols M, Hicks J (1995) Association of oral candidiasis with xerostomia-inducing medications and dentinal caries in HIV infection. J Dent Res 74: 137

Samaranayake LP (1992) Oral mycoses in human immunodeficiency virus infection: a review. Oral Surg Oral Med Oral Pathol 73: 171–180

Samaranayake LP, Holmstrup P (1989) Oral candidiasis and human immunodeficiency virus infection. J Oral Pathol Med 18: 554–564

Schiödt M (1992) HIV-associated salivary gland disease: a review. Oral Surg Oral Med Oral Pathol 73: 164–167

Schulten EAJM, Snijders PJF, Walboomers JMA, Snijders PJF, ten Kate RW, Mullink H, Walboomers JMM, Meijer CJLM, van der Waal I (1991) Oral hairy leukoplakia in HIV infection: a diagnostic pitfall. Oral Surg Oral Med Oral Pathol 71: 32–37

Syrjänen S (1995) Human papilloma viruses (HPV) and oral health and disease. In: Millard HD, Mason DK (eds) 2nd world workshop on oral medicine. University of Michigan, Ann Arbor, Michigan, pp 83–89

Tabata M, Langford A, Becker J, Reichart PA (1993) Distribution of immunocompetent cells in oral Kaposi's sarcoma (AIDS). Oral Oncol Eur J Cancer 3: 209–213

Zambon JJ, Reynolds HS, Genco RJ (1990) Studies of the subgingival microflora in patients with acquired immunodeficiency syndrome. J Periodontol 61: 699–704

Zhang X, Langford A, Gelderblom H, Reichart P (1988) Zur Ultrastruktur der Haarleukoplakie. Dtsch Z Mund Kiefer Gesichts Chir 12: 460–465

Zhang X, Langford A, Gelderblom H, Reichart P (1989) Ultrastuctural findings in clinically uninvolved oral mucosa of patients with HIV infection. J Oral Pathol Med 18: 35–41

Extranodal Non-Hodgkin's Lymphomas of the Oral Cavity

R.C.K. Jordan and P.M. Speight

1 Introduction

Lymphomas are malignant neoplasms of component cells of lymphoid tissues. A broad division of the group into Hodgkin's disease and non-Hodgkin's lymphoma (NHL) is widely accepted. Hodgkin's disease is primarily a nodal disease characterised by the presence of Reed-Sternberg cells and a lymphoid stroma composed of large numbers of non-neoplastic cells (BONADONNA et al. 1989). The condition rarely affects extranodal sites and will not be discussed here.

NHL comprise a heterogeneous group of lymphoid neoplasms with a spectrum of behaviour ranging from relatively indolent to highly aggressive and potentially fatal (SALHANY and PIETRA 1993). The classification of this diverse group of diseases has been based on the study of lymphomas arising in lymph nodes. Moreover, the biology and natural history has in large part been based upon the study of nodal disease, and only recently has more attention been directed at lymphomas arising at extranodal sites. Up to 40% of all NHL arise at extranodal sites, and the most common location is the gastro-intestinal tract. In the West, they most commonly occur in the stomach, but in the Middle East the intestine is the most common location. The head and neck is the second most common site for extranodal NHL, with the majority of cases arising in Waldeyer's ring, a band of lymphoid tissue which encircles the oropharynx.

Similar to lymphomas arising in lymph nodes, B cell lymphomas are the most common phenotype at extranodal sites (REGEZI et al. 1991). A spectrum of B cell lymphomas occurs in the head and neck with a wide range of biological behaviour.

Current Topics in Pathology
Volume 90, G. Seifert (Ed.)
© Springer-Verlag Berlin Heidelberg 1996

Although most are diffuse, large cell lymphomas, other types are seen in specific sites and populations of patients. These include Burkitt's lymphoma (BL), which occur in the facial bones of young patients, and T cell lymphomas, which occur in the nasofacial region, producing the clinical condition termed "midline lethal granuloma" (Ratech et al. 1989). Within the salivary glands, most lymphomas arise within lymph nodes embedded in the salivary tissues (Gleeson et al. 1986) and have clinical and histological features similar to lymphomas arising in lymph nodes at other sites. Lymphomas may also arise within the salivary gland parenchyma and resemble those arising in mucosa-associated lymphoid tissues (MALT) (Isaacson 1992). This group of tumours is genotypically and phenotypically unique and is characterised by a relatively long natural history. Others such as plasmacytoma and BL show a striking predilection for primary osseous involvement.

The clinical presentation of lymphomas of the oral regions varies with their site of origin and tumour type, but most patients present with a swelling or ulcerated mass which can bear striking resemblance to the most common oral malignancy, squamous cell carcinoma (Howell et al. 1987). Pain or dysphagia is the next most common symptom, but systemic manifestations are rare (McGurk et al. 1985) The characterisation of specific lymphoma types is important, because staging procedures and therapy may differ for each type. The only reliable method to distinguish and characterise these lesions is by biopsy coupled with immunological studies of biopsy tissue (Rooney and Ramsay 1994).

This chapter will review a number of extranodal NHL which occur in the oral cavity, including specific subtypes that affect Waldeyer's ring, salivary gland and the nasofacial region.

2 Classification

The classification of lymphoid neoplasms continues to be a source of controversy. At least eight classifications have been proposed over the past 30 years, but none have gained universal acceptance (Stein 1995). Currently, only two classifications are widely used, the Kiel system in Europe and the Working Formulation for Clinical Usage in North America (Rosenberg 1994).

The basis for many systems has been the morphological and immunological resemblance of lymphoma cells to their non-neoplastic lymphocyte counterparts. Lukes and Collins (1977) proposed a classification scheme based on B or T cell lineage of the neoplastic lymphocytes. A similar system based on functional lineage was proposed by Lennert (Lennert et al. 1975; Lennert and Feller 1990; Table 1) and further divides lymphomas into groups based on clinical behaviour.

A number of other classifications have flourished based on varying contributions of cell morphology, immunology and clinical behaviour. The Working Formulation is based on the placement of lymphomas into prognostic groups based

Table 1. Updated Kiel classification for lymphomas (STANSFELD et al. 1988; LENNERT and FELLER 1990)

B cell lymphomas	T cell lymphomas
Low grade	**Low grade**
Lymphocytic	Lymphocytic
Chronic lymphocytic leukaemia	Chronic lymphocytic leukaemia
Prolymphocytic leukaemia	Prolymphocytic leukaemia
Hairy cell leukaemia	Small, cerebriform
Lymphoplasmacytic/cytoid (LP	Mycosis fungoides, Sézary syndrome
immunocytoma	Lympho-epithelioid (Lennert's lymphoma
Plasmacytic	immunocytoma)
Centroblastic/centrocytic	Angio-immunoblastic (angioimmunoblastic
follicular ± diffuse, diffuse	lymphadenopathy, lymphogranulomatosis X)
Centrocytic	T zone lymphoma
	Pleomorphic, small cell (HTLV-1+ or HTLV-1-)
High grade	**High grade**
Centroblastic	Pleomorphic, medium-sized and large cell
Immunoblastic	(HTLV-1+ or HTLV-1-)
Large cell anaplastic (Ki-1+)	Immunoblastic (HTLV-1+ or HTLV-1-)
Burkitt's lymphoma	Large cell anaplastic (Ki-1+)
Lymphoblastic	Lymphoblastic
Rare types	**Rare types**

HTLV, human T lymphotrophic virus.

on morphological patterns of the tumour and the cytology of neoplastic cells. Although originally designed as a mechanism to translate between differing lymphoma classifications, the Working Formulation is now used as the primary classification system in many North American institutions. Since its introduction, it has been criticised for its poor immunological basis, its grouping together of heterogenous diseases and its omission of a number of important subtypes of lymphoma (ROSENBERG et al. 1982).

Most classifications of lymphomas have been based mainly on lesions arising within lymph nodes. Their application to extranodal lymphomas has been more problematic, since a number of entities which arise in these sites do not have obvious nodal counterparts and have not found their place in current schemes. The newest system for lymphoma classification, the Revised European American Lymphoma (REAL) scheme, proposed by the International Lymphoma Study Group, has attempted to remedy this situation (CHAN et al. 1994; HARRIS et al. 1994). This scheme divides lymphomas into T and B cell groups and includes a number of entities which arise at extranodal sites. However, it has received some criticism for its lack of clinical correlation and strong reliance on immunophenotyping to classify the conditions (ROSENBERG 1994; LENNERT 1995). Although it includes a number of newer lymphoma types, it remains to be seen whether this classification will gain universal acceptance.

3 Staging

The importance of proper staging for patients with lymphoma in the oral region cannot be overemphasised. Staging serves a number of important purposes, including the determination of the type and extent of therapy, the overall prognosis for the patient and the potential complications associated with the disease (Bonadonna et al. 1989).

The Ann Arbor method, although initially designed to stage Hodgkin's disease, is now widely used for NHL. Patients are generally assigned a stage between I and IV, depending on the site and extent of their tumour (Table 2). In addition, they are classified as having A- or B-type symptoms, depending on the presence of constitutional symptoms associated with the tumour (Bonadonna et al. 1989).

The staging procedure often differs for the type and site of lymphoma within the head and neck region. Gastro-intestinal assessment is performed for lymphomas of Waldeyer's ring, since these tumours are often accompanied by gastro-intestinal involvement. Lymphomas of MALT tend to remain localised for prolonged periods and have a relatively indolent clinical course hence less extensive investigation is often required. Assessment of the central nervous system (CNS) is performed for lymphomas of the nose and paranasal sinuses and for lymphoblastic lymphoma and undifferentiated types. Bone marrow biopsy is generally performed for all extranodal lymphomas of the head and neck, but staging laparotomy is rarely undertaken, since the yield is low (Cobleigh and Kennedy 1986).

4 B Cell Lymphomas

4.1 Lymphomas of the Salivary Gland
Including Mucosa-Associated Lymphoid Tissue

The incidence of lymphomas arising in salivary glands is controversial, since most lymphomas arise in lymph nodes embedded within the salivary tissues, whilst

Table 2. Ann Arbor staging system for non-Hodgkin's lymphoma

Stage	Definition
I	Involvement of single lymph node region or of a single extranodal organ or site (I_E)
II	Involvement of two or more lymph node regions on the same side of the diaphragm, or localised involvement of an extranodal site or organ (II_E) and one or more lymph node regions on the same side of the diaphragm
III	Involvement of lymph node regions on both sides of the diaphragm, which may also be accompanied by localised involvement of an extranodal organ or site (III_E) or spleen (III_S) or both (III_{SE})
IV	Diffuse or disseminated involvement of one or more distant extranodal organ with or without associated lymph node involvement

others arise within the salivary gland parenchyma (GLEESON et al. 1986). The former group are similar to lymphomas arising within lymph nodes at other sites and will not be discussed here. It is increasingly being shown that lymphomas which arise in salivary gland parenchyma resemble those which develop in MALT. This term defines a group of unencapsulated lymphoid tissues adapted to protect mucosae exposed to the external environment (ISAACSON and WRIGHT 1983). The best characterised MALT is in the gastro-intestinal tract represented by Peyer's patches. In contrast to lymph nodes, where antigens are exposed to lymphoid tissue via the afferent lymphatics, in MALT antigens access B cells across an epithelial surface. Antigen stimulation of B cells results in the formation of immunoglobulin A (IgA) blast cells, which leave Peyer's patches through efferent lymphatics. These cells freely circulate and then return to the MALT as memory B cells or plasma cells through a poorly understood homing mechanism (PALS et al. 1989).

ISAACSON and WRIGHT (1983) were the first to describe a low-grade B cell lymphoma of the gastro-intestinal tract which recapitulated the features of MALT. These features were later described in a number of lymphomas arising in other sites, including the thyroid (ISAACSON and WRIGHT 1984), thymus (TAKAGI et al. 1992), salivary gland (HYJEK et al. 1988), conjunctiva (WOTHERSPOON et al. 1993), Waldeyer's ring (PAULSEN and LENNERT 1994), kidney (PARVEEN et al. 1993) and lung (LI et al. 1990).

One of the difficulties with the MALT lymphoma concept is that most do not arise at sites where MALT is most abundant, specifically Peyer's patches. Lymphomas of MALT tend to arise most commonly in the stomach, a site usually lacking lymphoid tissues. Furthermore, many cases of MALT lymphomas in the stomach arise in the setting of *Helicobacter pylori*-associated chronic gastritis. This bacteria can be identified in almost all cases of gastric lymphomas of MALT. It was thus proposed that these lymphomas arise in acquired MALT, including *H. pylori* gastritis and autoimmune diseases such as Hashimoto's thyroiditis and Sjögren's syndrome (SS). The prerequisite for the development of acquired MALT is reactive, chronic inflammation at a mucosal site (ISAACSON 1990). The development of MALT lymphoma in the major salivary glands is preceded by a salivary lympho-epithelial lesion (SLEL) (HYJEK et al. 1988; JORDAN and SPEIGHT 1996). This lesion usually arises in association with SS, although it may be seen in other auto-immune disorders and may occasionally may arise de novo. The risk of lymphoma development in SS is high, estimated to be 44 times that of the general population (KASSAN et al. 1978).

The clinical presentation of MALT lymphomas differs from other low-grade B cell lymphomas and resembles a chronic inflammatory process rather than a neoplasm (ISAACSON 1992). In contrast to nodal B cell lymphomas, they tend to remain localised for long periods and are late to disseminate. When spread does occur, it is usually to local lymph nodes, with dissemination to bone marrow being an uncommon and late event. Moreover, their clinical course is relatively indolent, and they generally respond to local measures such as surgical excision (ISAACSON 1992). This is in contrast to other low-grade B cell lymphomas, which are essentially incurable. Evolution of low-grade lymphomas of MALT to a high-grade lymphoma is well recognised, but although the prognosis is less favourable, it is still better than for other high-grade B cell lymphomas (BATEMAN and WRIGHT 1993).

All low-grade lymphomas of MALT show similar histopathological features, irrespective of their site. The tumour is composed of a monotonous population of small to medium-sized lymphocytes which often have irregular nuclei and resemble centrocytes. Although these have been termed centrocyte-like cells (CCL cells), they can show a spectrum of morphology from resembling lymphocytes to monocytoid (ISAACSON and NORTON 1994; Fig. 1). In the salivary glands, lesions develop in salivary lympho-epithelial lesions (Fig. 2) and show "proliferation areas" of CCL cells, which typically invade and destroy the epithelium to form lympho-epithelial lesions which can be few or extensive (Fig. 3; BATEMAN and WRIGHT 1993). Monotypia can often be identified in these proliferation areas, ' which are considered to represent malignant lymphoma even in the absence of lymph node involvement (SCHMID et al. 1982). A large proportion of tumour cells may show plasmacytoid morphology, which in some cases can be so extensive as to resemble a plasmacytoma (WRIGHT 1994; Fig. 1b). The tumour cells begin in the marginal zone of MALT and gradually expand around reactive lymphoid follicles. With time, the neoplastic CCL cells may infiltrate reactive follicles in one of three patterns termed follicular colonisation (ISAACSON et al. 1991). Occasionally, this can give the tumours a vague nodularity, which can lead to a misdiagnosis of a follicular lymphoma (WRIGHT 1994).

The B cells of MALT lymphomas phenotypically express surface and cytoplasmic immunoglobulins, usually IgM, and show light-chain restriction. They usually express CD35 and CD21, but are CD10, CD23 and CD5 negative (ISAACSON 1993). The lack of CD5 is useful in differentiating the condition from mantle cell lymphomas, which invariably express this marker (ISAACSON 1992). Like follicle centre cell lymphomas, low-grade MALT lymphomas express the bcl-2 protein, but they consistently lack the chromosome translocation t(14;18) (WOTHERSPOON et al. 1990; DISS et al. 1995; JORDAN et al. 1995).

The term extranodal marginal zone B cell lymphoma has recently been proposed by the International Lymphoma Study Group as a pathologically more accurate designation for this group of lymphoid neoplasms (CHAN et al. 1994). Although it would appear that this better reflects the cell of origin of these tumours, for the time being the term MALT lymphoma is still more widely recognised and will continue to be used here.

A recently described condition termed monocytoid B cell lymphoma (MCBL) shares many similarities with lymphomas of MALT (ORTIZ-HIDALGO and WRIGHT 1992). MCBL occurs predominantly in lymph nodes, but a proportion has also been reported at extranodal sites, sometimes in association with SS (NGAN et al. 1991). When they occur at extranodal sites, they are indistinguishable from lymphomas of MALT (ORTIZ-HIDALGO and WRIGHT 1992). It is now thought that MCBL is a nodal, marginal zone lymphoma (CHAN et al. 1994) and represents the nodal equivalent of lymphomas of MALT. In many cases, a subclinical MALT lymphoma can be demonstrated at an adjacent mucosal or glandular site, such as the stomach or a salivary gland, suggesting that in some cases nodal MCBL may represent a secondary MALT lymphoma (NIZZE et al. 1991).

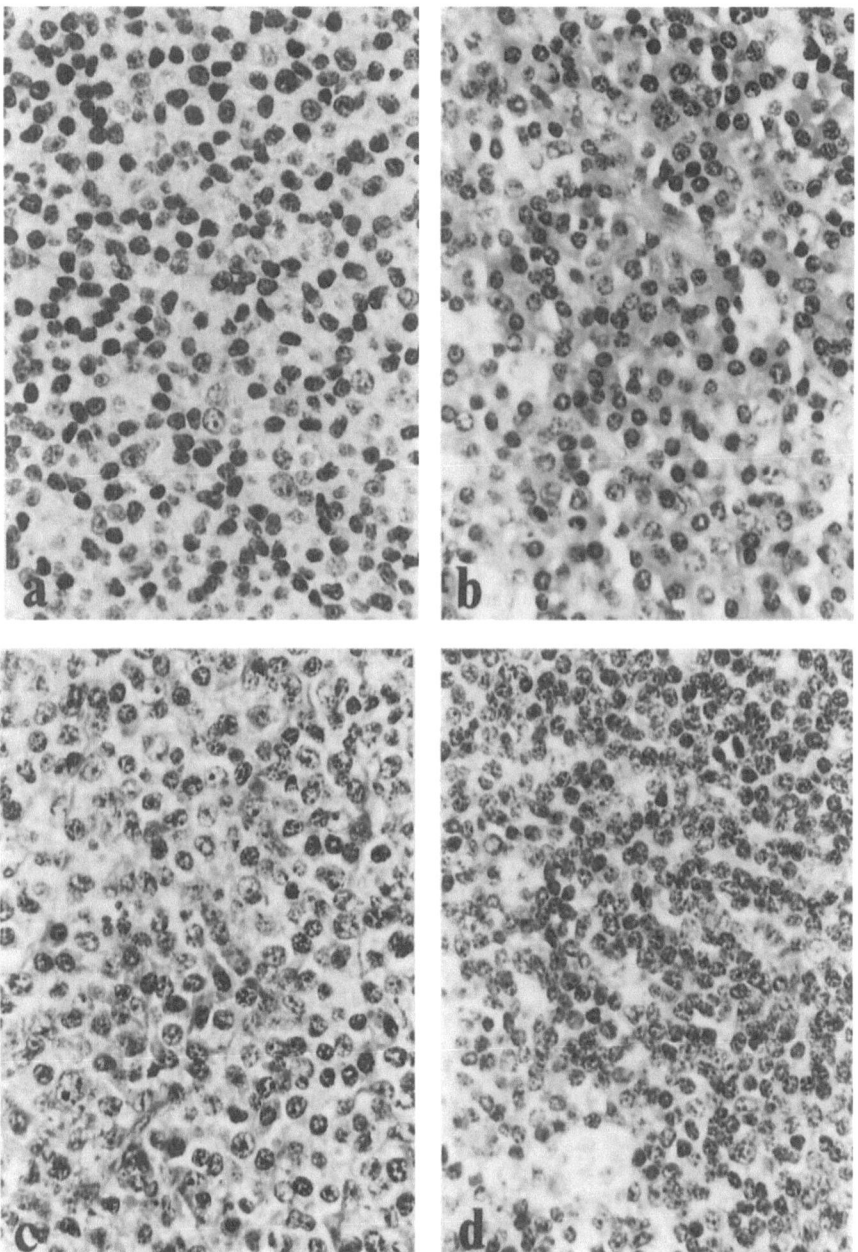

Fig. 1a–d. Cellular details from different mucosa-associated lymphoid tissue (MALT) lymphomas affecting the salivary glands, showing the variable morphology of the centrocyte-like cells. **a** The cells are quite small with irregular nuclei and resemble centrocytes. **b** Many cells show plasmacytoid differentiation. **c** Cells have abundant clear cytoplasm and resemble monocytoid B cells. **d** The cells resemble small lymphocytes. H&E, ×240

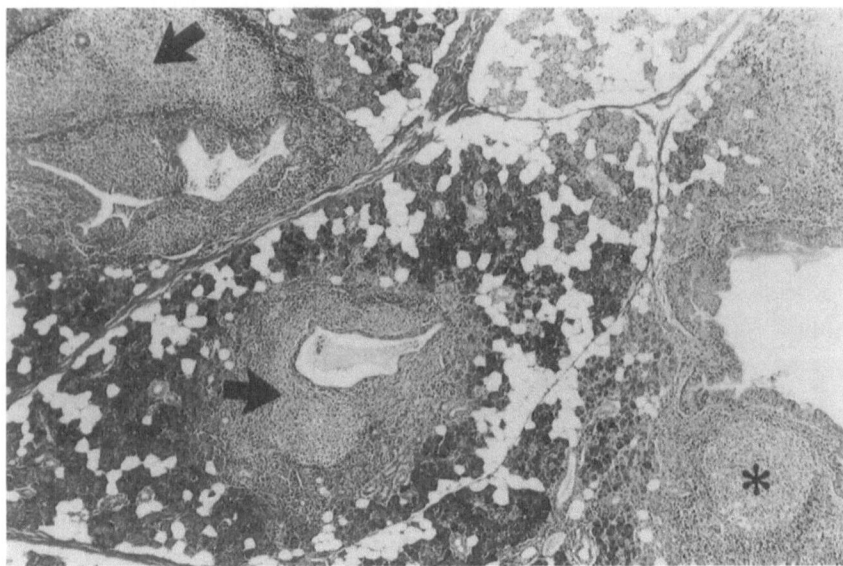

Fig. 2. An early mucosa-associated lymphoid tissue (MALT) lymphoma in a salivary lympho-epithelial lesion. Infiltrates of lymphocytes surround dilated ducts and islands of epithelium. In places follicle centres are seen (*asterisk*) adjacent to a duct, producing the typical MALT appearance. Elsewhere there are proliferation areas of clear centrocyte-like (CCL) cells. Those indicated (*arrows*) showed kappa light chain restriction on immunocytochemistry. H&E, ×15

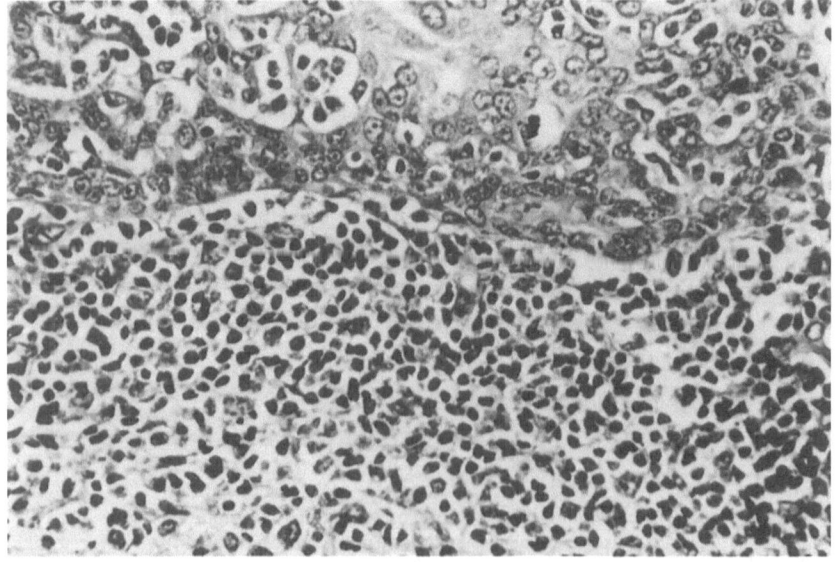

Fig. 3. A low-grade mucosa-associated lymphoid tissue (MALT) lymphoma from the parotid gland. Sheets of centrocyte-like cells have infiltrated and disrupted an island of proliferating epithelium to form a typical lympho-epithelial lesion. H&E, ×210

4.2 Lymphomas of Waldeyer's Ring

Waldeyer's ring is a band of lymphoid tissue which encircles the entrance of the aerodigestive tract and includes lymphoid tissues of the tonsils, nasopharynx and base of tongue. These tissues may represent a functional component of MALT, since they act as an interface between the systemic lymphoid tissues and the gut (WRIGHT 1994). Furthermore, studies have shown a morphological similarity between lymphoid tissues of Waldeyer's ring and those at other MALT sites, including a lack of sinusoids, a marginal zone of B lymphocytes and antigen presentation across an epithelial surface (MENARGUEZ et al. 1994). Although Waldeyer's ring shares many anatomical and functional similarities with MALT, the lymphomas arising at this site are more typical of lymphomas arising in lymph nodes (ISAACSON and NORTON 1994). The majority are centroblastic and centroblastic/centrocytic lymphomas.

However, Waldeyer's ring is still the second most common site for extranodal lymphomas after the gastro-intestinal tract. Most arise within the palatine tonsil, followed by the nasopharynx and then the base of tongue and soft palate (ECONOMOPOULOS et al. 1992). Multiple sites within Waldeyer's ring may be involved in about 4% of cases.

A total of 85% of lymphomas in Waldeyer's ring are high-grade B cell lymphomas, followed in order of frequency by extramedullary plasmacytoma and T cell lymphomas, including lympho-epithelioid lymphoma (Lennert's lymphoma) (BURKE and BUTLER 1992; ISAACSON and NORTON 1994; MENARGUEZ et al. 1994).

Histologically, high-grade lymphomas consist of cohesive sheets of pleomorphic lymphocytes and immunoblasts (Fig. 4) with a high rate of apoptosis and areas of necrosis. Only a minority of lymphomas at this site have been described as resembling lymphomas of MALT. PAULSEN and LENNERT (1994) reported that 12 of 329 lymphomas of Waldeyer's ring in their series were low-grade MALT lymphomas which predominantly affected the palatine tonsils. Histologically, two cases also contained high-grade elements. MENARGUEZ et al. (1994) reported only one MALT lymphoma in a series of 79 lymphomas of Waldeyer's ring. Three MCBL were also identified in this series, although they may now be classified as lymphoma of MALT.

The clinical and genotypic features of some high-grade lymphomas of Waldeyer's ring, including a good overall prognosis, epitheliotropism and lower bcl-2 protein expression, suggest that some of these tumours may represent high-grade MALT lymphomas. The diagnosis of a high-grade MALT lymphoma, however, requires the identification of low-grade areas within the same biopsy specimen. This can occasionally be difficult in small specimens, and it is not clear whether all series have been able to address this issue in all cases. It remains to be determined whether MALT lymphomas represent a larger proportion of lymphomas in Waldeyer's ring than has been previously reported.

Clinical staging is particularly important for lymphoma arising in Waldeyer's ring both from a therapeutic and prognostic standpoint. Lymphomas in this region are frequently associated with gastro-intestinal involvement, and a thorough

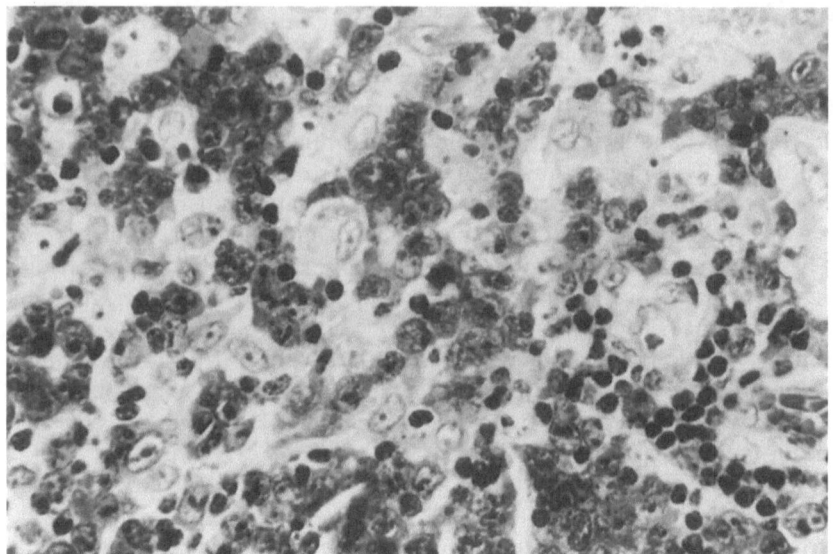

Fig. 4. High-grade B cell lymphoma. The tumour is composed of sheets of pleomorphic lymphocytes with many large immunoblasts. H&E, ×335

work-up will often result in upstaging of the patient's disease (Morton et al. 1992).

4.3 Burkitt's Lymphoma

BL is a high-grade B cell lymphoma which primarily affects children and adolescents (Burkitt 1958). Two forms of the disease are recognised, an endemic type in tropical climates where malarial infection is also common and a sporadic form occurring in North America and Europe (Patton et al. 1990). Involvement of the jaws is particularly common in endemic BL, with up to 50% of those affected having lesions of the maxilla or mandible. Multiple intra-oral sites can also be infiltrated simultaneously in up to one quarter of cases, and in up to one sixth of cases all four quadrants are affected simultaneously. Jaw lesions in sporadic BL are considerably less common than in the endemic form and occur in less than 6% of cases (Burkitt 1966). The small intestine and retroperitoneum are the most commonly affected sites in sporadic BL. A significant proportion of patients with BL will have bone marrow involvement at presentation, but leukaemic manifestations are rare (Minerbrook et al. 1982).

The Epstein-Barr virus (EBV), a member of the herpes group of DNA viruses, has been identified in a large proportion of endemic BL. Only 10%–20% of cases of sporadic BL are associated with EBV infection (Anderrson et al. 1976). The EBV genome is not integrated in BL, but persists in a circular, episomal state. Expression of EBV antigens is limited to EBV nuclear antigen (EBNA)-1, principally related to restricted promoter usage by the virus (SHAEFER et al. 1991).

Specific chromosome translations have been associated with BL. The translocation t(8;14) can be identified in up to three quarters of cases, juxtaposing the c-*myc* oncogene with the immunoglobulin heavy chain gene. Two other translocations have been described less frequently, but both involve translocation of the c-*myc* oncogene with either the kappa or the lambda immunoglobulin light chain gene. The translocation insertion sites differ in the endemic and sporadic forms of BL and are likely related to differences in B cell ontogeny in each form (PELICCI et al. 1986).

Microscopically, both forms of the disease show similar features, consisting of monomorphic sheets of densely packed, medium-sized neoplastic blast cells. The cytoplasm of the cells is deeply basophilic and often forms acute angles with neighbouring cells in well-fixed sections. The tumour has a very high mitotic rate, often with more than ten mitoses per high-power field, and it infiltrates widely through bone, occasionally involving the teeth (Fig. 5). Numerous macrophages containing cellular debris give the classical "starry sky" appearance to the tumour. Immunohistochemistry shows reactivity for many B cell markers, including CD19, CD20, CD22 and CD37. Over 90% of endemic BL express CD10, in contrast to variable expression in the sporadic type. Endemic BL does not express CD23, but expression can be identified in up to 50% of the sporadic form (ISAACSON and NORTON 1994).

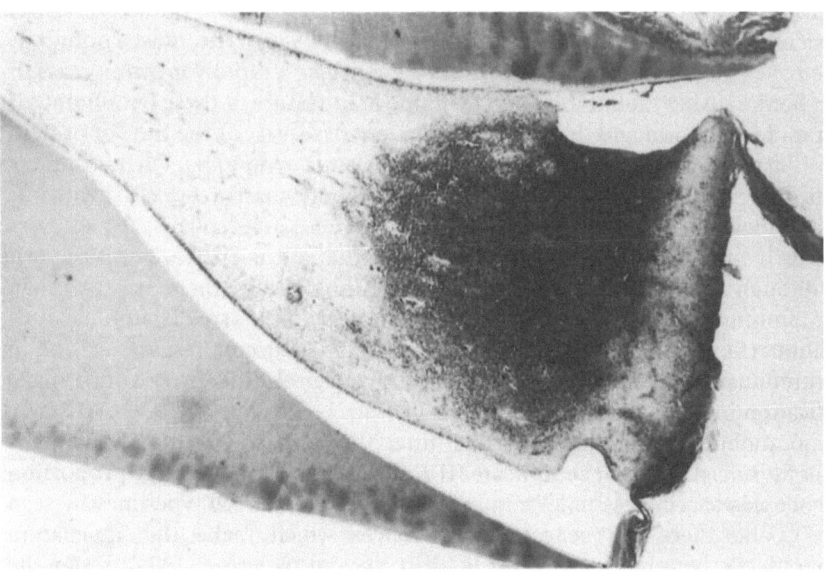

Fig. 5. This Burkitt's lymphoma in the jaw of a 6-year-old child has infiltrated into the pulp chamber of a partially formed incisor tooth. H&E, ×15

The tumour is particularly chemosensitive, with treatment often resulting in massive tumour lysis. Cure rates range from 54% to 59%, with relapses rare after 2 years (Ziegler 1981).

4.4 Lymphomas Associated with Human Immunodeficiency Virus Infection

The development of NHL has long been recognised as a rare complication of many congenital immunodeficiency states. The increase in organ transplantation coupled with immunosuppression techniques has also witnessed a marked increase in the development of many lymphoproliferative disorders. The development of lymphoma in the setting of the human immunodeficiency virus (HIV) is now seen as an important complication of acquired immunodeficiency.

NHL constitutes an AIDS-defining diagnosis in 3% of all patients (Serraino et al. 1992). It is a relatively late complication of HIV infection, with some lymphomas, particularly immunoblastic lymphoproliferations, occurring primarily when there is a marked depression of CD4-positive T cells (Levine 1992). All groups at risk for HIV infection are at risk of developing lymphoma, although some differences exist in the clinical and pathological features of individual risk groups (Serraino et al. 1992).

In contrast to lymphomas complicating other immunodeficiency states, up to 75% of those arising in HIV infection are extranodal and almost one fifth occur in the CNS (Carbone et al. 1995). Sites of involvement are relatively distinct in AIDS-related lymphomas and include the CNS, ano-rectal region and the oral cavity (Ioachim 1992). NHL account for 3% of all malignant tumours of the oral cavity in patients with HIV infection (Silverman et al. 1986). The most commonly affected sites include the tonsillar region or gingiva as a rapidly growing mass or within bone causing tooth mobility. One important feature of these lymphomas is their rapid infiltration and the widespread extent of disease at the time of presentation (Fig. 6) and the common presence of systemic symptoms. Furthermore, a large proportion of patients will develop CNS and bone marrow spread during the course of their disease (Ioachim 1992).

Most lymphomas complicating acquired immunodeficiency are of B cell origin, although T cell lymphomas also occur. Pathologically, there are two main types, immunoblastic lymphoma and Burkitt's-like (small non-cleaved) lymphoma (Levine 1992). Although both resemble their counterparts arising in non-immunosuppressed subjects, there are histological differences which make classification into conventional schemes difficult.

Immunoblastic lymphomas constitute the largest group of lymphoproliferative disorders that complicate HIV infection. Although a large proportion of the neoplastic cells resemble immunoblasts, many other cell types may be seen (Fig. 7), and there are genotypic differences which make the appellation immunoblastic lymphoma difficult. Isaacscon and Norton (1994) prefer the term polymorphous immunoblastic lymphoproliferation. This more accurately reflects the spectrum of pathology seen in these lesions, which includes a mixed

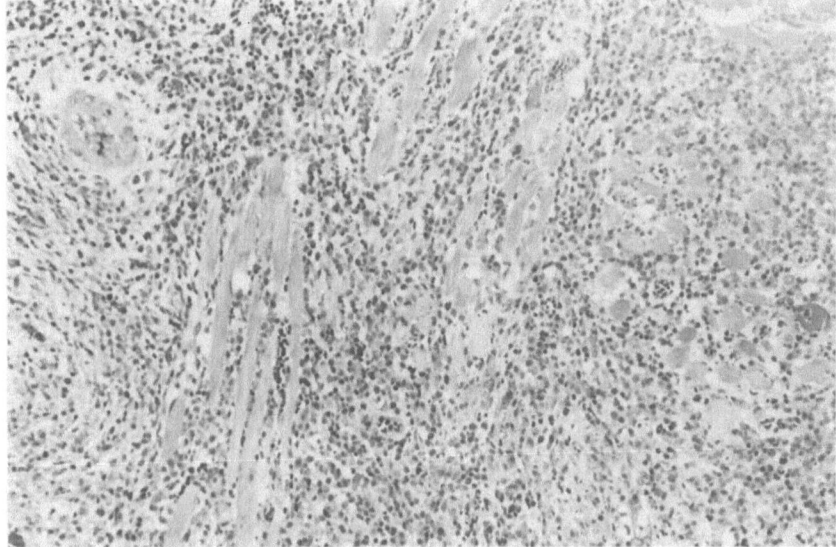

Fig. 6. High-grade B cell lymphoma associated with acquired immunodeficiency syndrome (AIDS). Pleomorphic immunoblasts and lymphocytes have infiltrated deeply into the muscle of the tongue. H&E, ×85

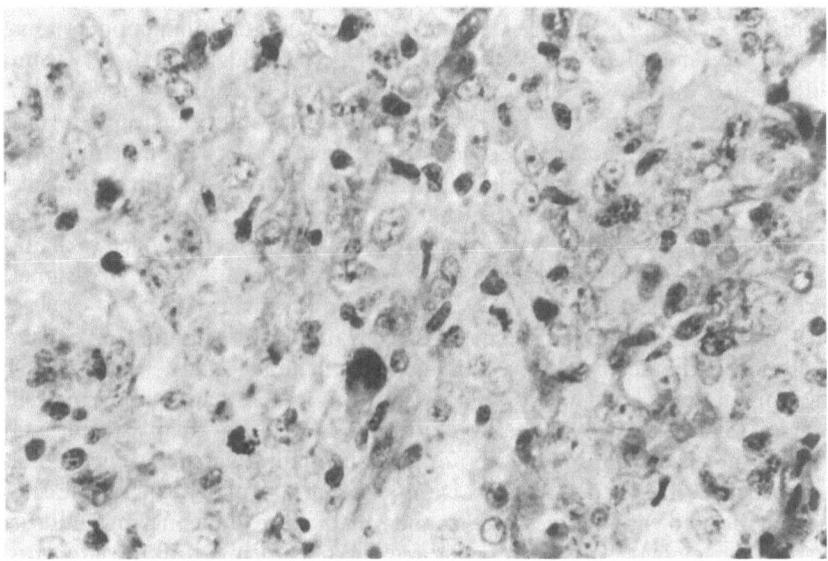

Fig. 7. A lymphoma of the gingiva associated with acquired immunodeficiency syndrome (AIDS). The tumour is composed primarily of pleomorphic immunoblasts with a high mitotic rate. Smaller lymphocytes, including inflammatory cells, are also seen. H&E, ×335

infiltrate of inflammatory cells with large pleomorphic immunoblasts, resembling florid infectious mononucleosis, and lesions with a predominance of centrocytes. Occasionally, more typical high-grade lymphomas, usually immunoblastic or anaplastic large cell lymphomas, may arise; these are rarely of T cell origin.

The other predominant lymphoproliferation to complicate HIV infection is a Burkitt's-like (small non-cleaved) lymphoma. Again, although these tumours bear a superficial resemblance to BL in non-immunosuppressed subjects, important histological differences also exist, including a greater degree of cellular pleomorphism and a high proportion of plasmacytic differentiation (ISAACSON and NORTON 1994).

The prognosis for lymphomas arising in HIV infection is generally very poor. The advanced stage at presentation, the aggressive behaviour of both low- and high-grade forms and the profound immunosuppression contribute to a poor outcome. The median survival for all patients with AIDS-associated lymphoma is 6.5 months (IRWIN and KAPLAN 1993).

4.5 Plasma Cell Tumours

The plasma cell dyscrasias include a number of diseases characterised by an expansion of a clone of immunoglobulin-secreting cells. These diseases are often characterised by the presence of immunoglobulin protein components in the serum or urine, termed M proteins. The spectrum of plasma cell dyscrasia includes multiple myeloma, solitary plasmacytoma of bone and extramedullary plasmacytoma. The biological behaviour of these conditions varies widely, although histologically all plasma cell tumours are similar and contain monotonous sheets of cells resembling plasma cells (Fig. 8). The cell population may vary from well-differentiated cells with an eccentric nucleus and basophilic cytoplasm to less-differentiated, atypical cells with occasional giant or multi-nucleated forms. Immunoblasts and plasmablasts are not seen, and there are very few inflammatory cells intermixed with the monotonous sheets of neoplastic plasma cells (WILTSHAW 1976). Immunohistochemical tests will show restriction of either kappa or lambda light chain and the presence of only one isotype of heavy chain, usually IgA or IgG (LENNERT and FELLER 1990; WAX et al. 1993). Occasional lesions contain extensive deposits of amyloid in the affected tissues.

The most common and important plasma cell dyscrasia is multiple myeloma. The condition is characterised by multiple osteolytic bone lesions, serum or urinary M proteins and a bone marrow biopsy showing greater than 10% plasma cell composition. Symptoms are related to infiltration of organs by neoplastic plasma cells and by the excessive production of immunoglobulins which have abnormal biochemical properties. Pathological fractures occur in 20% of patients. Advancing disease is associated with hypercalcaemia and renal failure. Bone marrow infiltration leads to anaemia, thrombocytopenia and leukocytopenia, with the latter resulting in an increased susceptibility to infection. Jaw lesions can be identified in 30% of cases of multiple myeloma and radiographically appear as non-corticated radiolucencies, more common in the mandible than maxilla. The posterior por-

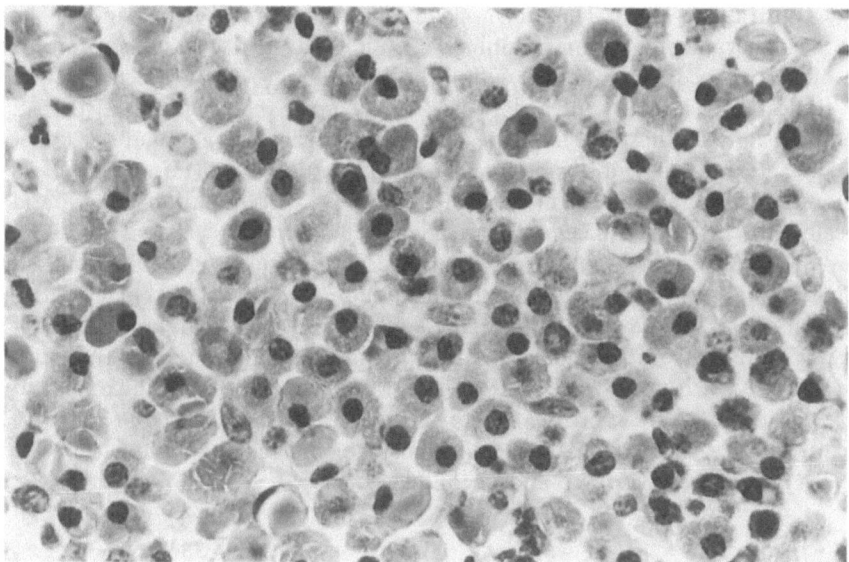

Fig. 8. A plasmacytoma from the gingiva. The tumour is composed of sheets of well-differentiated, although slightly atypical plasma cells. H&E, ×335

tions of the jaw are more commonly affected, as the marrow spaces are larger (BRUCE and ROYER 1953). The formation of amyloid from the aggregation of immunoglobulin light chain proteins is a common sequela of multiple myeloma and, when deposited in the tongue, can produce macroglossia (REINISH et al. 1994). Treatment of multiple myeloma is directed at reducing tumour burden and reversing complications of the disease, such as those related to renal failure. Single alkylating agent chemotherapy is the treatment of choice (ALEXANIAN and DIMOPOULOS 1994).

A solitary focus of lytic bone destruction showing a plasma cell tumour without bone marrow involvement is termed solitary plasmacytoma of bone. Detection of M proteins in the serum or urine does not exclude the diagnosis of solitary plasmacytoma of bone. This lesion comprises 3% of all plasma cell neoplasms and is believed to represent a localised form of myeloma (BATSAKIS 1983). Involvement of the facial bones is rare and, when present, typically represents more disseminated disease. Progression to myeloma occurs in many patients, with almost one half having done so by 2 years, although long-term survival is also common (CORWIN and LINDBERG 1979). Solitary lesions are typically treated with radiation therapy supplemented by chemotherapy (ABEMAYOR et al. 1988). When the disease is disseminated, it is treated in the same manner as multiple myeloma.

Isolated plasma cell tumours within soft tissues are termed extramedullary plasmacytoma. This does not include tumours that have arisen in bone and involved soft tissues secondarily, following perforation of the bone cortex. Over 80% of all extramedullary plasmacytomas arise in the upper respiratory tract and oral cavity (Wiltshaw 1976). They form 4% of all non-epithelial neoplasms of the nose, nasopharynx and paranasal sinuses (Fu and Perzin 1979) and account for 20% of all extranodal lymphomas within the oral cavity (Handlers et al. 1986). The clinical appearance is of a dark-red, fleshy mass that is rarely ulcerated. Multiple lesions at other sites in the head and neck may be present in up to 20% of patients, and regional lymph nodes may be involved in up to 40%. Unlike multiple myeloma and solitary plasmacytoma of bone, wide dissemination is rare and typically shows no preference for active haematopoietic sites (Wiltshaw 1976). Many investigators have reported that the progression of extramedullary plasmacytoma to myeloma is distinctly uncommon, in contrast to the behaviour of solitary plasmacytoma of bone. One group has suggested, however, that progression to myeloma is equally frequent in both these tumours and that both represent a spectrum of the same disease (Meis et al. 1987). Outcome and treatment options are not related to histological features of the tumour. Extramedullary plasmacytomas are radiosensitive, and regional control rates of 80% can be achieved (Corwin and Lindberg 1979).

5 Nasofacial T cell Lymphoma

Progressive, ulcerative destruction of the palate, nose and paranasal structures has long been recognised as a striking and potentially fatal condition. Stewart (1933) introduced the term mid-line lethal granuloma to describe the condition, but a number of other terms have been suggested, including polymorphous reticulosis, lymphomatoid granulomatosis, idiopathic destructive disease and mid-line malignant reticulosis (Ramsay and Rooney 1993). A number of diseases can produce destruction of mid-line facial structures, including Wegener's granulomatosis, infectious agents and lymphoma (Harrison 1987), but it is now recognised that the majority of cases previously described as mid-line lethal granuloma represent a lymphoproliferative disorder, commonly a T cell lymphoma (Ratech et al. 1989). The term nasofacial lymphoma will be used here to describe the heterogeneous group of lymphoproliferative diseases that affect and destroy the mid-line palate, nose and paranasal structures (Ramsay and Rooney 1993).

Nasofacial lymphoma is typically a disease of adults. Nasal symptoms are often the most common presenting feature, with epistaxis occasionally present. Some patients may present early with swelling of the soft or hard palate. With time, there is evolution to frank ulceration, with destruction of the palatal and nasal tissues leading to the development of an oro-nasal fistula. Infection is often a late feature (Ratech et al. 1989).

The histological appearance of nasofacial lymphoma is characterised by the presence of varying amounts of granulation tissue and extensive coagulative necrosis. There is usually an inflammatory infiltrate consisting of a mixture of acute and chronic inflammatory cells. Intermingled with this are atypical lymphocytes which are strikingly pleomorphic and can range in number from only a few to extensive, monotonous sheets (Fig. 9). These cells are medium-sized or large with a clear cytoplasm and an irregular nuclear outline. Some have prominent nucleoli

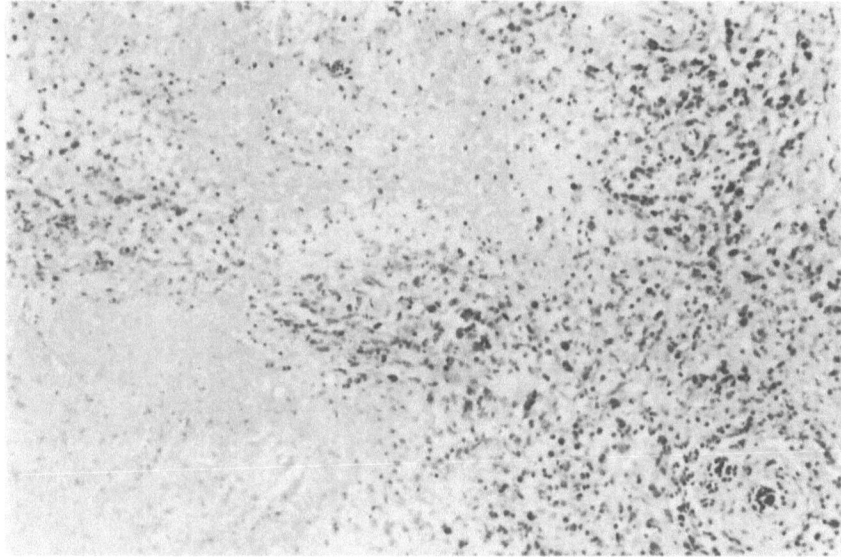

Fig. 9. A nasofacial T cell lymphoma. Sheets of pleomorphic lymphocytes are admixed with focal areas of necrosis. H&E, ×85

and may resemble immunoblasts. T cell lymphomas are the predominate type in the nasal region, and this is particularly true in Asian populations. Many of these cases resemble peripheral T cell lymphomas and phenotypically share many common features (LIEPERT et al. 1994). Angiocentricity (Fig. 10) and epitheliotropism are important and common histopathological features of nasofacial T cell lymphomas and provide evidence to support the contention that some of these tumours in the mid-face are related to angiocentric T cell lymphomas of the lung (LIPFORD et al. 1988).

Immunological staining shows that, in most cases of nasofacial lymphoma, the malignant cells express T cell markers, including CD45RO (UCHL-1), CD43 (MT1) and CD3 (CHAN et al. 1987; RAMSAY et al. 1988). A large number of macrophages can be demonstrated in the background, leading, in the past, to the erroneous conclusion that many nasofacial lymphomas were histiocytic in origin (RAMSAY and ROONEY 1993). A minority of nasofacial tumours are derived from B cells, and these will show the presence of B cell markers, with gene analysis showing heavy chain gene rearrangements (MAXYMIW et al. 1992).

Without treatment, the relentless destruction of mid-face structures by the lymphomatous infiltrate can lead to death from haemorrhage or secondary infection. Typically, the condition is treated using chemotherapy, radiation therapy or a combination of both (RATECH et al. 1989). Reports of long-term survival vary, in part because of the confusion regarding the nature of the condition and the unclear terminology used in the past. Previous reluctance to clearly define the condition as a lymphoma has led to inadequate treatment

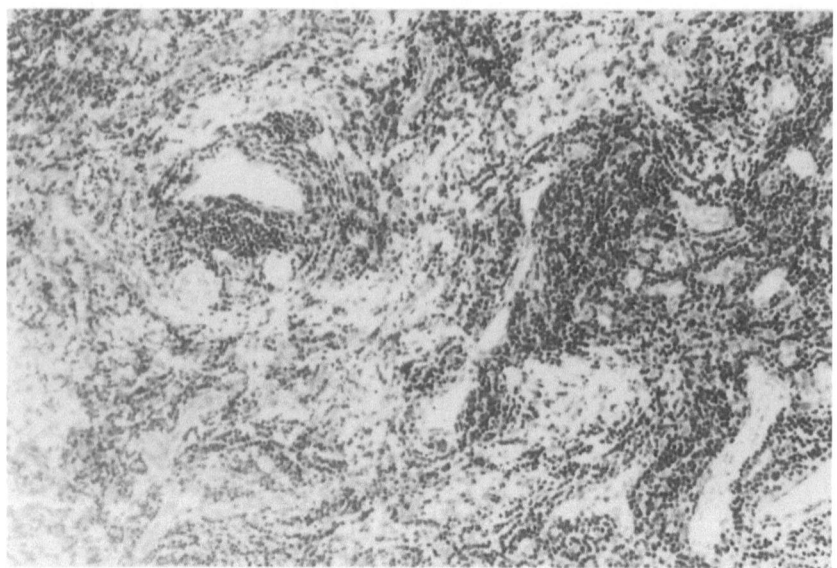

Fig. 10. A T cell lymphoma from the upper lip showing a prominent angiocentric pattern. H&E, ×85

and high recurrence rates. Overall survival from the time of diagnosis has been reported to be from 3 months to 14 years (Ramsay and Rooney 1993). More aggressive management in recent years has improved prognosis, with a 5-year disease-free survival of 78% for patients with early-stage lesions and 19% for those with more widely disseminated disease (Robbins et al. 1985). Others suggest that grade and stage of tumour do not affect survival for patients with nasofacial lymphoma, but this may reflect the heterogeneity of tumours that arise in this site (Ratech et al. 1989).

6 Conclusions

Extranodal lymphomas of the head and neck comprise a diverse collection of pathological entities. Although most are B cell neoplasms, other types are seen at specific sites, including MALT lymphomas arising in salivary glands and T cell lymphomas in the nasofacial area. The importance of identifying the subtle histological features of each, coupled with immunological and molecular biological studies of biopsy tissues, has been discussed. The clinical behaviour of these tumours varies greatly, as does management of the conditions. The requirement to properly categorise the specific lymphoma type further reinforces the need to have a thorough understanding of the biology of each condition.

References

Abemayor E, Canalis RF, Greenberg P, Wortham DG, Rowlands JP, Sun NCJ (1988) Plasma cell tumors of the head and neck. J Otolaryngol 17: 376-381

Alexanian R, Dimopoulos M (1994) The treatment of multiple myeloma. N Engl J Med 330: 484-489

Anderrson M, Klein G, Ziegler J, Henle W (1976) Association of Epstein-Barr viral genomes with American Burkitt lymphoma. Nature 260: 357-359

Bateman AC, Wright DH (1993) Epitheliotropism in high-grade lymphomas of mucosa-associated lymphoid tissue. Histopathology 23: 409-415

Batsakis JG (1983) Plasma cell tumours of the head and neck. Ann Otol Rhinol Laryngol 92: 311-313

Bonadonna G, Molinari R, Banfi A (1989) Hodgkin's and non-Hodgkin's lymphoma presenting in the head and neck. In: Suen Y, Myers EN (eds) Cancers of the head and neck, 2nd edn. Churchill Livingstone, New York, pp 877-896

Bruce KW, Royer RQ (1953) Multiple myeloma occurring in the jaws: a study of seventeen cases. Oral Surg 6: 729-744

Burke JS, Butler JJ (1992) Malignant lymphoma with a high content of epithelioid histiocytes (Lennert's lymphoma). Am J Clin Pathol 16: 156-162

Burkitt D (1958) A sarcoma involving the jaws in African children. Br J Surg 46: 218-233

Burkitt D (1966) Malignant lymphoma of the jaws. J Dent Res 45: 554-559

Carbone A, Vaccher E, Barzan L, Gloghini A, Volpe R, de Re V et al (1995) Head and neck lymphomas associated with human immunodeficiency virus infection. Arch Otolaryngol Hend Neck Surg 121: 210-218

Chan JKC, Ng CS, Lau WH, Lo STH (1987) Most nasal/nasopharyngeal lymphomas are peripheral T-cell neoplasms. Am J Surg Pathol 50: 418-429

Chan JKC, Banks PM, Cleary ML, Delsol G, De Wolf-Peeters C, Falini B et al (1994) A proposal for classification of lymphoid neoplasms (by the International Lymphoma Study Group). Histopathology 25: 517-536

Cobleigh MA, Kennedy JL (1986) Non-Hodgkin's lymphomas of the upper aerodigestive tract and salivary glands. Otolaryngol Clin North Am 19: 685-710

Corwin J, Lindberg RD (1979) Solitary plasmacytoma of bone vs. extramedullary plasmacytoma and their relationship to multiple myeloma. Cancer 43: 1007-1013

Diss TC, Wotherspoon AC, Speight PM, Pan L, Isaacson PG (1995) B-cell monoclonality, Epstein Barr virus and t(14;18) in myoepithelial sialadenitis and low-grade B-cell MALT lymphoma of the parotid gland. Am J Surg Pathol 19: 531-536

Economopoulos T, Asprou N, Stathakis N, Fountzilas G, Pavlidis N, Papaspyrou S et al (1992) Primary extranodal non-Hodgkin's lymphoma of the head and neck. Oncology 49: 484-488

Fu YS, Perzin KH (1979) Nonepithelial tumors of the nasal cavity, paranasal sinuses and nasopharynx: a clinicopathologic study. X. Malignant lymphomas. Cancer 43: 611-621

Gleeson MJ, Bennet MH, Cawson RA (1986) Lymphomas of salivary glands. Cancer 58: 699-704

Handlers JP, Howell RE, Abrams AM, Melrose RJ (1986) Extranodal oral lymphoma. 1. A morphologic and immunoperoxidase study of 34 cases. Oral Surg Oral Med Oral Pathol 61: 362-367

Harris NL, Jaffe ES, Stein H, Banks PM, Chan JKC, Cleary ML et al (1994) A revised European-American classification of lymphoid neoplasms: a proposal from the International Lymphoma Study Group. Blood 84: 1361-1392

Harrison DFN (1987) Midline lethal granuloma: fact or fiction. Laryngoscope 97: 1049-1053

Howell RE, Handlers JP, Abrams AM, Melrose RJ (1987) Extra-nodal oral lymphoma. II. Relationships between clinical features and the Lukes-Collins classification of 34 cases. Oral Surg Oral Med Oral Pathol 64: 597-602

Hyjek E, Smith WJ, Isaacson PG (1988) Primary B-cell Lymphoma of salivary glands and its relationship to myoepithelial sialadenitis. Hum Pathol 19: 766-776

Ioachim HL (1992) Lymphoma: an opportunistic neoplasia of AIDS. Leukemia 6: 305–335

Irwin D, Kaplan L (1993) Clinical aspects of HIV-related lymphoma. Curr Opin Oncol 5: 852–860

Isaacson PG (1990) Lymphomas of mucosa-associated lymphoid tissue (MALT). Histopathology 16: 617–619

Isaacson PG (1992) Extranodal lymphomas: the MALT concept. Verh Dtsch Ges Pathol 76: 14–23

Isaacson PG (1993) Lymphomas of mucosa-associated lymphoid tissue (MALT-type lymphomas). Forum Trends Exp Clin Med 3: 234–245

Isaacson PG, Norton AJ (1994) Extranodal lymphomas. Churchill Livingstone, Edinburgh

Isaacson PG, Wright DH (1983) Malignant lymphoma of mucosa-associated lymphoid tissues. A distinct type of B-cell lymphoma. Cancer 52: 1410–1416

Isaacson PG, Wright DH (1984) Extranodal malignant lymphoma arising from mucosa-associated lymphoid tissue. Cancer 53: 2515–2524

Isaacson PG, Wotherspoon AC, Diss T, Pan LX (1991) Follicular colonization in B-cell lymphoma of mucosa-associated lymphoid tissue. Am J Surg Pathol 15: 819–828

Jordan RCK, Speight PM (1996) Sjögren's syndrome: from histopathology to molecular pathology. Oral Surg Oral Med Oral Pathol 81: 308–320

Jordan RCK, Diss TC, Lench NJ, Isaacson PG, Speight PM (1995) Immunoglobulin gene rearrangements in lymphoplasmacytic infiltrates of labial salivary glands in Sjögren's syndrome. Oral Surg Oral Med Oral Pathol 79: 723–729

Kassan SS, Thomas TL, Moutsopoulos HM, Hoover R, Kimberly RP, Budman DR et al (1978) Increased risk of lymphoma in sicca syndrome. Ann Intern Med 89: 888–892

Lennert K (1995) The proposal for a Revised European American Lymphoma classification – a new start of a transatlantic discussion. Histopathology 26: 481–483

Lennert K, Feller AC (1990) Histopathology of non-Hodgkin's lymphomas. Based on the updated Kiel classification, 2nd edn. Springer, Berlin Heidelberg New York

Lennert K, Mohri N, Stein H, Kaiserling E (1975) The histopathology of malignant lymphoma. Br J Haematol 31: 193–203

Levine AM (1992) Acquired immunodeficiency syndrome-related lymphoma. Blood 80: 8–20

Li G, Hansmann ML, Zwingers T, Lennert K (1990) Primary lymphomas of the lung: morphological, immunohistochemical and clinical features. Histopathology 16: 519–533

Liepert DR, Kudryk WH, Jewell LD (1994) Nasal T-cell lymphoma: a case presentation. J Otolaryngol 23: 32–35

Lipford EH, Margolick JB, Longo DL, Fauci AS, Jaffe ES (1988) Angiocentric immunoproliferative lesions: a clinicopathologic spectrum of post-thymic T-cell proliferations. Blood 72: 1674–1681

Lukes RJ, Collins RD (1977) Lukes-Collins classification and its significance. Cancer Treat Rep 61: 971–979

Maxymiw WG, Patterson BJ, Wood RE, Meharchand JM, Munro AJ, Gorska-Flipot I (1992) B-cell lymphoma presenting as a midfacial necrotizing lesion. Oral Surg Oral Med Oral Pathol 74: 343–347

McGurk M, Goepel JR, Hancock BW (1985) Extranodal lymphoma of the head and neck: a review of 49 consecutive cases. Clin Radiol 36: 455–458

Meis JM, Butler JJ, Osbourne BM, Ordonez NG (1987) Solitary plasmacytomas of bone and extramedullary plasmacytomas. Cancer 59: 1475–1485

Menarguez J, Mollejo M, Oliva H, Balla C, Forteza J, Martin C et al (1994) Waldeyer's ring lymphomas. A clinicopathological study of 79 cases. Histopathology 24: 13–22

Minerbrook M, Schulman P, Budman DR, Teichberg S, Vinciguerra V, Kardon N et al (1982) Burkitt's leukemia: a re-evaluation. Cancer 49: 1444–1448

Morton RP, Sillars HA, Benjamin CS (1992) Incidence of "unsuspected" extranodal head and neck lymphoma. Clin Otolaryngol 17: 373–375

Ngan B, Warnke RA, Wilson M, Tagaki K, Cleary ML, Dorfman RF (1991) Monocytoid B-cell lymphoma: a study of 36 cases. Hum Pathol 22: 409–421

Nizze H, Cogliatti SB, von Schilling C, Feller AC, Lennert K (1991) Monocytoid B-cell lymphoma: morphological variants and relationship to low-grade B-cell lymphoma of the mucosa-associated lymphoid tissue. Histopathology 18: 403–414

Ortiz-Hidalgo C, Wright DH (1992) The morphological spectrum of monocytoid B-cell lymphoma and its relationship to lymphomas of mucosa-associated lymphoid tissue. Histopathology 21: 555–561

Pals ST, Horst E, Scheper RJ, Meijer CLMJ (1989) Mechanisms of human lymphocyte migration and their role in the pathogenesis of disease. Immunol Rev 108: 111–133

Parveen T, Navarro-Roman L, Medeiros LJ, Raffeld M, Jaffe ES (1993) Low-grade B-cell lymphoma of mucosa-associated lymphoid tissue arising in the kidney. Arch Pathol Lab Med 117: 780–783

Patton LL, McMillan CW, Webster WP (1990) American Burkitt's lymphoma: a 10 year review and case study. Oral Surg Oral Med Oral Pathol 69: 307–316

Paulsen J, Lennert K (1994) Low-grade B-cell lymphoma of mucosa-associated lymphoid tissue type in Waldeyer's ring. Histopathology 24: 1–11

Pelicci PG, Knowles DM, Magrath I, Dalla-Favera R (1986) Chromosomal breakpoints and structural alterations of the c-myc locus differ in endemic and sporadic forms of Burkitt lymphoma. Proc Natl Acad Sci USA 83: 2984–2988

Ramsay AD, Rooney N (1993) Lymphomas of the head and neck. 1. Nasofacial T-cell lymphoma. Oral Oncol Eur J Cancer [B] 29B: 99–102

Ramsay AD, Michaels L, Isaacson PG (1988) Lethal midline granuloma – a T-cell lymphoma? J Pathol 154: 56

Ratech H, Burke JS, Blayney DW, Sheibani K, Rappaport H (1989) A clinicopathologic study of malignant lymphomas of the nose, paranasal sinuses, and hard palate, including cases of lethal midline granuloma. Cancer 64: 2525–2531

Regezi JA, Zarbo RJ, Stewart JCB (1991) Extranodal oral lymphomas: histologic subtypes and immunophenotypes (in routinely processed tissue). Oral Surg Oral Med Oral Pathol 72: 702–708

Reinish EI, Raviv M, Srolovitz H, Gornitsky M (1994) Tongue, primary amyloidosis, and multiple myeloma. Oral Surg Oral Med Oral Pathol 77: 121–125

Robbins KT, Fuller LM, Vlasak M, Osborne B, Jing BS, Velasquez WS et al (1985) Primary lymphomas of the nasal cavity and paranasal sinuses. Cancer 56: 814–819

Rooney N, Ramsay AD (1994) Lymphomas of the head and neck. 2. The B-cell lymphomas. Oral Oncol Eur J Cancer 30B: 155–159

Rosenberg SA (1994) Classification of lymphoid neoplasms. Blood 5: 1359–1360

Rosenberg SA, Berard CW, Brown BWJ, Burke J, Dorfman RF, Glatstein E et al (1982) National Cancer Institute sponsored study of classifications of non-Hodgkin's lymphomas. Cancer 49: 2112–2135

Salhany KE, Pietra GG (1993) Extranodal lymphoid disorders. Am J Clin Pathol 99: 472–485

Schmid U, Helbron D, Lennert K (1982) Development of malignant lymphomas in myoepithelial sialadenitis (Sjögren's syndrome). Virchows Arch [A] Pathol Anat Histopathol 395: 11–43

Serraino D, Salamina G, Franceschi S, La Vecchia C, Brunet JB, Ancelle-Park R (1992) The epidemiology of AIDS-associated non-Hodgkin's lymphoma in the World Health Organization European region. Br J Cancet 66: 912–916

Shaefer BC, Woisetchlaeger M, Strominger JL, Speck SH (1991) Exclusive expression of Epstein-Barr virus nuclear antigen 1 in Burkitt lymphoma arises from a third promoter, distinct from promoters used in latently infected lymphocytes. Proc Natl Acad Sci USA 88: 6550–6554

Silverman S, Migliorati CA, Lazada-Nur F, Greenspan D, Conant MA (1986) Oral findings in people with or at high risk for AIDS: a study of 375 homosexual males. JADA 112: 187–192

Stansfeld AG, Diebold J, Kapanci Y, Kelenyi G, Lennert K, Mioduszewska O et al (1988) Updated Kiel classification for lymphomas. Lancet 1: 292–293

Stein H (1995) Critique of the critique. Ann Oncol 6: 109–111

Stewart JP (1933) Progressive lethal granulomatous ulceration of the nose. J Laryngol Otol 48: 657–701

Takagi N, Nakamura S, Yamamoto K, Kunishima K, Takagi I, Suyama M et al (1992) Malignant lymphoma of mucosa-associated lymphoid tissue arising in the thymus of a patient with Sjogren's syndrome. A morphologic, phenotypic, and genotypic study. Cancer 69: 1347–1355

Thompson SH, Altini M (1989) Gigantiform cementoma of the jaws. Head Neck 11: 538–544

Wax MK, Yun KJ, Omar RA (1993) Extramedullary plasmacytomas of the head and neck. Otolaryngol. Head Neck Surg 109: 877–885

Wiltshaw E (1976) The natural history of extramedullary plasmacytoma and its relation to solitary myeloma of bone and myelomatosis. Medicine 55: 217–238

Wotherspoon AC, Pan LX, Diss TC, Isaacson PG (1990) A genotypic study of low grade B-cell lymphomas, including lymphomas of mucosa-associated lymphoid tissue (MALT). J Pathol 162: 135–140

Wotherspoon AC, Diss TC, Pan LX, Schmid C, Kerr-Muir MG, Hardman Lea S et al (1993) Primary low-grade B-cell lymphoma of conjunctiva: a mucosa-associated lymphoid tissue type lymphoma. Histopathology 23: 417–424

Wright DH (1994) Lymphomas of Waldeyer's ring. Histopathology 24: 97–99

Ziegler JL (1981) Burkitt's lymphoma. N Engl J Med 305: 735–745

Importance of Proliferation Markers
in Oral Pathology

K.A.A.S.Warnakulasuriya and N.W. Johnson

1 Introduction

Disturbances in growth, including the carcinogenic process, are often linked with an increased rate of cell proliferation, usually combined with sustained hyperplasia (Iverson 1992). As a result, over the past three decades, there has been considerable interest in markers of cell proliferation that can be used as indicators of the clinical aggressiveness of human neoplasms, additional to what can be judged from histology alone. The hope is that such markers will have value in prognosis and treatment planning. It is necessary at the outset to understand that the significance of "proliferative activity" depends on the number of cells undergoing programmed cell death or apoptosis (Wyllie 1993) in a given compartment of cells. Aspects of cell proliferation have, however, been studied more extensively, and data taking apoptosis into account are limited.

Current Topics in Pathology
Volume 90, G. Seifert (Ed.)
© Springer-Verlag Berlin Heidelberg 1996

In this chapter we review, mainly in quantitative terms, the major parameters useful in understanding the kinetics of cell proliferation and look critically at the methodology used, with particular reference to epithelial systems and to oral mucosal disease. Data derived from many studies examining the cell kinetics of both oral and some other head and neck malignancies (particularly squamous cell carcinomas, SCC), potentially malignant lesions of the oral mucosa and a few other oral diseases of interest are presented. The usefulness of such investigations in understanding the pathogenesis of oral diseases and their potential value as diagnostic and prognostic markers in the discipline of oral pathology is addressed.

2 Methods of Studying Cell Proliferation

Methods of studying cell proliferation and growth in human neoplasms, together with their pitfalls, were reviewed by QUINN and WRIGHT (1990), HALL and LEVISON (1990) and, with particular relevance to oral mucosa in health and disease, by SCRAGG and JOHNSON (1980a, 1982). Considerable advances in techniques have been reported since the latter report, and these are reviewed here.

Cell proliferation markers attempt to identify and measure the proportion of cells undergoing the particular phases of cell cycle. Studies involving dual parameter estimates over a period of time incorporate a measurement of time spent in each phase or in transit, thereby allowing not only assessment of the *state* of proliferation but also providing information about the *rate* of proliferation (BARNES and GILLETT 1995).

The cell cycle is well described; the demonstrable stages are mitosis (M) and the DNA synthesis phase (S), during which replication of DNA in the nucleus occurs and is demonstrable by DNA labelling techniques. There is a time lapse (G_2 phase) between completion of DNA synthesis and beginning of mitosis. Similarly, daughter cells produced by mitosis do not start replicating DNA immediately, and this is referred to as G_1 phase. During this phase, cells may exit the cell cycle, and this "out of cycle" phase is referred to as G_0. Several cell cycle check points or restriction points exist mostly in G_0/G_1 phases, where a cell is able to integrate internal and external signals, allowing entry or exit of cells into and out of the cycle (MORGAN 1992; SCHNEIDER et al. 1991). Factors which influence cell proliferation by operation through these check points are discussed in Sect. 5. Our knowledge on selection of markers to identify proliferating cells relates largely to those cells participating in the cell cycle; we do not yet have any means of accurately establishing any subpopulations of cells in resting G_1 or G_0 phases, so that the true growth fraction of a neoplasm cannot yet accurately be determined.

The majority of cell cycle estimates are known to be influenced by circadian rhythms (PILGRIM et al. 1963). WARNAKULASURIYA and MACDONALD (1993, 1995a) have quantified the range of circadian variations expected in several cell kinetic parameters in human buccal mucosa. Human clinical studies need to control for this effect by appropriate sampling techniques.

2.1 Mitotic Counts

Mitoses can be counted in conventionally stained sections (Fig. 1), but the method identifies only a small fraction of the cycling population, because the time spent by cells in mitosis is relatively short – of the order of less than 1 h to a maximum of 2 h in oral epithelia – compared to other phases of the cell cycle. As mentioned earlier, the method allows only an assessment of the state of proliferation, and not the rate of proliferation. Standardizing mitotic counting techniques is important to achieve reproducibility. The selection of the counting field, criteria for identification of mitotic figures and other variables such as level of (microscope) focus all need to be taken into account (AHERNE et al. 1977; BAAK 1990). Delay in fixation, particularly of large specimens, can result in a reduction of mitotic figures, because cells move out of M phase ex vivo, thus lowering the count (CROSS et al. 1990). Nevertheless, despite the methodological problems of assessing mitotic count in human neoplasms (QUINN and WRIGHT 1990), when correctly measured and given as a fraction of interphase nuclear population, the *mitotic index* thus derived can be a useful marker of cell proliferation (GILLETT et al. 1993).

Mitotic arrest techniques provide more accurate data by increasing the number of figures available to be counted and introduce a longitudinal (time) component (SCRAGG and JOHNSON 1980b), but are rarely applicable to oral lesions in humans for ethical and safety reasons.

2.2 S-Phase Indices

The most commonly used cell proliferation marker method in experimental studies has been to establish the proportion of cells in DNA synthesis (S) phase, referred to as the *labelling index* (LI), quantified on the basis of nucleic acid precursor incorporation using (usually) tritiated thymidine [³H]dT or bromodeoxyuridine (BrdUrd).

2.2.1 Thymidine Labelling

Before the 1980s, cell proliferation status was mostly studied using [³H]dT, and this technique continues to have a well-established role. Methods of in vitro incorporation into DNA by incubating freshly biopsied mucosal fragments over a short period of time (15 min) in a medium containing [³H]dT have been standardised (RENNIE et al. 1984) and can achieve reliable results. Autoradiographs prepared from pre-labelled tissues allow assessment of LI by counting labelled cells and expressing these as a proportion of 100 total cell population, or to a unit of surface length or of basement membrane length of the tissue, when covering epithelia are examined. In the past, linear measurements using microscope graticules or stereological techniques for morphometric estimates (AHERNE and DUNHILL 1982) have been used to denominate such indices; more recently, interactive computer

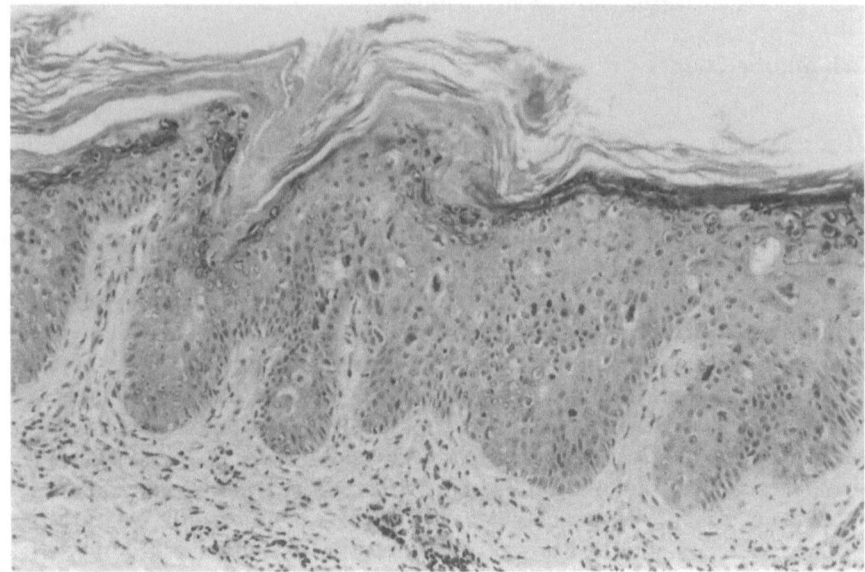

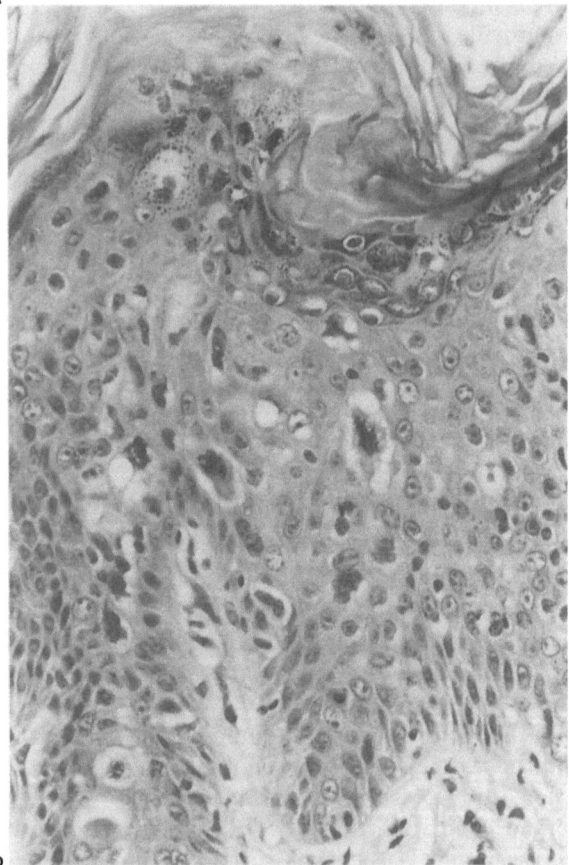

Fig. 1a,b. Increased mitotic activity in dysplastic oral epithelium from an in situ carcinoma. Numerous atypical mitotic figures and mitoses in superficial epithelial layers are apparent. **a** ×130. **b** ×330

systems with drawing devices and image digitisation have been a major advance (HAMILTON and ALLEN 1995).

A LI derived by a single-pulse label in vivo or in vitro allows an assessment of a static index, but with the introduction of double labelling techniques (WARNAKULASURIYA 1976) the time spent in S phase or the rate of cell influx and efflux can be calculated. This also allows an estimation of turnover time of a tissue or a compartment. In vitro incorporation of thymidine analogues has considerable methodological problems in that small pieces of fresh tissue trimmed to 1-2 mm³ are required for incubation, and the representative nature of data derived from such small fragments of tissue has been questioned (LAMBERT 1986).

Data derived from pulse labelling also have the disadvantage – shared by many other similar techniques referred to later – that only cells in the actively dividing cell cycle are ascertained, and we do not know the actual compartment size of the growth fraction of the tissue which is represented by such data. This seriously limits the usefulness of such indices.

2.2.2 Bromodeoxyuridine Labelling

As an alternative to thymidine labelling, non-radioactive markers have been developed. Immunohistochemical or flow cytometric (FCM) detection of BrdUrd (or other halagonated pyrimidines) incorporated into DNA either in vivo or in vitro (WYNFORD-THOMAS and WILLIAMS 1986), made possible by the introduction of a monoclonal antibody which recognises BrdUrd (GRATZNER 1982), has revolutionised the study of cell kinetics. BROWMAN et al. (1991) showed a dose response in uptake of BrdUrd when biopsies from oral carcinomas were incubated in vitro, with a mean BrdUrd index rising from 1.6 (±0.05) to 8.8 (±0.9), with a 50-fold rise in incubating concentration (2–100 μM). Thus optimal conditions for in vitro incubation must be determined before using the technique widely. Many laboratories incorporate BrdUrd under high oxygen tensions (BRITTO et al. 1992) to improve diffusion of the label (Fig. 2). BrdUrd and iododeoxyuridine (IrdUrd) are cytotoxic drugs and may be used in vivo in patients with an established malignancy in a single, low dose (200 mg in 20 ml normal saline) via the intravenous route (WILSON 1991). Although little toxicity has been reported in animal studies, use in humans should be undertaken with caution and certainly with ethical approval. In vivo double labelling using BrdUrd and IrdUrd – both approved for clinical use – allows estimation of potential doubling times of solid tumours (POLLACK et al. 1995).

2.3 Immunohistochemical Methods

The principle underlying assessment of cell proliferation by immunohistochemical methods is that there are cell cycle-associated alterations in the amount or distribution of cellular proteins that are recognised as antigens (HALL and WOODS 1990). A wide range of molecules are potential targets for immunohistochemical

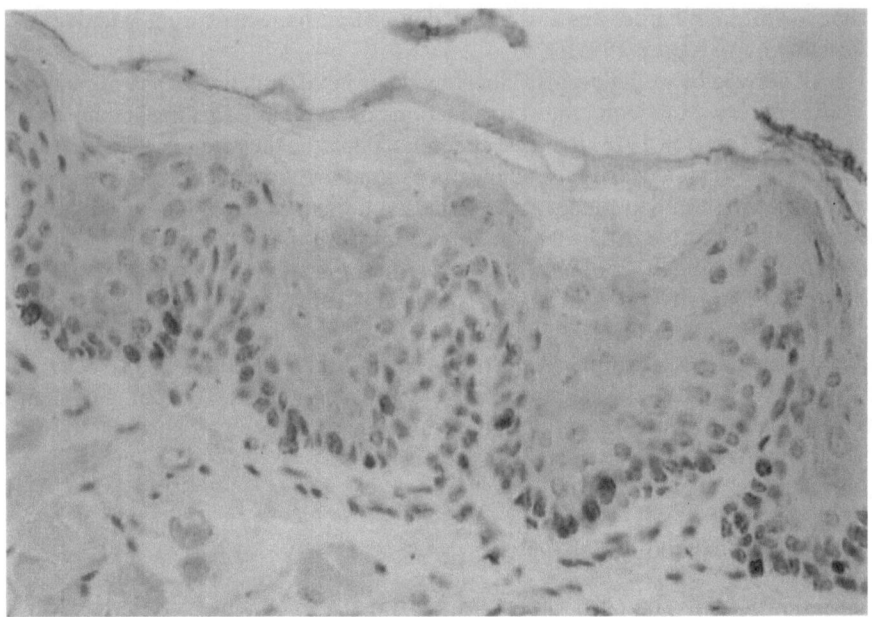

Fig. 2. Dorsal mucosa of hamster tongue labelled in vitro with bromodeoxyuridine. There is uniform incorporation of the label in the progenitor compartment across the full width of specimen. ×180

assessment. Here we will focus on two well-characterised antigens, Ki-67 and proliferating cell nuclear antigen (PCNA).

2.3.1 Ki-67

Ki-67 antigen is expressed in all phases of the cell cycle except G_0 and early G_1 (Gerdes et al. 1984), and staining with Ki-67 antibody is widely used as an operational marker of cell proliferation (Yu et al. 1992). Although the half-life of detectable antigen is recognised to be 1h or less, and Ki-67 expression correlates with other cell proliferation indices, it has been said that it may overestimate the growth fraction (Scott et al. 1991). The first widely available monoclonal antibody against Ki-67 was reactive only on frozen sections (Fig. 3), but genetically engineered MIB-1 and MIB-3 antibodies and polyclonal Ki-67 antibodies can now be used on archival tissues following microwave antigen retrieval (Catterotti et al. 1992). It has been recently shown, by counting MIB-1-stained cells in breast cancer, that some judgement is needed in selecting only moderately-heavily stained MIB-1-positive cells if comparable labelling indices are to be obtained on formalin-fixed, wax-embedded versus frozen tissues (Gee et al. 1995).

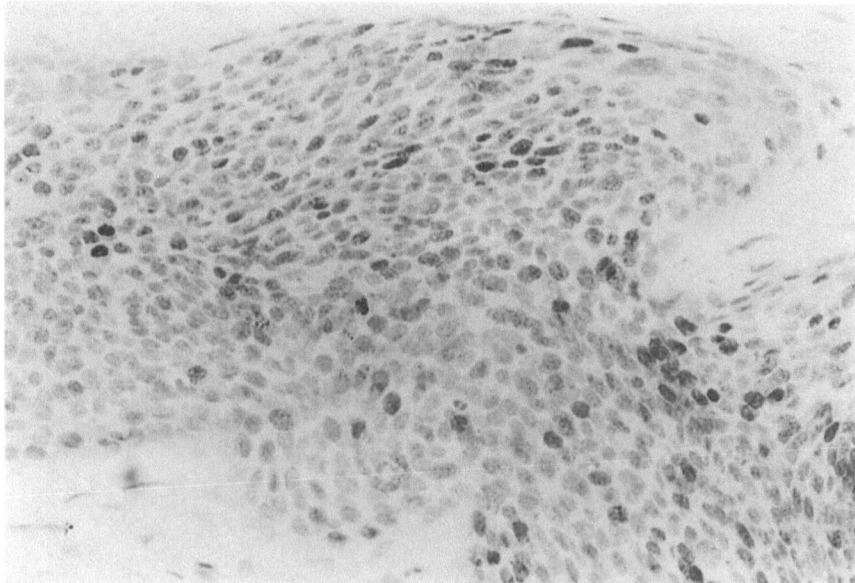

Fig. 3. Ki-67 labelling of a frozen section from oral squamous cell carcinoma (SCC) showing strong nuclear labelling of proliferating cells. ×180

2.3.2 Proliferating Cell Nuclear Antigen

PCNA is a 36-kDa nuclear protein associated with the cell cycle. A monoclonal antibody that has been generated to genetically engineered PCNA (WASEEM and LANE 1990), designated PC10, demonstrates the proliferative compartment (Fig. 4) in conventionally fixed and processed tissues (HALL et al. 1990). The time of fixation affects PCNA immunostaining; good results are observed after 24–36h, while more than a 48-h fixation is associated with significant reduction in staining intensity (HALL et al. 1990; LÖRZ et al. 1994). In optimally fixed tissues, positive staining is predominantly nuclear, but cytoplasmic staining is occasionally observed in cells with mitotic nuclei. A gradation of staining intensity is seen from basal to suprabasal cells in stratified epithelia, and criteria for differentiating darkly labelled cells from lightly labelled cells need to be defined. WELSGERBER et al. (1993), by enumerating strongly stained PCNA cells using a strictly standardised enumeration method, have shown the PCNA index to be comparable to the BrdUrd index. On the other hand, if all positively stained cells are counted irrespective of the intensity, the PC10 labelling index could be almost fourfold that derived by [³H]dT or BrdUrd labelling (WARNAKULASURIYA and JOHNSON 1993a). This poor correlation with other indices has been confirmed in many studies (for a review, see YU et al. 1992) and may reflect the long half-life of PCNA (about 20h), resulting in the labelling of some cells that have actually left the cell cycle recently (HALL et al. 1990). Furthermore, very small levels of PCNA may

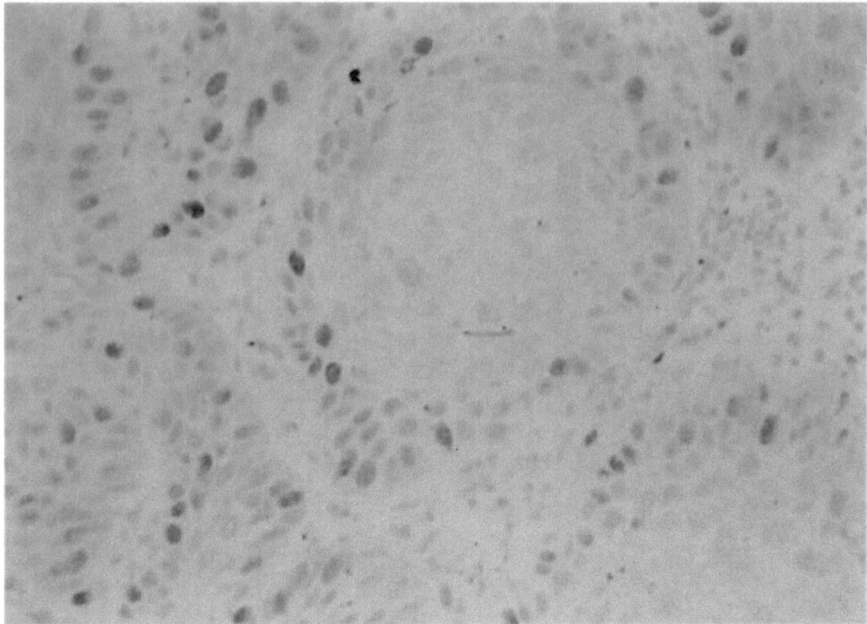

Fig. 4. Islands of well-differentiated oral squamous cell carcinoma (SCC) stained against prolif-erating cell nuclear antigen (PCNA). PC10 immunoreactivity is more frequent in basal cell populations and nearly absent in the central, more differentiated areas. ×180

be found in non-cycling cells with up-regulation occurring on entry to the cell cycle (Bravo and MacDonald-Bravo 1985). Authors using mouse monoclonal antibody 19A2 against PCNA in methanol-fixed tissues claim this immune label is specific for marking S-phase cells (Galand and Degraef 1989; Berlingin et al. 1992).

2.4 Argyrophilic Nucleolar Organisation Region Protein Enumeration

The location of nucleolar organisation regions (NOR) is easily demonstrable by the silver-staining method described by Ploton et al. (1986). The argyrophilic NOR proteins (AgNOR) appear as small, dark, intranuclear dots (Fig. 5) in routine histological sections treated with a colloid composed of gelatin and silver formate at room temperature. Their number (per nucleus) has been shown to be correlated with the rate of ribosomal RNA transcription, cell proliferation and DNA ploidy. While the counting of AgNOR is tedious (Crocker et al. 1989), an increased number has been documented in human malignant neoplasms in many tissues (Egan and Crocker 1992). A higher frequency and scattered distribution of AgNOR are hallmarks of increased cell proliferation (Underwood and Giri 1988). For the estimate to be reliable – as with all quantitative assessments – a sufficient and representative number of nuclei have to be counted; Ruschoff et al.

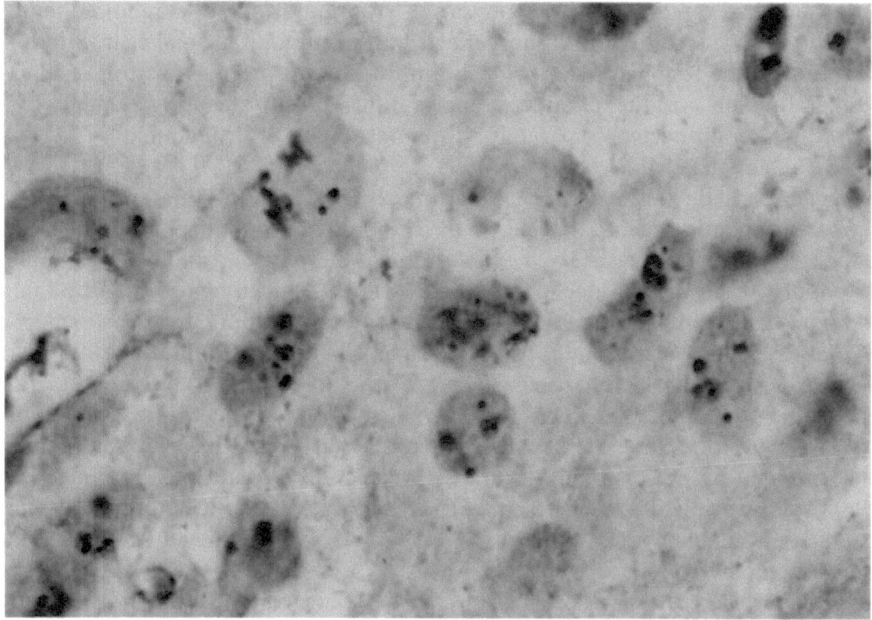

Fig. 5. A squamous cell carcinoma with a high number of silver-stained agyrophilic nucleolar organisation regions (AgNOR) per nucleus. AgNOR are widely dispersed throughout the nuclei. ×3580

(1990) recommend the standardised continuous (or running) mean method to arrive at an optimal nuclear count, rather than arbitrarily deciding to estimate 100 or 200 nuclei, as is done in most studies.

2.5 Flow Cytometry

DNA analysis by FCM is emerging as an important clinical tool in cell prliferation. In DNA analysis, the fluorochrome most commonly used is propidium iodide (PI). PI binds stoichiometrically to the DNA of cells, and under laser excitation the intensity with which a cell nucleus emits light is directly proportional to its DNA content. Cancer cells often have an abnormal chromosome number that is not a multiple of 23. These aneuploid cells thus emit an abnormal fluorescent intensity. FCM techniques readily divide neoplasms into two categories: diploid cells and aneuploid cells. Broad chromosome numbers, e.g. tetraploidy or other hyper-diploidy, can be recorded with reasonable accuracy. This information can be obtained from single cell suspensions prepared from fresh tissue or thick sections (30–50 μm) from routinely prepared paraffin-embedded material (HEDLEY et al. 1983). Using currently available fluorescence-activated cell sorter (FACScan) FCM machines and accompanying computer programmes, about 10 000 cells per sample can be analysed rapidly. However, physical disruption of tissues is required, and results are influenced by the dilution effects of non-tumour/stromal cells. Micro-dissection of the lesional area obviously improves the specificity of the results. Cytokeratin labels in dual parameter analyses further improve the specificity by recording keratinocytes separately from stromal or inflammatory cells (NYLANDER et al. 1994b).

Several kinetic parameters, i.e. DNA index (DI), denoting the ratio of DNA fluorescence of abnormal to normal G_1/G_0 cell populations, S-phase and potential doubling time (t_{pot}), a measure of the theoretical poliferative capability of a tumour cell population in the absence of cell loss (STEEL 1977), can be obtained by this method. The technique to estimate t_{pot} is based on the procedure first described by BEGG et al. (1985), whereby a biopsy is taken several hours after incorporation of a label. This method has been used widely to estimate cell proliferation of oral and head and neck tumours in the CRC Gray Laboratory in the United Kingdom (WILSON 1991), and these results are discussed below. With proper sampling time, t_{pot} assessment by FCM is reported to be precise and reproducible (HOYER et al. 1994). The principle advantage of the FCM technique is that it is rapid and the results are available within a day of surgery, allowing the clinician to utilise the information derived in treatment planning.

Using FCM, DNA parameters can also be recorded in parallel with other markers, such as the expression of oncogene (e.g. c-*myc*) or tumour suppressor gene (e.g. p53) proteins, growth factor receptors (e.g. epidermal growth factor receptor, EGFR) or growth factors themselves (e.g. transforming growth factor, TGF; tumour necrosis factor, TNF). These markers are discussed further in Sect. 5.

3 Comparison of Methods Used in the Study of Cell Proliferation

Whilst the methods for estimation of cell proliferation described above attempt to measure several different parameters, they are closely interrelated in biological terms. Furthermore, different techniques aimed at measuring the same parameters do not produce strictly comparable results. Nevertheless, kinetic information derived from different approaches using [³II]dT LI, BrdUrd LI and Ki-67 LI were shown to be more or less concordant in non-Hodgkin's lymphomas (SILVESTRINI et al. 1988) and in several other human and mouse neoplasms (WILSON et al. 1985). A more detailed investigation in our laboratory (WARNAKULASURIYA and JOHNSON 1993a) using hamster tongue showed that proliferative indices of simple, flat lining mucosae such as ventral tongue derived by in vivo and in vitro labelling using [³H]dT or BrdUrd were very similar. However, dorsal tongue epithelium, which is thicker, has an undulating morphology, and a complex cell renewal pattern gives markedly and significantly different results with the different methods. There are also potential differences between the information on proliferative status derived by PCNA immunostaining and other established cell cycle markers (see Sect. 2.3). This is not surprising, as it has been shown that PCNA (as detected by PC10) is expressed in non-cycling cells (HALL et al. 1992). The latter authors concluded that PCNA immunoreactivity can occur without cell proliferation in association with neoplasia. Such methodological differences need to be taken into account when comparing data from different studies.

Other practical difficulties also exist. Techniques such as mitotic and AgNOR counting are time-consuming and are prone to introduce inter- and intra-observer variations, particularly if sampling is inadequate. Measurement of the number of mitoses per ten high-power fields, though quick, easy and inexpensive, has attracted criticism (QUINN and WRIGHT 1990) due to lack of reproducibility. Despite these difficulties, careful work has shown that mitotic activity recorded in this way can be a powerful prognostic marker in breast and ovarian carcinomas (BAAK et al. 1985, 1986; COLLAN et al. 1988; HAAPASALO et al. 1989). DNA FCM is an objective method, which can be performed rapidly on archival tissues. Several mathematical models to estimate the S-phase fraction have been described (SCOTT et al. 1992), and a high variability of S-phase values may result by the use of different methods (SILVESTRINI 1994). There is also conflicting evidence on the correlation between S-phase index determined by FCM and by other labelling methods (STANTON et al. 1991; SILVESTRINI 1994; WALKER and CAMPLEJOHN 1988). Much work on standardisation of methods remains to be done before measures of cell proliferation become routine in clinical practice.

4 Clinical Applications in Diagnosis and Prognosis of Oral Lesions

It seems evident from the methodologies described in Sect. 2 that most techniques used to study cell proliferation are complex and time-consuming. As a result, such methods primarily remain research tools. Their value and utility in routine clinical practice remains to be determined. In this section, we examine the evidence from reported studies to highlight the importance of these techniques in diagnosis and grading of oral lesions and, where possible, in predicting the outcome or prognosis.

4.1 Cancer

4.1.1 Diagnosis and Grading

Mitotic counting is regarded as useful in differentiating certain malignancies from their benign counterparts, e.g. leiomyosarcoma from leiomyoma (ELLIS and WHITEHEAD 1981). In routine practice, histopathologists *grade* the degree of differentiation of squamous cell carcinomas of the oral cavity in terms of features seen in the microscope image, one of the key features being the so-called mitotic "activity" of the tissue. BRYNE et al. (1991) include the number of mitoses per high-power field as one of the five morphological features used to grade oral cancer. Many of the reports which have used such grading systems do not present data on individual morphological features, giving only the total malignancy grading score. Data on actual mitotic counts are, as a consequence, meagre for oral cavity carcinomas.

Among the range of proliferative markers, LI appears to be the most researched technique for oral lesions. Data from 12 studies reported between 1974 and 1995 are presented in Table 1, the first five using [³H]dT and the remainder the BrdUrd labelling method, in both cases either in vivo or in vitro. A wide range of mean values are reported (LI, 2.6%–22.4%) and, where both oral and head and neck squamous cell carcinomas were analysed, no consistent differences by site are apparent. Studies which used advanced-stage cancers (T3 or T4) report higher LI values (SAKUMA 1980; MOLINARI et al. 1991). The LI is reported not to be correlated with histology of the tumour (degree of differentiation; HEMMER 1990; CHAUVEL et al. 1983; WILSON et al. 1988), but significant increases are noted of the LI distribution with regard to tumour size as well as lymph node involvement (HEMMER 1990; CHAUVEL et al. 1989; SAKUMO 1980). A higher LI is also recorded in aneuploid tumours (BOURHIS et al. 1994a; NYLANDER et al. 1994a). In the latter study, the mean LI of diploid tumours was 8.7%, compared to 15.6% in aneuploid tumours. Two studies by BENNETT et al. (1992) and NYLANDER et al. (1994), respectively, noted marked differences in LI when measured by histology (14.9%, 13.6%) compared to the FCM technique (6.8%, 9.1%) following BrdUrd incorporation in vivo. Comparison of LI values derived from different studies is fraught with danger because of different reference units used in the estimations. Nevertheless LI for oral carcinomas are considerably higher than those reported for both normal human buccal mucosa (2.48% ± 0.47%) following [³H]dT in vitro labelling (WARNAKULASURIYA and MACDONALD 1993) or for oral leukoplakias reported later in this chapter. LI determination has, however, failed to separate keratoacanthoma from cutaneous squamous cell carcinoma (RANDALL et al. 1990).

Several studies utilising immunohistochemical markers of cell cycle antigens to derive LI in oral carcinomas have been reported recently (Table 2). A strong correlation between PCNA and Ki-67 expression ($p < 0.0001$) was reported by JONES et al. (1994) for head and neck carcinomas. These result in much higher indices and probably overestimate the proliferative fraction (Table 1). A wide range of mean values are reported, particularly for the PCNA index. Recent studies have shown, not surprisingly, that the proportion of Ki-67-positive cells increases with histopathological grade (STRÖKEL et al. 1993; STEINBECK et al. 1993; ZOELLER et al. 1994). These immunolabelling methods are now widely accepted, as they obviate the need for either in vivo and in vitro pre-labelling of tissues; however, before they are adopted for routine use, it is necessary to have a better understanding of how the results obtained compare with previously used techniques.

An increased number of AgNOR counts has been documented in many human malignant neoplasms from various sites, compared to their normal tissue of origin or to benign lesions arising therefrom (EGAN and CROCKER 1992). We reported a higher AgNOR count (8.37 ± 6.11 per cell) in oral squamous cell carcinomas compared to epithelial dysplasia (5.61 ± 4.63) or benign keratosis (4.51 ± 2.57) (WARNAKULASURIYA and JOHNSON 1993b). Although these differences were sig-

Table 1. Reported labelling index (LI) of oral and other head and neck carcinomas

Reference	Carcinomas (n)	Tool	Method of labelling	Detection	Mean LI (%) Oral	Mean LI (%) Head and neck
BRESCIANI et al. 1974	5	[³H]dT	In vivo	Autoradiography	–	17.6
SAKUMA 1980	–	[³H]dT	?	Autoradiography	22.4[a]	–
SILVESTRINI et al. 1984	92	[³H]dT	In vitro	Autoradiography	11	–
CHAUVEL et al. 1989	–	[³H]dT	?	Autoradiography	12.9	8.0
MOLINARI et al. 1991	35	[³H]dT	In vitro	Autoradiography	14.0[a]	–
WILSON et al. 1988	9	BrdUrd	In vivo	Histology	5.7	6.3
HEMMER 1990	33	BrdUrd	In vitro	Histology	2.6[b]	–
BENNETT et al. 1992	123	BrdUrd	In vivo	Histology	–	14.9
WILSON et al. 1995	99	BrdUrd	In vivo	Histology	–	8.1
FORSTER et al. 1992	82	BrdUrd	In vivo	FCM	–	8.0
LOCHRIN et al. 1992	38	BrdUrd	In vivo	FCM	–	7.1
BOURHIS et al. 1994a	49	BrdUrd	In vivo	FCM	8.5[c]	–
NYLANDER et al. 1994a	31	BrdUrd	In vivo	FCM	–	13.6
JONES et al. 1994	75	BrdUrd	In vivo	FCM	–	8.9

[³H]dt, tritiated thymidine; BrdUrd, bromodeoxyuridine; FCM, flow cytometry.
[a] Only advanced stage (T3, T4) tumours were included.
[b] Some cancers recorded 0% LI, leading to a low mean value; the range was 0%–23%.
[c] Included some oropharyngeal tumours.

Table 2. Mean labelling indices (LI) for oral and head and neck carcinomas derived by immunolabelling techniques

Reference	Carcinomas (n)	Labelling index (%)	
		Ki-67[b]	PCNA[c]
KEARSLEY et al. 1990	42	2–52	–
TSUJI et al. 1992	48	–	11.6
GÜNZL et al. 1993	40	–	3.9–7.6
STÖRKEL et al. 1993[a]	100	–	40–78
WARNAKULASURIYA et al. 1994	20	27.1	67.4
ROLAND et al. 1994	79	27.8	–
GIROD et al. 1994	144	–	29–50
LÖRZ et al. 1994	53	–	17.5
JONES et al. 1994	75	29.8	56.0
TSAI and JIN 1995	38	–	29.2

PCNA, proliferating cell nuclear antigen.
[a] Lower mean LI (40%) in grade 1 and higher value (78%) in grade 3 (Bryne's malignancy grading).
[b] For Ki-67 LI monoclonal antibody against Ki-67 in frozen sections.
[c] For PCNA, most studies report use of PC10 antibody.

nificant, counts in each diagnostic group overlapped so much that they were of no practical value in distinguishing between individual lesions. However, the higher counts found in many carcinomas were due to dispersion of AgNOR within the nucleoplasm (Fig. 5), so that AgNOR *type* is more useful in making a diagnosis of malignancy than the actual *count*. Several other laboratories have confirmed these results (CHUNGPANICH and SMITH 1989; PICH et al. 1992; CHATTOPADHYAY et al. 1994).

Many studies on oral squamous cell carcinomas have reported on the measurement of DNA content (ploidy status) by FCM. The biological rationale behind the measurement of nuclear ploidy is that deviation from normal nuclear complement of DNA is likely to reflect cellular aberration and resistance to growth control (MILLER 1992). The ploidy status of oral and head and neck carcinomas has been examined rather extensively (Table 3). Close to 50% of oral and head and neck cancers have aneuploid DNA patterns. A higher percentage of aneuploid tumours are noted in oral cavity and tongue cancers compared to lip cancers (STEINBECK et al. 1993). Aneuploidy appears to be associated with less well differentiated tumours (TYTOR et al. 1987; SUZUKI et al. 1994) and more advanced clinical stages, including lymph node metastasis (TYTOR et al. 1987; BALSARA et al. 1994; SUZUKI et al. 1994).

Examining the ploidy status, CHEN et al. (1993) confirmed that the incidence of lymph node metastasis in the aneuploid tumours (70%) was significantly higher than for diploid tumours (24%). A comparison of the ploidy status of primary and metastatic squamous cell carcinomas (SUZUKI et al. 1994) revealed that most metastatic lymph nodes were in fact diploid. This may suggest that a primary neoplasm may have increased incidence of aneuploidy with the increase in size of the tumour, but that diploid cells rather than aneuploid cells are responsible for causing lymph node metastasis.

Table 3. Ploidy states and potential doubling time (t_{pot}) in oral and head and neck carcinomas by flow cytometry (FCM)

Reference	Carcinomas (n)	Aneuploid (%)	t_{pot} (days)
WILSON et al. 1988	9	–	6.2 ± 2.7[b]
FORSTER et al. 1992	82	63	6.2
NYLANDER et al. 1994	31	65	4.6
VAN HEERDEN et al. 1995	50	44	–
SICKLE-SANTANELLO et al. 1986	15	66	–
TYTOR et al. 1987	88	48	–
GOLDSMITH et al. 1987	48	48	–
BENNETT et al. 1992	123	41	1.8–41.2
LOCHRIN et al. 1992	38	–	3.9
BOURHIS et al. 1994a	49	59	5.07
WILSON et al. 1995	99	49	3.9
SUZUKI et al. 1994	41	39	–
BALSARA et al. 1994	68	42[a]	–
BENAZZO et al. 1995	52	20	5.7

[a] Includes tetraploid tumours.
[b] Estimated from author's own data.

Recent FCM studies also attempt to estimate the potential doubling times (t_{pot}). Mean t_{pot} values recorded by FCM in six studies on head and neck carcinomas range from 4 to 6 days (Table 3), but a wide range is reported for individual tumours: 1.8–41.2 days by BENNETT et al. (1992) and 1.3–12.2 days by NYLANDER et al. (1994a). Aneuploid tumours have shorter median t_{pot} values and higher LI indices than diploid tumours (BOURHIS et al. 1994a; NYLANDER et al. 1994a). Proposals for combining these three variables in prognostication is discussed in Sect. 4.1.2.

4.1.2 Prognosis

At present most institutions use a range of static descriptors of the primary neoplasm (JONES 1994; BRYNE et al. 1991), as well as a range of host factors, in determining the prognosis and treatment plan for patients with oral carcinoma (JOHNSON et al. 1996). However, in order to obtain a better approximation of biological potential, the morphological grade should be supplemented by functional attributes, such as proliferation markers. Contrary to this observation, JOHNSON (1976), employing a multifactorial analysis based on 39 different histological features on 100 cases of oral carcinomas, found many of the variables, including the degree of mitotic activity, had little or no prognostic value. The reason for expecting that features of cellular proliferation will be useful in prognosis is that they reflect the rate of tumour growth. The faster the velocity of the tumour, the quicker it will spread (EVANS et al. 1982).

LI derived from [³H]dT/BrdUrd or from immune labelling have value in predicting the short-term clinical response to radiotherapy (SILVESTRINI et al. 1984; GÜNZL et al. 1993) and chemotherapy (MOLINARI et al. 1991); this is not surprising, as rapidly dividing cells are more vulnerable to the effects of ionising radiation or cytotoxic agents. BETTINGER et al. (1991) and BOURHIS et al. (1994b) used kinetic methods to assess success or failure of induction chemotherapy in head and neck squamous cell carcinomas. Rapid cell proliferation was noted among patients who had responded poorly to therapy. Immune markers have not been examined in large-scale retrospective or prospective studies to determine their value in relation to recurrence rates or survival times. Two recent studies of PC10 and Ki-67 indices did not find the data useful as predictors of lymph node metastasis or of survival (JONES et al. 1994; ROLAND et al. 1994). Contradicting results were reported by STÖRKEL et al. (1993) and GIROD et al. (1995). SANO et al. (1991), who examined the prognostic implication of AgNOR enumeration in 39 patients with oral carcinoma, showed that the 5-year survival rate of patients with high AgNOR (>6.5) was 38% and significantly lower than the group with an AgNOR count of less than 6.5 (5-year survival rate, 67%). PICH et al. (1992) also claim that a lower mean AgNOR count per nucleus may reflect an improved survival.

KEARSLEY and THOMAS (1993), examining a range of potential proliferation markers, showed ploidy status to be of value in head and neck cancer; their review suggests that patients with aneuploid tumours had substantially worse prognosis. Aneuploid tumours are also known to have a shorter t_{pot} than diploid tumours (FORSTER et al. 1992) and, as observed above, because t_{pot} measures the velocity of tumour growth, it is likely to prove valuable in predicting both relapse and survival. A complete response reported for many tumours with a long t_{pot} (>7.0 days) by NYLANDER et al. (1994) provides some promise for future studies. Many small retrospective studies have yielded inconsistent results, and larger prospective studies are needed to validate the proliferation markers developed so far. A subset of oral squamous cell carcinomas characterised by an LI greater than 15%, , DNA aneuploidy and a t_{pot} of less than 5 days may benefit from more aggressive therapies, such as accelerated regimes of radiotherapy and/or other multimodal therapies compared to slow-growing tumours (LI, <15%; t_{pot}, >5 days) showing DNA diploidy. Further multicentric studies are needed to test kinetic parameters which – either alone or in combination – may provide useful and accurate prognostic information. The cell kinetics data used for treatment planning should also be subjected to external quality assessment in one central laboratory.

It is also worth reiterating that a true understanding requires concomitant measures of apoptosis and of a large number of host response variables, together with absence or continuous presence of aetiological agents, notably tobacco and alcohol use.

4.2 Potentially Malignant Lesions

4.2.1 Leukoplakia

There is considerable interest in the characterisation of cellular and molecular markers that may actually predict which potentially malignant lesions of the oral cavity may, with time, transform to cancer (BURKHARDT 1985; JOHNSON et al. 1993, 1996). Although the majority of proliferating cells in a keratinising epithelium may contribute little, if any, to the process of malignant transformation in vivo (HUME 1981) most, but not all, "precancerous" lesions and conditions are associated with periods of increased cell proliferation (IVERSON 1992). Some of the histological features commonly recognised as components of oral epithelial dysplasia (SMITH and PINDBORG 1969) relate to the proliferation state of the tissue. Mitotic index is reported to be higher in parakeratotic than in orthokeratotic oral lesions (RENSTRUP 1963; MAIN 1965; EL-LABBAN et al. 1971); the former metaplastic variety of keratosis is more often associated with malignant potential, suggesting that increased cell proliferation may indirectly have a role in transformation to cancer. Kramer's group, in a discriminant analysis of histological features of oral dysplasia, recognised three factors as important determinants of subsequent malignant transformation (KRAMER et al. 1970): (1) presence of abnormal mitoses, (2) increased mitotic activity and (3) mitosis in superficial layers of the epithelium (Fig. 1). Regrettably, long-term, follow-up studies of oral leukoplakia concerning "histopathological risk markers" are scarce.

During the 1970s, a few studies attempted to determine the LI of oral leukoplakia by in vitro incorporation of $[^3H]dT$. Available data on the cell proliferation status of leukoplakias compared to control tissues are shown in Table 4. Although the criteria used for the selection of leukoplakias and the methods of determining reference indices are likely to be different in these various studies, there is an interesting small, but significant rise of LI in leukoplakia specimens compared to normal tissues. A shift in labelling of proliferative cells from the suprabasal to the basal compartment was reported in leukoplakias by MAIDHOF and HORNSTEIN (1979). This was confirmed by WARNAKULASURIYA and MACDONALD (1995b), who showed that the rise in LI was related to an increase in the proportion of the cells in the basal cell layer engaged in cell production. In one of these studies (WARNAKULASURIYA 1976), in vitro double labelling showed that the time spent by cells in S phase (t_s) is not significantly altered in leukoplakia. The LI itself was, therefore, regarded as a sufficient indicator of cell proliferation. The observation by WARNAKULASURIYA and MACDONALD (1995b) that the ranking of LI in leukoplakia specimens correlated (r, 0.50; p = 0.019) with the severity of epithelial dysplasia scored by the method of SMITH and PINDBORG (1969) lends support to the importance of individual features classically assumed to indicate

Table 4. Labelling indices of oral leukoplakia and normal mucosa

Reference	Reference index	Labelling index (%)		Lesion to control ratio	p value
		Leukoplakia	Controls		
ALVARES et al. 1972	LC/TNC	4.75	2.72	1.75	<0.01
WARNAKULASURIYA 1976	LC/TNC	6.01	3.39	1.77	<0.005
MAIDHOF and HORNSTEIN 1979	LC/BC	6.62	5.53	1.20	<0.01
CRISCUOLO et al. 1989	LC/TNC	5.3	2.6	2.0	<0.004

LC/TNC, labelled cells per 100 total nucleated cells; LC/BC, labelled cells per 100 basal cells.

proliferation state in histology grading systems. Conversely, LI as determined by [³H]dT may prove to be an important objective criterion to assess the probability/ risk of transformation to cancer.

STEINBECK et al. (1993) observed that PCNA immunoreactivity in basal cell layers of oral precancerous lesions increased with increasing grade of dysplasia. Mean PCNA LI values recorded in their study were as follows: normal, 17%; mild, 49%; moderate, 54%; and severe dysplastia, 73%. With increase in severity of dysplasia grade, PCNA-immunoreactive cells increased in number in the basal cell layer. In severe dysplasia, however, PCNA-positive cells were abundant in superficial cell layers. No follow-up information was given on these oral lesions, so the predictive value of the kinetic indices remain unknown. Cell proliferation detected by PCNA LI is also reported to be increased in *Candida*-associated leukoplakia (WARNAKULASURIYA et al. 1994). The mean PC10 count in this study for the *Candida* group was 33.8% ± 12.2% compared to 23.6% ± 14.4% in control leukoplakia samples ($p = 0.057$). Whether this rise in LI in the *Candida*-associated lesions was caused by factors released by the organisms or cytokines from the immune/inflammatory responses is unknown, but both are certain to be involved, directly or indirectly.

AgNOR enumeration, commonly used for neoplastic discrimination (see Sect. 4.1.1), has also been applied to oral precancer by several groups. Leukoplakia lesions with histologically defined dysplasia have been shown to have a higher mean AgNOR count per nucleus compared to normal mucosa or simple keratoses (WARNAKULASURIYA and JOHNSON 1993b; CHATTOPADHYAY et al. 1994). The range of the scatter of the AgNOR values is, however, too wide for this information to be of any potential value in detecting oral leukoplakia with poor prognosis. RAJENDRAN and NAIR (1992), applying the AgNOR technique to oral submucous fibrosis (OSF) cases from India, reported a two- to threefold increase of AgNOR numbers in the OSF epithelium compared to normal mucosa. This is surprising, since moderate and advanced OSF cases included in their study demonstrate marked epithelial atrophy compared to normal controls.

DNPA ploidy status of oral leukoplakia has been examined by FCM to a limited degree. GRÄSSEL-PIETRUSKY et al. (1982), SAITO et al. (1991) and KAHN et al. (1992), utilising small sample sizes, described aneuploidy in eight out of 24, two out of 11 and six out of 19 leukoplakia lesions, respectively. All these studies provide examples of aneuploidy being more frequently observed in severely dysplastic lesions than in simple keratoses. Further studies are needed to clarify whether determination of ploidy status has a value in diagnosis of more serious lesions and in predicting likelihood of malignant transformation.

4.2.2 Lichen Planus

Malignant development in oral lichen planus is reported. This, however, is a very rare event (see D.M. WILLIAMS, this volume) but full assessment of subjects at risk is of considerable value in clinical practice. Oral lesions with "lichenoid dysplasia" have been reported, but follow-up information on these is very meagre. Few attempts have been made to characterise cell kinetics of oral lichen planus. WALKER and DOLBY (1974), examining the in vitro [³H]dT labelling indices of 17 lichen planus lesions compared to normal controls ($n = 10$), reported a significant rise in basal LI in both atrophic and acanthotic lesions. No differences were found when the LI was plotted by the total cell count of the epithelium. A more recent study of oral lichen planus has confirmed this shift of proliferation to the basal compartment (SARDELLA et al. 1991). This may reflect the loss or liquefaction of non-dividing basal cells. Basal cell proliferation, on the other hand, may be induced by cytokines derived from the immune inflammatory response at and below the basement membrane. More work is needed to understand the implications of these preliminary findings.

4.3 Salivary Neoplasms

Malignant salivary gland neoplasms are rare, consitute a heterogenous group and are often difficult to diagnose histologically. Immunohistochemical methods that are useful in diagnosis of malignant salivary gland tumours were reviewed by SEIFERT (1992). AgNOR enumeration in salivary neoplasms has been reported by many authors to be of potential diagnostic value (Table 5). The differences between mean NOR counts in malignant salivary neoplasms (×4.5) and benign adenomas (×1.5) is about two- to threefold in most studies (KAMATH and SASTRY 1994). LANDINI (1990), examining NOR in pleomorphic adenomas, reported that cells in solid/ductal areas had a higher NOR count than chrondroid cells. Application of AgNOR enumeration to examine its potential value in determining prognosis of muco-epidermoid carcinoma was described by CHOMETTE et al. (1991). AgNOR in 15 cases with poor prognosis (fatal outcome or early recurrence and/or metastasis) were 2.8–6.2 per nucleus compared to 1.0–3.6 per nucleus in a group with good prognosis (no recurrence in 5 years). The AgNOR count seemed better than histological criteria for establishing the prognosis of muco-epidermoid tumours.

Application of other methods to investigate cell proliferation has been meagre. Poliferative activity of pleomorphic adenomas and myo-epitheliomas were compared by PCNA labelling and no significant differences were reported, suggesting that the method has no potential value in discrimination (OGAWA et al. 1993). Not surprisingly, marked differences in PCNA index were shown between carcinomas in expleomorphic adenomas (22.9 ± 6.2) and pleomorphic adenoma (6.9 ± 3.4) by YANG et al. (1994). Using Ki-67 antibody on six malignant salivary tumours, MURAKAMI et al. (1992) demonstrated a high proliferation status (18.3% cells positive compared to 4.7% in normal salivary gland tissue).

An FCM study on a series of muco-epidermoid, acinic and adenoid cystic carcinomas revealed very few aneuploid DNA stem-lines; when present, this feature was seen largely in undifferentiated carcinomas. The survival time of these patients with aneuploid tumours was considerably reduced compared to those with diploid tumours (BANG et al. 1994).

A cytophotometric analysis of DNA to assess the aggressiveness of adenoid cystic carcinomas of salivary and lacrimal glands revealed that the method is useful to define the ploidy status. Tumours with diploid histograms had the longest survival, and those with aneuploidy had the worst prognosis (HAMPER et al. 1990).

Table 5. Mean argyrophilic nucleolar organisation region (AgNOR) counts per nucleus in salivary neoplasms

Histology	Mean AgNOR values					
	Morgan et al. (1988)	Van Heerden and Raubenheima (1991)	Matsumura et al. (1989)	Cardillo (1991)	Chomette et al. (1991)[a]	Landini (1990)[b]
Pleomorphic adenoma	1.47	1.52	1.62–1.68	1.67	–	1.30–2.06
Clear cell adenoma	–	–	1.47	–	–	–
Warthin's tumour	–	–	1.72	–	–	–
Adenocystic carcinoma	3.93	2.83	2.78	3.38	–	–
Adenocarcinoma	–	–	2.25	2.07	–	–
Mucoepidermoid carcinoma	4.25	1.93	2.59	–	1.0–3.6 2.8–6.2	–
Squamous cell carcinoma	–	–	–	4.31	–	–
Carcinoma (originally pleomorphic adenoma)	–	–	–	4.87	–	6.05

[a] 16 cases with poor prognosis and 15 cases with good prognosis.
[b] Range shown is for chondroid versus solid/ductal areas in pleomorphic adenoma.

4.4 Jaw Lesions

Following Toller's original description of high rates of epithelial proliferation in the lining of odontogenic keratocysts (TOLLER 1971), immunohistochemical markers have recently been applied to this issue. Using immunohistochemistry, LI et al. (1994) demonstrated that PCNA-positive cells were mostly located in the suprabasal layers of odontogenic keratocysts (OKC), with less than 5% labelled cells distributed in the basal layers. OKC also had a much higher LI (in some instances of the order of ten- to 20-fold) compared to radicular or dentigerous cysts. Greater proliferative activity of OKC is in accord with their aggressive clinical behaviour. Subsequent studies by the same group using Ki-67 antibody showed that LI in simple and recurrent OKC were not different. OKC associated with basal cell naevus syndrome, however, had a markedly elevated Ki-67 index. Jaw cysts associated with the syndrome had a LI which was nearly twice that of single or recurrent OKC. The Ki-67 method does not appear to allow detection of a subgroup of OKC which are more likely to recur, and it was concluded that recurrence following surgery may be linked to incomplete excision rather than any differences attributable to intrinsic biological behaviour of such cysts. Significant differences in proliferative indices in different cyst types have now been confirmed by other studies (LOMBARDI and MORGAN 1994; SLOOTWEG 1995). Comparing the published data on odontogenic cyst linings (LI et al. 1994) with PCNA LI derived for unicystic ameloblastoma, it was shown that the latter group contained significantly more PCNA cells (LI et al. 1995b). This study also demonstrated significant differences in the proportions of labelled cells between unicystic and solid ameloblastomas and between unicystic lesions with and without invading tumour islands. These differences in proliferative capacity may explain the differences in behaviour between ameloblastomas that are basically cystic and those which, in addition, contain tumour islands invading the fibrous wall and which are known to have a greater potential to recur.

The other pathological entity among jaw lesions which has received some attention is the giant cell lesion. WHITAKER et al. (1993) applied AgNOR techniques to differentiate aggressive/recurrent lesions and reported significant differences in mean AgNOR counts in both mononuclear and multinucleate cell populations of clinically aggressive/recurrent compared to non-aggressive lesions. Close examination of these data shows that most of the mean AgNOR counts derived fall between one and two dots per nucleus for all groups of lesions and are therefore unlikely to be of practical diagnostic value.

5 Interaction of Cell Proliferation Assessment with Oncogenes and Tumour Suppressor Genes that Control the Cell Cycle

The relatively uncontrolled proliferation that characterises neoplastic cell populations is now recognised to result from specific gene mutations, amplifications or losses. It has recently been suggested that *all* human neoplasms have aberrations of one or more cell cycle genes (CLURMAN and ROBERTS 1995). Activation of several proto-oncogenes and the overproduction of growth factors and their receptors (e.g. *ras*, PRAD-1, *c-myc*, EGF/*c-erbB*) may result in persistent mitogenic signalling or, conversely, loss of tumour suppressor genes (e.g. *p53*, *Rb*) may result in a cell becoming less responsive to negative growth factors. The genes which control mitosis and apoptosis in oral squamous cell carcinoma were reviewed by SCULLY (1993), SUGERMAN et al. (1995) and JOHNSON et al. (1996). Lack of control of these molecular mechanisms are the fundamental stigmata of the malignant phenotype. In this section, we briefly review the current knowledge on associations of proliferation markers and oncogene/tumour suppressor gene alterations in oral and salivary neoplasms.

It has been proposed that the autocrine production of growth factors is an essential element of tumourigenesis (PUSZTAI et al. 1993). EGFR is a transmembrane glycoprotein (Fig. 6) whose expression is important in the growth regulation of many neoplasms, particularly in breast cancer, where in some studies it is suggested to be a significant and independent indicator of a likely recurrence (GASPARINI et al. 1992). Strong EGFR expression in oral squamous cell carcinoma has been associated with a comparatively short survival time (STÖRKEL et al. 1993), and this group recommend it as a valuable tool in estimating the patient's prognosis. The amplification of an associated proto-oncogene, *c-erbB*, has been linked to carcinogenesis in the hamster cheek pouch, with the amplified product being expressed at the time of early invasion and increasing in parallel with the increased

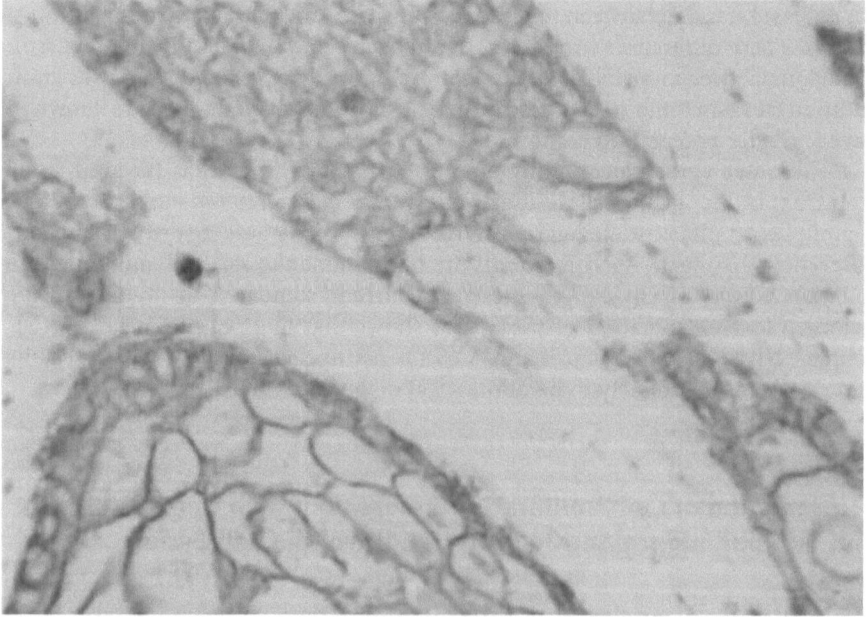

Fig. 6. Epidermal growth factor receptor (EGFR) staining in oral squamous cell carcinoma (SCC). The immunoreactivity is strong and mostly membranous. ×990

tumour burden (WONG and BISWAS 1987). The c-erb2 oncoprotein is known to be infrequently expressed in salivary gland tumours (KERNOHAN et al. 1991) and was reported to be confined to malignant cells of carcinoma of expleomorphic adenoma (SHRESTHA et al. 1992). When present, c-erb2 amplification may be associated with more aggressive tumour behaviour (BIREK et al. 1994).

The G_1 to S phase and also G_2 to M transitions require prior synthesis and accumulation of cyclins to critical threshold levels. There are at least eight distinct cyclin genes in the mammalian genome (HUNTER 1993). Of these, the cyclin D1 (PRAD-1) gene is shown consistently to be amplified in many human tumours (HINDS et al. 1994). Overexpression of D-type cyclins was recently described in 25 out of 52 human head and neck carcinomas (48%; BARTKOVA et al. 1995) using a monoclonal antibody (DCS6) on archival specimens. These authors' observations on antibody-mediated neutralisation of cyclin D1 and D2 in five head and neck squamous cell carcinoma cell lines has provided evidence for the cooperative roles played by cyclin D1 and D2 in persistent regulation of G_1/S entry. Although there is no proof that this effect, when stimulated, is causal in squamous cell carcinoma, comparative analysis of cell cycle markers and D-type cyclin expression may further explain the G_1 dysregulation in cancers of the oral/head and neck region. Such dual assessment may, perhaps, allow us to identify a subset of neoplasms that are rapidly and uncontrollably proliferating and, therefore, aggressive in nature.

Expression of c-myc is rapidly induced by a variety of growth factors, and this is critical in deciding whether a cell is to grow or die in response to external stimuli (HUNTER 1993; IVAN and LITTLEWOOD 1993). Although it has been shown that c-myc alone may drive quiescent cells into the cell cycle, few data exist to prove any variation in the level of c-myc in continuously growing cells. In oral squamous cell carcinoma, c-myc expression may indicate poor prognosis (FIELD et al. 1989). Nuclear labelling of c-myc has been shown to reflect progressive histological changes in pre-cancer and early cancerous lesions of the oral cavity (EVERSOLE and SAPP 1993).

Wild-type p53 is a growth suppressor protein, the expression of which inhibits the growth of both normal and transformed cells. The p53 checkpoint controls entry to S phase by cells containing damaged DNA. Delaying S-phase entry allows the cell time to repair DNA damage in an extended G_1 phase, thereby avoiding propogation of permanent genetic damage. Overexpression of p53 protein (presumptively mutated or otherwise inactivated) has been reported in 11%–80% of oral squamous cell carcinoma. Three recent studies have examined the relationship of overexpression of p53 oncoprotein with the state of cell proliferation in oral carcinoma (WARNAKULASURIYA and JOHNSON 1994; SLOOTWEG et al. 1994; BOURHIS et al. 1994a). Cell proliferation was found to be significantly higher in p53-positive neoplasms. WARNAKULASURIYA and JOHNSON (1994) argue that inactivated p53 probably confers a growth advantage to the p53-positive neoplasms. It has emerged that the p53 protein is a sequence-specific DNA-binding protein that can activate or repress transcription of other genes such as p16/waf-1 which participate in the cell cycle. Deactivation of p53 by mutation or deletion may therefore, through complex molecular pathways, result in blocking apoptosis and allow cell proliferation to proceed unabated, a change also necessary for malignant transformation (SUGERMAN et al. 1995). Overexpression of p53, now known to be a hallmark of neoplasia and for which detection systems are routine in many laboratories, may itself reflect the cell proliferation status because of its close interaction with cell proliferation/apoptosis balance.

6 Conclusions

The methods commonly employed for the assessment of cell proliferation have been critically considered. As interest in the assessment of proliferative activity has grown, so has the number of techniques devised to extract proliferation-related information from processed tissues. The availability of monoclonal and polyclonal antibodies for immunohistochemical detection of antigens related to the cell cycle – particularly Ki-67 and PCNA – have opened up new possibilities with fixed tissues, obviating the need for in vivo and in vitro pulse labelling. Oral pathology laboratories need to utilise these tools, particularly to facilitate staging and grading of oral lesions, so that objective assessments can be introduced in defining lesions at risk.

The pathological assessment, i.e. malignant grading, of oral squamous cell carcinoma has remained unchanged for decades. The measurement of cellular DNA content by FCM is emerging as a prognostic aid in many human tumours. The value of FCM in diagnosis and prognosis of oral cancer needs clarification. Prospective clinical trials are needed to examine the usefulness of combinations of cell kinetic markers (e.g. LI, ploidy and t_{pot}) in prognostication and in the choice of the most effective therapy for the individual patient.

Acknowledgements. We thank Mrs Linda Fleming for typing the manusript and also Miss Katherine Paterson and Mr Robert Harely for assistance with the illustrations. K.A.A.S. Warnakulasuriya is supported by the Dunhill Medical Trust.

References

Aherne WA, Dunhill MS (1982) Morphometry. Arnold, London, pp 46–59
Aherne WA, Camplejohn RS, Al-Wiswazy M, Ford D, Kellerer M (1977) Assessment of inherent fluctuations of mitotic and labelling indices of human tumours. Br J Cancer 36: 577–591
Alcalde RE, Shintani S, Yoshihama Y, Matsumura T (1995) Cell proliferation and tumor angiogenesis in oral squamous cell carcinoma. Anticancer Res 15: 1417–1422
Alvares O, Skougaard MR, Pindborg JJ, Roed-Petersen B (1972) In vitro incorporation of tritiated thymidine in oral homogeneous leukoplakias. Scand J dent Res 80: 510–514
Baak JPA (1990) Mitosis counting in tumours. Hum Pathol 21: 683–685
Baak JPA, van Dep H, Kurver PHJ, Hermans J (1985) The value of morphometry to classic prognosticators in breast cancer. Cancer 56: 374–382
Baak JPA, Wise-Brekelmans ECM, Langley FA, Talerman A, Delamarre JFM (1986) Morphometric data to FIGO stage and histological type and grade for prognosis of ovarian tumours. J Clin Pathol 39: 1340–1346

Balsara BR, Borges AM, Pradhan SA, Rajpal RM, Bhisey AN (1994) Flow cytometric DNA analysis of squamous cell carcinomas of the oral cavity: correlation with clinical and histopathological features. Oral Oncol Eur J Cancer 30: 98–101

Bang G, Donath K, Thoresen S, Clausen OP (1994) DNA flow cytometry of reclassified subtypes of malignant salivary gland tumors. J Oral Pathol Med 23: 291–297

Barnes DM, Gillett CE (1995) Determination of cell proliferation. J Clin Pathol Mol Pathol 48: M2–M5

Bartkova J, Lukas J, Müller H, Strauss M, Gusterson B, Bartek J (1995) Abnormal patterns of D-type cyclin expression and G_1 regulation in human head and neck cancer. Cancer Res 55: 949–956

Begg AC, McNally NJ, Shrieve DC, Karcher H (1985) A method to measure the duration of DNA synthesis and the potential doubling time from a single sample. Cytometry 6: 620

Benazzo M, Mevio E, Occhini A, Franchini G, Danova M (1995) Proliferative characteristics of head and neck tumors. In vivo evaluation by bromodeoxyuridine incorporation and flow cytometry. J Otorhinolaryngol Relat Spec 57: 39–43

Bennett MH, Wilson GD, Dische S, Saunders MI, Martindale CA, Robinson BM, O'Halloran AE, Leslie MD, Laing JHE (1992) Tumour proliferation assessed by combined histological and flow cytometric analysis: implications for therapy in squamous cell carcinoma in the head and neck. Br J Cancer 65: 870–878

Berlingin E, Heenen M, Galand P (1992) Measurement of S phase duration in human epidermis using cyclin immunostaining and ³H-thymidine pulse labelling. Arch Dermatol Res 284: 238–241

Bettinger R, Loerz M, Meyer-Breiting E (1991) Proliferative activity following induction chemotherapy in squamous cell carcinoma of the head and neck. A histopathological and immunohistochemical study using monoclonal antibodies. Eur Arch Otorhinolaryngol 248: 236–241

Birck C, Lui E, Jordan RCK, Dardick I (1994) Analysis of c-erbB-2 amplification in salivary gland tumours by differential polymerase chain reaction. Oral Oncol Eur J Cancer 30: 47–50

Bourhis J, Bosq J, Wilson GD, Bressac B, Talbot M, Leridant AM, Dendale R, Janin N, Armand JP, Luboinski B, Malaise EP, Wibault P, Eschwege F (1994a) Correlation between p53 gene expression and tumor-cell proliferation in orophayngeal cancer. Int J Cancer 57: 458–462

Bourhis J, Wilson G, Wibault P, Janot F, Bosq J, Armand JP, Luboinski B, Malaise EP, Eschwege F (1994b) Rapid tumor cell proliferation after induction chemotherapy in oropharyngeal cancer. Laryngoscope 104: 468–472

Bravo R, MacDonald-Bravo H (1985) Changes in the nuclear distribution of cyclin (PCNA) but not its synthesis depend upon DNA replication. EMBO J 4: 655–661

Bresciani F, Paoluzi R, Benassi M, Nervi C, Casale C, Ziparo E (1974) Cell kinetics and growth of squamous cell carcinomas in man. Cancer Res 34: 2405–2415

Britto MJ, Filipe MI, Morris RW (1992) Cell proliferation study on gastric carcinoma and non involved gastric mucosa using bromodeoxyuridine (Brd U) labelling technique. Eur J Can Prev 1: 429–435

Browman GP, Kanclerz A, Booker L, Daya D, Archibald SD, Young JEM, Goldsmith CH (1991) Optimal concentration for immunohistochemical determination of the in vitro DNA synthesis labelling index with bromodeoxyuridine in head and neck cancer. Cell Prolif 24: 579–585

Bryne M, Nielsen K, Koppang HS, Dabelsteen E (1991) Reproducibility of two malignancy grading systems with reportedly prognostic value for oral cancer patients. J Oral Pathol Med 20: 369–372

Burkhardt A (1985) Advanced methods in the evaluation of premalignant lesions and carcinomas of the oral mucosa. J Oral Pathol 14: 751–778

Cabrini RL, Schwint AE, Mendex A, Femopase F, Lanfranchi H, Itoiz ME (1992) Morphometric study of nucleolar organizer regions in human oral normal mucosa, papilloma and squamous cell carcinoma. J Oral Pathol Med 21: 275–279

Cardillo MR (1991) Ag-NOR technique in fine needle aspiration cytology of salivary gland masses. Acta Cytol 36: 147–151

Cattoretti G, Becker MHG, Key G, Duchrow M, Schulter C, Galle J, Gerdes J (1992) Monoclonal antibodies against recombinant parts of the Ki-67 antigen (MIB1 and MIB3) detect proliferating cells in microwave processed formalin-fixed paraffin sections. J Pathol 168: 357–363

Chattopadhyay A, Chawda JG, Doshi JJ (1994) Silver-binding nucleolar organizing regions: a study of oral leukoplakia and squamous cell carcinoma. Int J Oral Maxillofac Surg 23: 374–377

Chauvel P, Courdi A, Gioanni J, Vallicioni J, Santini J, Demard F (1989) The labelling index: a prognostic factor in head and neck carcinoma. Radiother Oncol 14: 231–237

Chen RB, Suzuki K, Nomura T, Nakajima T (1993) Flow cytometric analysis of squamous cell carcinomas of the oral cavity in relation to lymphnode metastasis. J Oral Maxillofax Surg 51: 397–401

Chomette GP, Auriol MM, Labrousee F, Vaillant JM (1991) Mucoepidermoid tumors of salivary glands: histoprognostic value of NORs stained with AgNOR technique. J Oral Pathol Med 20: 130–132

Chungpanich S, Smith CJ (1989) Nucleolar organizer regions (NORs) in hyperplastic lesions and squamous cell carcinomas of the oral mucosa. J Dent Res 68: 579

Clurman BE, Roberts JM (1995) Cell cycle and cancer. J Nat Cancer Inst 87: 1499–1501

Collan Y, Kunpusalo L, Pesonen E, Eskelinen M, Pajarinen P, Kettumen K (1988) Prediction of prognosis of breast cancer: multivariate analysis of mitotic index, lymph node status and tumour size. Acta Clinic Med 174: 8 (abstract)

Criscuolo M, Malagoli G, Falchi AM, Ancora M, Ancora R, De Pol A (1989) Kinetic features of the oral cavity epithelium in leukoplakia. Cell Tissue Kinet 22: 137

Crocker J, Boldy DAR, Egan MJ (1989) How should we count AgNOR's? Proposals for a standardized approach. J Pathol 158: 185–188

Cross SS, Start RD, Smith JHF (1990) Does delay in fixation affect the number of mitotic figures in processed tissue. J Clin Pathol 43: 597–599

Egan MJ, Crocker J (1992) Nucleolar organiser regions in pathology. Br J Cancer 65: 1–7

El-Labban N, Lucas RB, Kramer IRH (1971) The mitotic values for the epithelium in oral keratoses and lichen planus. Br J Cancer 25: 411–416

Ellis SJ, Whitehead R (1981) Mitoses counting: a need for reappraisal. Hum Pathol 12: 3–4

Evans SJ, Langdon JD, Rapidis AD, Johnson NW (1982) Prognostic significance of STNMP and velocity of tumor growth in oral cancer. Cancer 49: 773–776

Eversole LR, Sapp JP (1993) c-myc oncoprotein expression in oral precancerous and early cancerous lesions. Oral Oncol Eur J Cancer 29: 131–136

Field JK, Spandidos DA, Stell PM, Vaughan ED, Evan GI, Moore JP (1989) Elevated expression of the c-myc oncoprotein correlates with poor prognosis in head and neck squamous cell carcinoma. Oncogene 4: 1463–1468

Forster G, Cooke TG, Cooke LD, Stanton PD, Bowie G, Stell PM (1992) Tumour growth rates in squamous carcinoma of the head and neck measured by in vivo bromodeoxyuridine incorporation and flow cytometry. Br J Cancer 65: 698–702

Galand P, Degraef C (1989) Cyclin/PCNA immunostaining as an alterative to tritiated thymidine pulse labelling for marking S phase cells in paraffin sections from animal and human tissues. Cell Tissue Kinet 22: 383–392

Gasparini G, Gullick WJ, Bevilacqua P, Sainsbury JRC, Meli S, Boracchi P, Testolin A, La Malfa G, Pozza F (1992) Human breast cancer: prognostic significance of the c-erbB-2 oncoprotien compared with epidermal growth factor receptor, DNA ploidy, and conventional pathologic features. J Clin Oncol 10: 686–695

Gee JMW, Douglas-Jones A, Hepburn P, Sharma AK, McClelland RA, Ellis IO, Nicholson RI (1995) A cautionary note regarding the application of Ki-67 antibodies to paraffin-embedded breast cancers. J Pathol 177: 285–293

Gerdes J, Levike H, Baisch H, Walker HH, Schwab V, Stein H (1984) Cell cycle analysis of a cell proliferation associated human nuclear antigen defined by the monoclonal antibody Ki67. J Immunol 133: 1710–1715

Gillett CE, Smith P, Camplejohn RS, Mills RR (1993) Mitotic activity index – a useful marker of prognosis in breast carcinoma. J Pathol 169: 199 (abstract)

Girod SC, Pape HD, Krueger GRF (1994) p53 and PCNA expression in carcinogenesis of the oropharyngeal mucosa. Oral Oncol Eur J Cancer 30: 419–423

Girod SC, Leitner I, Fischer U, Junk M, Krueger GRF (1995) p53 overexpression and cell proliferation as prognostic markers in oral cancer. In: Varma AK, Mori M (eds) Oral oncology, vol IVB. Macmillan India, pp 3–7.

Goldsmith MM, Gresson DH, Arnold LA, Postma DS, Askin FB, Pillsbury HC (1987) DNA flow cytometry as a prognostic indicator in head and neck cancer. Otolaryngol Head Neck Surg 96: 307–318

Grässel-Pietrusky R, Deinlein E, Hornstein OP (1982) DNA-ploidy rates in oral leukoplakias determined by flow-cytometry. J Oral Pathol 11: 434–438

Gratzner HG (1982) Monoclonal antibody to 5-bromo- and 5-iododeoxyuridine: a new reagent for detection of DNA replication. Science 218: 474–475

Günzl HJ, Horn H, Schücke R, Donath K (1993) Prognostic value of PCNA and cytokeratins for radiation therapy of oral squamous cell carcinoma. Oral Oncol Eur J Cancer 29B: 141–145

Haapasalo H, Collen Y, Atkin NB, Pesonen E, Seppa A (1989) Prognosis of ovarian carcinomas: prediction of histo quantitative methods. Histopathology 15: 167–168

Hall PA, Levison DA (1990) Assessment of cell proliferation in histological material. J Clin Pathol 43: 184–192

Hall PA, Woods AL (1990) Immunohistochemical markers of cellular proliferation: achievements, problems and prospects. Cell Tissue Kinet 23: 505–522

Hall PA, Levison DA, Woods AL, Yu CCW, Kellock DB, Watkins JA, Barnes DM, Gillet GE, Camplejohn R, Dover R, Waseman NH, Lane DP (1990) Proliferating cell nuclear antigen (PCNA) immunologicalization in paraffin sections: an index of cell proliferation with evidence of deregulated expression in some neoplasms. J Pathol 162: 285–294

Hall PA, Hart I, Goodlad R, Coates PJ, Lane DP (1992) Expression of proliferating cell nuclear antigen in non-cycling cells. J Pathol 168: 97A (abstract)

Hamilton PW, Allen DC (1995) Morphometry in histology. J Pathol 175: 369–379

Hamper K, Lazar F, Dietel M, Caslitz J, Berger J, Arps H, Falkmer U, Auer G, Seifert G (1990) Prognostic factors for adenoid carcinoma of the head and neck: a retrospective evaluation of 96 cases. J Oral Pathol Med 19: 101–107

Hedley DW, Friedlander ML, Taylor IW, Rugg CA, Musgrove EA (1983) Method for analysis of cellular DNA content of paraffin-embedded pathological material using flow cytometry. J Histochem Cytochem 31: 1333–1335

Hemmer J (1990) In vitro bromodeoxyuridine labelling of squamous cell carcinomas of the oral cavity. Eur J Cancer 26: 113–115

Hinds PW, Dowdy SF, Eaton EN, Arnold A, Weinberg RA (1994) Function of a human cyclin gene as an oncogene. Proc Natl Acad Sci USA 91: 709–713

Hoyer M, Bentzen SM, Salling LN, Overgaard J (1994) Influence of sampling time on assessment of potential doubling time. Cytometry 16: 144–151

Hume WJ (1981) A theoretical consideration of some biological parameters involved in cell kinetic investigations of oral leukoplakia and abnormal states in stratified squamous epithelium. J Oral Pathol 10: 375–385

Hunter T (1993) Oncogenes and cell proliferation. Current Opinion Gene Devel 3: 1–4

Ivan GI, Littlewood TD (1993) The role of c-myc in cell growth. Curr Opin Gene Dev 3: 44–49

Iverson OH (1992) Role of cell proliferation in carcinogenesis: is increased cell proliferation in itself a carcinogenic hazard. In: Iverson OH (ed) New frontiers in cancer causation. Taylor and Francis. Washington, pp 97–107

Johnson NW (1976) The role of histopathology in diagnosis and prognosis of oral squamous cell carcinoma. Proc R Soc Med 69: 740–747

Johnson NW, Ranasinghe AW, Warnakulasuriya KAAS (1993) Potentially malignant lesions and conditions of the mouth and oropharynx: natural history – cellular and molecular markers of risk. Eur J Cancer Prev 2: 31–51

Johnson NW, Warnakulasuriya KAAS, Tavassoli M (1996) Hereditary and environmental risk factors: clinical and laboratory risk markers for oral cancer and precancer. Eur J Cancer Prev 5: 5–17

Jones AS (1994) Prognosis in mouth cancer: tumour factors. Oral Oncol, Eur J Cancer 30: 8–15

Jones AS, Roland NJ, Caslin AW, Cooke TG, Cooke LD, Forster G (1994) A comparison of cellular proliferation markers in squamous cell carcinoma of the head and neck. J Laryngol Otol 108: 859–864

Kahn MA, Dockter ME, Hermann-Petrin JM (1992) Flow cytometer analysis of oral premalignant lesions: a pilot study and review. J Oral Pathol Med 21: 1-6

Kamath VV, Sastry KARH (1994) Nucleolar organizer regions (NORs) in oral lesions. Indian J Oral Pathol 1: 1-11

Kearsley JH, Thomas S (1993) Prognostic markers in cancers of the head and neck region. Anti Cancer Drugs 4: 419-429

Kearsley JH, Furlong KL, Cooke PA, Waters MJ (1990) An immunohistochemical assessment of cellular proliferation markers in head and neck squamous cell carcinoma. Br J Cancer 61: 821-827

Kernohan NM, Blessing K, King G, Corbett IP, Miller ID (1991) Expression of c-erbB-2 oncoprotein in salivary gland tumours: an immunohistochemical study. J Pathol 163: 77-80

Kramer IRH, Lucas RB, El-Labban N, Lister L (1970) The use of discriminant analysis for examining the histological features of oral keratoses and lichen planus. Br J Cancer 24: 673-686

Lambert M (1986) Tritiated thymidine labelling in vitro for human cancer of the breast: counting error and sampling error. Eur J Cancer Clin Oncol 22: 781-785

Landini G (1990) Nucleolar organizing regions (NORs) in pleomorphic adenomas of the salivary glands. J Oral Pathol Med 19: 257-260

Li TJ, Browne RM, Matthews JB (1994) Quantification of PCNA⁺ cells within odontogenic jaw cyst epithelium. J Oral Pathol Med 23: 184-189

Li TJ, Browne RM, Matthews JB (1995a) Epithelial cell proliferation in odontogenic keratocysts: a comparative immunocytochemical study of Ki67 in simple, recurrent and basal cell naevus syndrome (BCNS)-associated lesions. J Oral Pathol Med 24: 221-226

Li TJ, Browne RM, Matthews JB (1995b) Expression of proliferating cell nuclear antigen (PCNA) and Ki-67 in unicystic ameloblastoma. Histopathology 26: 219-228

Lochrin CA, Wilson GD, McNally NJ, Dische S, Saunders MI (1992) Tumor cell kinetics, local tumor control, and accelerated radiotherapy: a preliminary report. Int J Radiat Oncol Biol Phys 24: 87-91

Lombardi T, Morgan PR (1994) Comparison of PCNA and P34^{cdc2} in the epithelium of odontogenic cysts. Proceedings of the VIIth international association of oral pathologists, York p 30, abstract no P38

Lörz M, Meyer-Breiting E, Bettinger R (1994) Proliferating cell nuclear antigen counts as markers of cell proliferation in head and neck cancer. Eur Arch Otorhinolaryngol 251: 91-94

Maidhof R, Hornstein OP (1979) Autoradiographic study on some proliferative properties of human buccal mucosa. Arch Dermatol Res 265: 165-172

Main DMG (1965) Mitotic activity in buccal keratoses. J Dent Res 44: 1182

Matsumua K, Sasaki K, Tsuji T, Shirozaki F (1989) Nucleolar organizer regions associated proteins (AgNORs) in salivary gland tumors. Int J Oral Maxillofac Surg 18: 76-78

Miller WR (1992) Prognostic factors in breast cancer. Br J Cancer 66: 775-776

Mulinari R, Costa A, Veneroni S, Mattavelli F, Salvatori P, Silvestrini R (1991) Cell kinetics and response to primary intra-arterial chemotherapy in patients with advanced oral cavity tumors. J Oral Pathol Med 20: 32-36

Morgan DO (1992) Cell cycle control in normal and neoplastic cells. Curr Opin Genet Dev 2: 33-37

Morgan DW, Crocker J, Watts A, Shenoi PM (1988) Salivary gland tumors studied by means of AgNOR technique. Histopathology 13: 553-560

Murakami M, Ohtani I, Hojo H, Wasaka H (1992) Immunohistochemical evaluation with Ki-67: an application to salivary gland tumours. J Laryngol Otol 106: 35-38

Nylander K, Anneroth G, Gustafsson H, Roos G, Stenling R, Zackrisson B (1994a) Cell kinetics of head and neck squamous cell carcinomas. Acta Oncol 33: 23-28

Nylander K, Sterling R, Gustafsson H, Ross G (1994b) Application of dual parameter analysis in flow cytometric DNA assessments of paraffin-embedded samples. J Oral Path Med 28: 190-192

Ogawa I, Miyauchi M, Takata T, Vuhahula E, Ijuhin N, Nikai H (1993) Proliferative activity of salivary gland pleomorphic adenomas and myoepitheliomas as evaluated by the proliferating cell nuclear antigen (PCNA) labeling index (LI). J Oral Pathol Med 22: 447-450

Pich A, Chiusa L, Pisani P, Krengli M, Pia F, Navone R (1992) Argyrophilic nucleolar organizer region counts and proliferating cell nuclear antigen scores are two reliable indicators of survival in pharyngeal carcinoma. J Cancer Res Clin Oncol 119: 106–110

Pilgrim C, Erb W, Maurer W (1963) Diurnal fluctuations in the number of DNA synthesizing nuclei in various mouse tissues. Nature 199: 863

Ploton D, Menager M, Jeannesson P, Himber G, Pigeon F, Adnet JJ (1986) Improvement in the staining and in the visualization of the argyrophilic proteins of the nucleolar organiser region at the optical level. Histochem J 18: 5–14

Pollack A, Terry NH, Wu CB, Wise BM, White RA, Meistrich ML (1995) Specific staining of iododeoxyuridine and bromodeoxyuridine in tumours double labelled in vitro: a cell kinetic analysis. Cytology 20: 61–63

Pusztai L, Lewis CE, Lorenzen J, McGee JO'D (1993) Growth factors: regulation of normal and neoplastic growth. J Pathol 169: 191–201

Quinn CM, Wright NA (1990) The clinical assessment of proliferation and growth in human tumours: evaluation of methods and applications as prognostic variables. J Pathol 160: 93–102

Rajendran R, Nair SM (1992) Silver binding nucleolar organiser region proteins as a possible prognostic markers in oral submucous fibrosis. Oral Surg 74: 481–486

Randall MB, Geisinger KR, Kute TE, Buss DH, Prichard RW (1990) DNA content and proliferative index in cutaneous squamous-cell carcinoma and keratoacanthoma. Am J Clin Pathol 93: 259–262

Rennie JS, MacDonald DG, Warnakulasuriya KAAS (1984) Oral epithelial cell kinetics: evaluation of an in vitro method of study. Med Lab Sci 41: 121–126

Renstrup G (1963) Studies in oral leukoplakias. IV. Mitotic activity in oral leukoplakias. A preliminary report. Acta Odontol Scand 21: 333–340

Roland NJ, Caslin AW, Bowie GL, Jones AS (1994) Has the cellular proliferation marker Ki67 any clinical relevance in squamous cell carcinoma of the head and neck? Clin Otolaryngol 19: 13–18

Ruschoff J, Plate KH, Contractor H, Kern S, Zimmerman R, Thomas C (1990) Evaluation of nucleolus organizer regions (NORS) by automatic image analysis. A contribution to standarization. J Pathol 161: 113–118

Saito T, Notani K-I, Miura H, Fukuda H, Mizuno S, Shindoh M, Amemiya A (1991) DNA analysis of oral leukoplakia by flow cytometry. Int J Oral Maxillofaci Surg 20: 259–263

Sakuma J (1980) Cell kinetics of human squamous cell carcinoma in the oral cavity. Bull Tokyo Med Dent Univ 27: 43–54

Sano K, Takahashi H, Fujita S, Inokuchi T, Pe MB, Okabe H, Tsuda N (1991) Prognostic implication of silver-binding nucleolar organizer regions (AgNORS) in oral squamous cell carcinoma. J Oral Pathol Med 20: 53–56

Sardella A, Abati S, Carrassi A (1991) Valutazione dell-attivita proliferativa del lichen planus orale. Minerva Stomatol 40: 557–561

Schneider C, Gustincich S, Del Sal G (1991) The complexity of cell proliferation control in mammalian cells. Curr Opin Cell Biol 3: 276–281

Scott N, Cross D, Plumb MI, Dixon MF, Quirke P (1992) An investigation of different methods of cell cycle analysis by flow cytometry in rectal cancer. Br J Cancer 65: 8–10

Scott RJ, Hall PA, Haldane JS, Price Y, Van Noorden S, Price Y, Lane DP, Wright NA (1991) A comparison of immunohistochemical markers of cell proliferation with experimentally determined growth fraction. J Pathol 165: 173–178

Scragg MA, Johnson NW (1980a) Epithelial cell kinetics – a review of methods of study and their application to oral mucosa in health and disease. A. Methods for studying cell proliferation and some sources of variation. J Oral Pathol 9: 309–341

Scragg MA, Johnson NW (1980b) A comparison of in vivo and in vitro stathmokinetic methods for the study of cell proliferation in hamster oral epithelia. Cell Tissue Kinet 13: 359–369

Scragg MA, Johnson NW (1982) Epithelial cell kinetics. A review of methods of study and their application to oral mucosa in health and disease. B. Comparison of cell kinetics in normal and abnormal epithelia. J Oral Pathol 11: 102–137

Scully C (1993) Oncogenes, tumour suppressors and viruses in oral squamous carcinoma. J Oral Pathol Med 22: 337–347

Seifert G (1992) Histopathology of malignant salivary gland tumours. Oral Oncol Eur J Cancer 28: 49–56

Shrestha P, Huang JW, Tsuji T, Shinozaki F, Maeda K, Sasaki K, Ueno K, Yamada K, Mori M (1992) Rare expression of the c-erbB-2 oncoprotein in salivary gland tumors: an immuno-histochemical study. J Oral Pathol Med 21: 477–480

Sickle-Santanello BJ, Farrar WB, Dobson JL, O'Toole RV, Keyhani-Rofagha S (1986) Flow cytometric analysis of DNA content as a prognostic indicator in squamous cell carcinoma of the tongue. Am J Surg 152: 393–395

Silvestrini R (1994) Cell kinetics: prognostic and therapeutic implications in human tumours. Cell Prolif 27: 579–596

Silvestrini R, Molinari R, Costa A. Volterrani F, Gardani G (1984) Short-term variation in labeling index as a predictor of radiotherapy response in human oral cavity carcinoma. J Radiat Oncol Biol Phys 10: 965–970

Silvestrini R, Costa A, Veneroni S, Del Bino G, Persici P (1988) Comparative analysis of different approaches to investigate cell kinetics. Cell Tissue Kinet 21: 123–131

Slootweg PJ (1995) p53 protein and Ki-67 reactivity in epithelial odontogenic lesions. An immu-nohistochemical study. J Oral Pathol Med 24: 393–397

Slootweg PJ, Koole R, Hordijk GJ (1994) The presence of p53 protein in relation to Ki-67 as cellular proliferation marker in head and neck squamous cell carcinoma and adjacent dysplastic mucosa. Oral Oncol Eur J Cancer 30: 138–141

Smith C, Pindborg JJ (1969) Histological grading of oral epithelial atypia by the use of photo-graphic standards. Hamburgers Bogtrykkeri, Copenhagen, pp 1–35

Stanton PD, Oakes SJ, McArdle CS, Forster G, Cooke TG (1991) Reliability of flow cytometric measurements of cell kinetics. Br J Surg 78: 750 (abstract)

Steinbeck RG, Moege J, Heselmeyer KM, Klebe W, Neugebauer W, Borg B, Auer GU (1993) DNA content and PCNA immunoreactivity in oral precancerous and cancerous lesions. Oral Oncol Eur J Cancer 29B: 279–284

Steel GG (1977) Growth kinetics of tumours. Clarendon, Oxford

Störkel S, Reichert T, Reiffen KA, Wagner W (1993) EGFR and PCNA expression in oral squa-mous cell carcinomas – a valuable tool in estimating the patient's prognosis. Oral Oncol Eur J Cancer 29B: 273–277

Sugerman PB, Joseph BK, Savage NW (1995) The role of oncogenes, tumour suppressor genes and growth factors in oral squamous cell carcinoma: a case of apoptosis versus proliferation. Oral Dis 1: 172–188

Suzuki K, Chen RB, Nomura T, Nakajima T (1994) Flow cytometric analysis of primary and metastatic squamous cell carcinoma of the oral and maxillofacial region. J Oral Maxillofac Surg 52: 855–861

Toller PA (1971) Autoradiography of explants from odontogenic cysts. Br Dent J 131: 57–61

Tsai ST, Jin YT (1995) Proliferating cell nuclear antigen (PCNA) expression in oral squamous cell carcinomas. J Oral Pathol Med 24: 313–315

Tsuji T, Shrestha P, Yamada K, Takagi H, Shinozaki F, Sasaki K, Maeda K, Mori M (1992). Proliferating cell nuclear antigen in malignant and pre-malignant lesions of epithelial origin in the oral cavity and the skin: an immunohistochemical study. Virchows Arch [A] Pathol Anat 420: 377–383

Tytor M, Franzén G, Olofsson J (1987) DNA pattern in oral cavity carcinomas in relation to clinical stage and histological grading. Pathol Res Pract 182: 202–206

Underwood JCE, Giri DD (1988) Nucleolar organiser regions as diagnostic discriminants of malignancy. J Pathol 155: 95–96 (editorial)

van Heerden WFP, Raubenheimer EJ (1991) Evaluation of the nucleolar organizer region associ-ated proteins in minor salivary gland tumours. J Oral Pathol Med 20: 291–295

van Heerden WFP, Raubenheimer EJ, van Rensburg EJ, le Roux R (1995) Lack of correlation between DNA ploidy, Langerhans cell population and grading in oral squamous cell carci-noma. J Oral Pathol Med 24: 61–65

Walker DM, Dolby AE (1974) Labelling index in the mucosal lesions of lichen planus. Br J Dermatol 91: 549–556

Walker RA, Camplejohn RS (1988) Comparison of monoclonal antibody Ki-67 reactivity with grade and DNA flow cytometry of breast carcinomas. Br J Cancer 57: 281–283

Warnakulasuriya KAAS (1976) Cell proliferation of human oral mucosa. PhD thesis, University of Glasgow

Warnakulasuriya KAAS, Johnson NW (1993a) Comparison of isotopic and immunohistochemical methods of studying cell proliferation in hamster tongue. Cell Prolif 26: 545–555

Warnakulasuriya KAAS, Johnson NW (1993b) Nucleolar organiser region (NOR) distribution as a diagnostic marker in oral keratosis, dysplasia and squamous cell carcinoma. J Oral Pathol Med 22: 77–81

Warnakulasuriya KAAS, Johnson NW (1994) Association of overexpression of p53 oncoprotein with the state of cell proliferation in oral carcinoma. J Oral Pathol Med 23: 246–250

Warnakulasuriya KAAS, MacDonald DG (1993) Diurnal variation in labelling index in human buccal epithelium. Arch Oral Biol 38: 1107–1111

Warnakulasuriya KAAS, MacDonald DG (1995a) The influence of rate of cell entry to S phase on the labelling index of human buccal epithelium. Arch Oral Biol 40: 107–110

Warnakulasuriya KAAS, MacDonald DG (1995b) Epithelial cell kinetics in oral leukoplakia. J Oral Pathol Med 24: 165–169

Warnakulasuriya KAAS, Ahmed MS, Penhallow J, Johnson NW (1994) Increased cell proliferation and dysplasia in candida associated oral keratoses. Proceedings of the VIIth international association of oral pathologists, York meeting, abstract no PO6

Waseem NH, Lane DP (1990) Monoclonal antibody analysis of the proliferating cell nuclear antigen (PCNA). Structural conservation and the detection of a nucleolar form. J Cell Sci 96: 121–129

Welsgerber VIM, Boeing H, Neunitz R, Ruedasih R, Waldehen R (1993) Proliferation cell nuclear antigen (clone 19A2) correlates with 5-bromo-2-deoxyuridine labelling in human colonic epithelium. Gut 34: 1587–1592

Whitaker SB, Vigneswaran N, Budnick SD, Waldron CA (1993) Giant cell lesions of the jaws: evaluation of nucleolar organizer regions in lesions of varying behavior. J Oral Pathol Med 22: 402–405

Wilson GD (1991) Assessment of human tumour proliferation using bromodeoxyuridine – current status. Acta Oncol 30: 903–910

Wilson GD, McNally NJ, Dunphy E, Karcher H, Pfragner R (1985) The labelling index of human and mouse tumours assessed by bromodeoxyuridine staining in vitro and in vivo and flow cytometry. Cytometry 6: 641

Wilson GD, McNally NJ, Dische S, Saunders MI, Des Rochers C, Lewis AA, Bennett MH (1988) Measurement of cell kinetics in human tumours in vivo using bromodeoxyuridine incorporation and flow cytometry. Br J Cancer 58: 423–431

Wilson GD, Richman PI, Dische S, Saunders MI, Robinson B, Daley FM, Ross DA (1995) p53 status of head and neck cancer: relation to biological characteristics and outcome of radiotherapy 71: 1248–1252

Wong DTW, Biswas DK (1987) Expression of c-erbB proto-oncogene during dimethylbenzanthracene-induced tumorigenesis in hamster cheek pouch. Oncogene 2: 67–72

Wyllie AH (1993) Apoptosis (the 1992 Frank Rose Memorial Lecture). Br J Cancer 67: 205–208

Wynford-Thomas D, Williams ED (1986) Use of bromodeoxyuridine for cell kinetic studies in intact animals. Cell Tissue Kinet 19: 179–182

Yang L, Liu B, Qin C, Hashimura K, Yamada T, Sumitoma S, Mori M (1994) Comparison of proliferating cell nuclear antigen index in benign and malignant salivary pleomorphic adenoma. Oral Oncol Eur J Cancer 30: 56–60

Yu CCW, Woods AL, Levison DA (1992) The application of immunohistochemistry in assessment of cellular proliferation. In: Hall PA, Lawson DA, Wright DA (eds) Assessment of cell proliferation in clinical practice. Springer, Berlin Heidelberg New York, pp 141–157

Zhao FY (1992) Flow cytometric analysis of squamous cell carcinoma of the oral and maxillofacial region. Chung Hua Kou Chiang Hsueh Tsa Chih 27: 222–224

Zoeller J, Flentje M, Sinn P, Born IA (1994) Evaluation of AgNOR and Ki-67 antigen as cell kinetic parameters in oral dysplasias and carcinomas. Anal Cell Pathol 7: 77–88

Suppressor Protein p53 and Its Occurrence in Oral Tumours

P.J. Slootweg

1 Introduction

As summarised by Levine and Momand (1990), a cancer cell is the result of a multistep process in which multiple sequential mutations occur. In this process, two distinct categories can be discerned: the inappropriate activation of proto-oncogenes to become oncogenes and the inactivation of tumour suppressor genes, both of which may lead to disturbed cell proliferation and the development of tumours (Chang et al. 1993). One of the most intensely studied tumour suppressor genes is the *p53* gene. The protein encoded by this gene appears to act as "the guardian of the genome" (Lane 1994) by blocking the division of cells that have sustained DNA damage, resulting in either a delay in progress through the cell cycle to permit repair or triggering cell death by apoptosis, thus eliminating abnormal cells that could lead to cancer (Levine et al. 1994). Moreover, p53 appears to play a role during embryogenesis, as mice lacking the *p53* gene exhibited an increased incidence of neural tube defects (Sah et al. 1995) and an increased sensitivity to an environmental teratogen (Nicol et al. 1995).

This contribution will focus upon the occurrence of p53 alterations in oral tumours and their significance; before this, historical background, more general aspects and the various means currently available for analysis of the *p53* gene will be briefly discussed.

Current Topics in Pathology
Volume 90, G. Seifert (Ed.)
© Springer-Verlag Berlin Heidelberg 1996

2 Historical Background

The story of the discovery of the p53 protein is connected with the production of the Salk polio vaccine in monkey kidney cells. From a shift from rhesus monkeys to African green monkeys, it became apparent that the extract of cells of the former had a cytopathic effect on the kidney cells of the latter kind of monkey. Subsequent analysis revealed this effect to be due to a virus that initiated cancers in hamsters. This virus was named SV40 (simian vacuolating virus 40). SV40 expressed a viral protein, the large T antigen, which was shown to form a tight complex with a nuclear phosphoprotein, the p53 protein. Subsequent studies revealed that the p53 protein was present in minute amounts in normal cells, but in high levels in tumour cells. Initially, the protein was classified as a tumour antigen and thereafter as an oncogene product but finally, as all p53 protein in neoplastic cells turned out to be the product of a mutated gene, *p53* appeared to represent a tumour suppressor gene (Lane and Benchimol 1990; Levine et al. 1991; Levine 1994).

3 Role of *p53* in Tumourigenesis

Evidence that *p53* is a tumour suppressor gene is twofold. Firstly, *p53* mutations in human cancers commonly take the form of a missense mutation in one allele and the loss of the other. This complete loss of both wild-type alleles is typical of a tumour suppressor gene. Secondly, mice with both *p53* alleles mutated develop cancers within 6–9 months, showing that absence of *p53* function predisposes to cancer (Berns 1994; Levine et al. 1994; Picksley and Lane 1994). Mutation of one allele in the germ line results in cancers occurring at unusually early age, a condition known as the Li-Fraumeni syndrome (Birch 1992, 1994).

However, there is some evidence that in some aspects the *p53* gene behaves differently from an ordinary tumour suppressor gene, in which the loss of function is responsible for tumour development. This evidence comes from observations that indicate that the mutant protein may block the function of the wild-type protein if one allele is mutated and one is wild-type *p53*. Moreover, mutant p53 proteins may be actively involved in cell transformation. Therefore, the *p53* gene has features of an oncogene as well as of a tumour suppressor gene. Mutations resulting in loss of function and acquisition of new activities may both be responsible for tumour development (Lane and Benchimol 1990; Levine et al. 1994).

Normally, the p53 protein acts as a checkpoint control in the cell cycle, inhibiting progression of cells in G_1 by inducing expression of genes that block the cell cycle (El-Deiry et al. 1993) and preventing entry into S phase in the event of damaged DNA. Moreover, the p53-mediated DNA damage response includes an inducible DNA repair component (Smith et al. 1994). Thus the duplication of damaged DNA is prevented. This normal function of p53 can be abolished in several ways. Firstly, no normal protein is present due to a loss of one *p53* allele together with a missense mutation of the other *p53* allele. Secondly, the product of a mutated *p53* allele blocks the activity of the wild-type protein encoded by the remaining normal allele. Thirdly, the normal protein is blocked in its activity by binding to another protein; this may be a viral protein from SV40, from human adenovirus or from human papillomavirus (HPV), but binding to a cellular gene product such as the murine double minute-2 (MDM-2) may also lead to inactivation of p53 protein (MOMAND et al. 1992; MELTZER 1994).

4 Analysis of *p53* and Its Protein

The *p53* gene encompasses 20 kilobases (kb) of DNA on the short arm of chromosome 17 at position 17p13.1. The product of the gene is a 393-amino acid nuclear phosphoprotein of about 53kDa (hence its name p53 protein) (LEVINE and MOMAND 1990). The gene consists of 11 exons; exons 2–11 code for the p53 protein. There are five regions of the p53 protein in which amino acid sequence in several species is similar over lengths of up to 20 amino acids. These are the so-called conserved regions I–V. These correspond to codons 13–19, 120–143, 172–182, 238–259 and 271–290, respectively; 86% of mutations are located between codons 120 and 290, and a high frequency of mutations are found at the "hotspots", codons 175, 248 and 273 (LEVINE et al. 1994).

At present, more than 2500 mutations of the *p53* gene in human cancers or cell lines have been reported (GREENBLATT et al. 1994).

Most *p53* gene alterations are missense mutations. The mutant p53 proteins mostly have a much longer half-life than the wild-type protein, which permits detection by immunohistochemistry with the aid of the appropriate antibodies (Fig. 1). This finding has led to an immense amount of data on the occurrence of the p53 protein in human cancer (SOUSSI et al. 1994). However, uncritically equating presence of immunohistochemically detectable p53 protein with a mutant genotype is unwarranted, as it seems that stabilisation of the p53 protein may occur without *p53* gene mutations (WYNFORD-THOMAS 1992; BATTIFORA 1994; HALL and LANE 1994).

The discrepancies between the presence of *p53* mutations and negative p53 protein staining may be due to a mutation leading to a premature stop codon or to mutations without amino acid substitution. The presence of immunohistochemically detectable p53 protein without detectable *p53* gene mutations has been explained as follows. Firstly, it is possible that mutations are located outside of the most commonly analyzed part of the *p53* gene, exons 5–8. Secondly, the p53 protein may accumulate at levels sufficient to be detected by immunohistochemistry due to stabilisation induced by viral or cellular proteins. Thirdly, defects in other p53-responsive cell cycle regulators, such as the cyclin-dependent kinase inhibitor gene *p21* WAF-1/CIP-1, may lead to cell division not inactivated by p53 protein produced at a normal level, which the cell attempts to compensate by overexpression (MELHEM et al. 1995).

Obtaining real insight into the status of the *p53* gene and its protein in an individual lesion requires molecular biological analysis of the gene, which includes amplifying the gene by polymerase chain reaction (PCR) followed by the use of

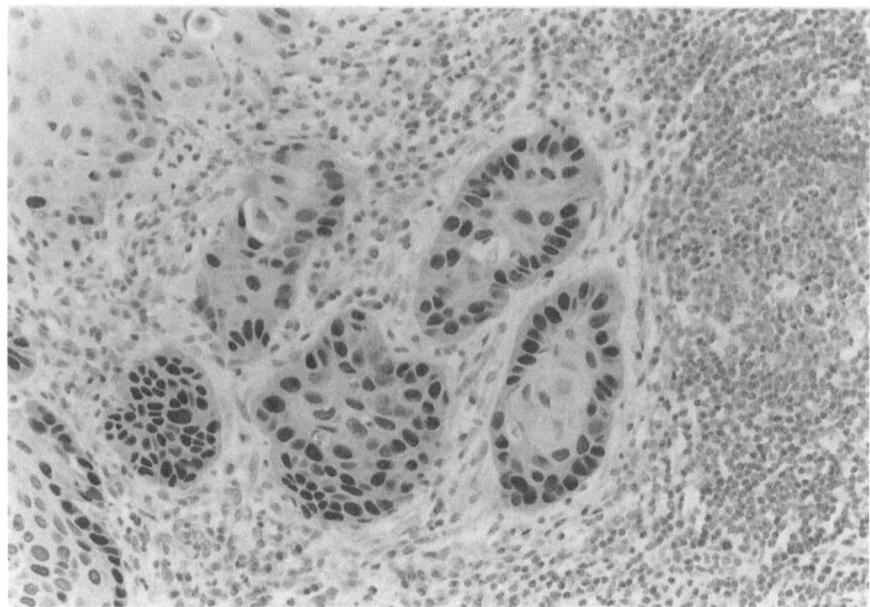

Fig. 1. Photomicrograph shows strong positivity for p53 protein in the nuclei of this squamous cell carcinoma. Haematoxylin–anti-p53 protein peroxidase–anti-peroxidase stain

techniques aimed at detecting altered electrophoretic mobility patterns, such as single-strand conformation polymorphism analysis (SSCP) or denaturant gradient gel electrophoresis (DGGE), followed by sequencing to detect the site of the mutation and detection of the protein by immunohistochemistry (GREENBLATT et al. 1994; SOUSSI et al. 1994). Analysis for loss of heterozygosity at the *p53* locus completes the picture (ADAMSON et al. 1994).

5 p53 and Oral Tumours

5.1 Expression of p53 and *p53* Mutations

Data on *p53* gene alterations in oral tumours mainly concern squamous cell carcinomas (SCC) and their cell lines (SAKAI et al. 1992; SAKAI and TSUCHIDA 1992). In these tumours, *p53* gene mutations and the presence of p53 protein are consistent findings, although the proportion of SCC exhibiting these features varies in different series (FIELD et al. 1993a). The relationship between expression of detectable p53 protein and gene mutations has been investigated by combined immunohistochemical and molecular biological analysis. Some of these studies provided support for the assumption that expression of a stabilised and therefore detectable p53 protein is indeed correlated with a gene mutation (GUSTERSON et al. 1991;

SOMERS et al. 1992; BURNS et al. 1993; CAAMANO et al. 1993; AHOMADEGBE et al. 1995). In other studies, however, discrepancies between protein immunohistochemistry and gene analysis became apparent, indicating overexpression of p53 protein without apparent gene mutations (RANASINGHE et al. 1993a; XU et al. 1994a,b; MELHEM et al. 1995) as well as occurrence of gene mutations without p53 protein overexpression (CHEN et al. 1994; MELHEM et al. 1995).

Thus overexpression of p53 protein in oral SCC is not necessarily synonymous with *p53* gene mutations. Nevertheless, in general there is a correlation between detectable expression of p53 protein and neoplasia (HALL and LANE 1994), and therefore both data concerning p53 protein overexpression and studies in which gene alterations have been investigated will be reviewed.

5.2 Association of p53 Status with Risk Factors for Oral Cancer

Elevated p53 protein expression has been attributed to gene alterations induced by smoking, a well-known risk factor for oral SCC in Western countries (FIELD et al. 1991, 1994; LANGDON and PARTRIDGE 1992; OGDEN et al. 1992; GALLO et al. 1995a; GALLO and BIANCHI 1995; TSUJI et al. 1995). These findings agree very well with similar data obtained for SCC of the lung, another tobacco-induced cancer, in which *p53* gene alterations play a prominent role (GREENBLATT et al. 1994). In contrast, no association between p53 protein overexpression and tobacco smoking was reported by MATTHEWS et al. (1993), HÖGMO et al. (1994), FRANCESCHI et al. (1995) and NAKANISHI et al. (1995). Differences in studied populations or anti-p53 antibodies used cannot explain these contradictory results, as similar divergent data come from molecular biological studies. By sequencing the *p53* gene, it was demonstrated that smoking increased the frequency of *p53* gene mutations found in head and neck SCC (BRENNAN et al. 1995a; KOCH et al. 1995) and in pre-malignant lesions (LAZARUS et al. 1995), whereas it was also found that the spectrum of types of *p53* gene mutations in non-smokers was limited to sites characteristically seen with spontaneous mutations, the hotspots, while those seen in smokers were more widely distributed (BRENNAN et al. 1995a; KOCH et al. 1995). On the other hand, YEUDALL et al. (1995), who performed studies on SCC cell lines, failed to observe this correlation between the nature of *p53* gene mutations and the use of tobacco by the patients from which the cell lines were derived.

Nevertheless, after combining the high proportion of *p53* gene mutations in head and neck SCC with the epidemiological evidence that smoking is an aetiological factor in this kind of tumour, one is led to the conclusion that the induction of *p53* gene alterations might be a way by which tobacco exerts its deleterious influence on the oral mucosa.

Whether *p53* gene mutations may be caused by betel quid chewing, a habit considered to play a prominent role in causing oral SCC in Asian populations, is also a subject of debate. Investigations in patients from Sri Lanka (RANASINGHE et al. 1993a,b) and from Papua New Guinea (THOMAS et al. 1994) showed a low prevalence of *p53* gene alterations and p53 protein overexpression in betel-associated oral cancers. However, in a study on patients from Northern India, the opposite was found (KAUR et al. 1994). Different chewing habits and differences in the ingredients of the quid in the various populations are probably responsible for the divergent data on the aetiological significance of betel quid chewing and *p53* gene alterations in the development of oral SCC (KUTTAN et al. 1995).

Abrogation of p53 function may also be caused by HPV, another risk factor associated with the development of oral SCC (YEUDALL 1992), as it has been shown that HPV-16 and HPV-18 E6 proteins form a complex and promote the degradation of cellular p53 protein (SCHEFFNER et al. 1990; WERNESS et al. 1990; LI et al. 1992). These observations prompted several authors to study the association between p53 status and HPV in oral SCC. BRACHMAN et al. (1992) were the first to investigative head and neck SCC for both *p53* gene mutations and the presence of HPV DNA and, as they did not find *p53* gene mutations and HPV DNA in the same tumour, they concluded that alteration of *p53* gene function in oral SCC may occur through gene mutations as well as HPV infection. MIN et al. (1994) found an inverse relationship between *p53* gene mutations and the presence of HPV in oral cancer cell lines; moreover, these authors reported a lower level of p53 protein than normal in cell lines expressing HPV-18 E6/E7 genes. Finally, an inverse relationship between p53 protein overexpression and HPV antigen detection in oral SCC has been reported by MUKHOPADHYAY et al. (1994).

Although these data do indeed suggest the involvement of HPV-triggered p53 protein degradation in oral carcinogenesis, matters may be more complicated, as SNIJDERS et al. (1994) and LEWENSOHN-FUCHS et al. (1994) found evidence for p53 protein stabilisation rather than increased degradation in some cases of tonsillar SCC containing HPV. Therefore, it might well be that HPV can interfere with normal p53 functioning by protein degradation as well as by binding to an HPV-derived viral protein. Evidence of HPV-mediated p53 protein stabilisation has also been provided by DEMERS et al. (1994). Finally, YEUDALL et al. (1995) demonstrated that SCC cell lines may express mutant p53 protein and also harbour HPV DNA, and they speculate that cells transformed by HPV may become further transformed by co-expression of mutant p53.

In summary, HPV may be a risk factor associated with oral SCC by disturbing p53 function, but its mode of operation is still far from clear.

5.3 Alterations of *p53* in Carcinogenesis

5.3.1 Timing

There is ample evidence that oral SCC may be preceded by pre-malignant mucosal changes, but the molecular events associated with the development of malignancy are poorly understood. Determination of the timing of p53 changes during the multistage process of progression from normal epithelium through dysplasia to invasive carcinoma may be helpful in understanding the genetic alterations which give rise to pre-malignant oral mucosal lesions and which influence their progression.

Timing of *p53* changes in the development of SCC has mainly been investigated by immunohistochemical analysis of p53 protein overexpression in oral mucosal dysplasia found adjacent to invasive carcinoma or in dysplastic lesions without an invasive component. GUSTERSON and colleagues (1991) were the first to report expression of p53 protein in oral SCC as well as in areas of adjacent mucosal dysplasia, with cytologically normal epithelial cells being negative (Figs. 2, 3). These findings have since been confirmed several times (WARNAKULASURIYA and JOHNSON 1992; NEES et al. 1993; PAVELIC et al. 1992, 1994; SLOOTWEG et al. 1994; XU et al. 1994a; GALLO et al. 1995a; LAVIEILLE et al. 1995). Moreover, expression of p53 protein has been observed in dysplastic lesions without a concomitant invasive component (COLTRERA et al. 1992; LANGDON and PARTRIDGE 1992; WARNAKULASURIYA and JOHNSON 1992; NAKANISHI et al. 1993; NISHIOKA et al. 1993; KAUR et al. 1994; PAVELIC et al. 1994) and in dysplastic lesions that subsequently developed into SCC (REGEZI et al. 1995). SAUTER et al. (1994) and SHIN et al. (1994) contributed to these data by reporting that the frequency of p53 protein expression was increased in lesions showing moderate or severe dysplasia compared to mildly dysplastic lesions. Occurrence of p53 overexpression in normal epithelium adjacent to tumour was reported by NEES et al. (1993), SAUTER et al. (1994), SHIN et al. (1994), AHOMADEGBE et al. (1995), GALLO and Bianchi (1995) and NAKANISHI et al. (1995).

Occurrence of p53 protein overexpression in normal control epithelium taken from cancer-free individuals was reported by GIROD et al. (1993, 1994a,b), who observed p53 protein positively in patients with lichen planus. However, lichen

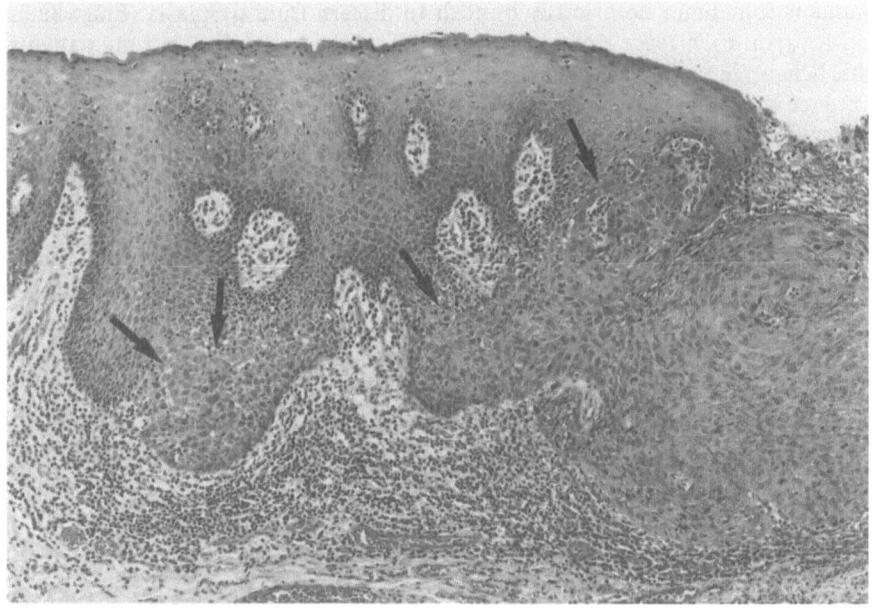

Fig. 2. Photomicrograph shows border between dysplastic and healthy oral epithelium; border indicated by *arrows*. H&E

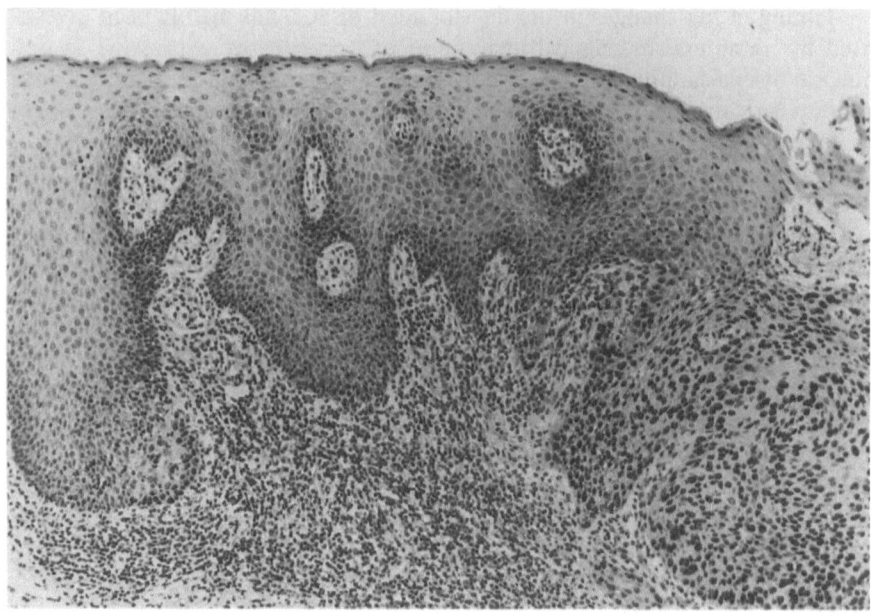

Fig. 3. Same area as shown in Fig. 2. Cells in the dysplastic epithelium exhibit positivity for p53 protein, which indicates protein overexpression. Haematoxylin–anti-p53 protein peroxidase-anti-peroxidase stain

planus is sometimes notoriously difficult to discern from dysplasia (EISENBERG and KRUTCHKOFF 1992; HOLMSTRUP 1992), and the possibility that the patients with lichen planus in reality suffered from lichenoid dysplasia may explain the presence of p53-positive cells in these cases. Overexpresion of p53 protein in cancer-free control tissue was also observed by GALLO and BIANCHI(1995), who observed a few positive cells in patients with chronic inflammation. To clarify this issue, more studies on the association between p53 protein positivity and inflammatory mucosal disorders are needed.

All these data from which a derangement of p53 function early in cancer development can be inferred come from studies in which overexpression of p53 protein has been employed as an indication for *p53* gene mutations which are not necessarily synonymous with each other, as illustrated by the observation that a positive immunoreaction in dysplasia might reflect nuclear accumulation of wild-type p53 protein (NAKANISHI et al. 1995). However, evidence that *p53* gene mutations, and not merely wild-type p53 protein overexpression, are associated with the development of dysplasia comes from several molecular biological studies. BOYLE et al. (1993) and LAZARUS et al. (1995) observed *p53* gene mutations in non-invasive lesions, from which they inferred that *p53* mutations could precede invasion in oral SCC. These observations were extended by NEES et al. (1993), who found *p53* gene mutations in histologically inconspicuous epithelia at a significant distance from the primary tumour, thus demonstrating that an occasional p53 protein-positive cell in an otherwise normal epithelium from a patient with oral

SCC may indeed harbour a mutated *p53* gene. Both the observations of BOYLE et al. (1993) and LAZARUS et al. (1995) that *p53* mutations occur in pre-invasive lesions and the finding of NEES et al. (1993) that tumour-distant epithelial areas may harbour *p53* mutations different from the invasive tumour argue against the idea that the presence of p53 protein-positive cells in tumour-adjacent mucosa may be due to intra-epithelial lateral spread of tumour cells and demonstrated that p53 protein positivity in non-invasive lesions may indeed denote the presence of gene mutations.

Moreover, evidence that *p53* gene mutations already occur during the transition from normal epithelium to dysplastic epithelium comes from a study by BURNS et al. (1994a) on the p53 status of cultured human pre-malignant keratinocytes in which they demonstrated elevated levels of p53 protein together with gene mutations.

Two studies suggest that *p53* gene changes are a late event in oral carcinogenesis. The first of these was carried out by CAAMANO et al. (1993), who base their opinion on the observation that the clinically furthest advanced tumours exhibit the most intense p53 protein immunostaining and that tumours showing the most invasive growth in an vivo assay employing growth of tumour explants in rat tracheal grafts also exhibit the most intense p53 protein expression. The other study providing support for *p53* alterations as a late event comes from LEE et al. (1993), who were only able to demonstrate *p53* gene mutations in invasive tumours, but not in adjacent tissue. However, no dysplasias were investigated.

In spite of these two reports, data from other studies mentioned above provide overwhelming evidence that *p53* alterations are an early event in oral carcinogenesis, involved in the development of pre-malignant mucosal changes.

Studies on the association between p53 protein overexpression in oral pre-malignant lesions and other histologically detectable features indicative of disturbed proliferation and differentiation are scarce. GIROD et al. (1994a,b) reported that proliferating cell nuclear antigen (PCNA) expression in pre-malignant lesions of the oral mucosa correlated with the dysplasia grade but did not quantify PCNA expression in correlation with p53 protein expression. NEES et al. (1993) observed p53 protein expression in tumour-adjacent epithelium to be associated with increased proliferation, as measured by analysis of expression of the histone H3 gene. However, whether this phenomenon also occurred in p53 protein-negative specimens of tumour-adjacent epithelium was not mentioned. As SLOOTWEG et al. (1994) found no quantitative differences in proliferation, as measured by Ki-67 reactivity between p53 protein-positive and p53 protein-negative tumour-adjacent dysplastic epithelia, it can be argued that p53 protein expression is related to dysplasia-associated increased cellular proliferation and development of cytological atypia but is not a condition sine qua non, as histologically similar epithelial dysplastic changes can be found without p53 protein expression.

To obtain more insight in the role of *p53* alterations in the development of mucosal pre-malignancies, studies are needed in which p53 protein expression is compared with changes in proliferation rates and DNA ploidy, as was done for bronchial mucosa, in which DNA aneuploidy was preceded by increased proliferation and followed by p53 protein immunoreactivity (HIRANO et al. 1994).

Moreover, the recently described association between *p53* gene changes and angiogenesis needs to be explored. As reviewed by WEIDNER (1995), angiogenesis plays a key role in tumour growth, progression and metastasis, and there are some indications that a normal *p53* gene inhibits angiogenesis (GASPARINI 1995). As angiogenesis is more related to advanced tumour growth than to early cellular events, an involvement of the *p53* gene with this phenomenon would mean that *p53* disturbances play a role not only in tumour initiation, but also in tumour progression and development of metastatic deposits. Up to now, only one report has paid attention to the relationship between p53 protein overexpression and intratumoral microvessel density; in this study, a significant association between the two features was observed (GASPARINI et al. 1993). One other study has also been devoted to p53 protein overexpression and tumour angiogenesis (LEEDY et al. 1994), but without investigating their mutual association. Whether *p53* gene changes are important in more advanced SCC will be an important item for future investigations; at present, their role in early stages of carcinogenesis has been better analyzed.

5.3.2 Use as a Biomarker

As concluded in the previous section, *p53* gene alterations occur early in oral carcinogenesis and may be visualised by immunohistochemical demonstration of p53 protein. Whether p53 protein serves as a useful biomarker will now be discussed.

A useful biomarker should fulfil two requirements. Firstly, the purported biomarker should be present in cells which do not yet show conventional histological signs of malignancy, such as cytonuclear atypia, but nevertheless are already at risk for malignant degeneration, as shown by subsequent development of dysplasia or carcinoma. As most studies indicate p53 protein overexpression in cells already exhibiting atypia or in normal cells from patients already suffering from SCC (references as cited in the previous section), p53 protein does not appear to be a useful biomarker in predicting the occurrence of oral SCC in patients not yet showing dysplasia or SCC. Matters may be different with patients already suffering from oral SCC, as there are some indications that in this group p53 protein overexpression in tumour-adjacent normal epithelium may indicate an increased risk for the development of multiple primary SCC of the upper aerodigestive tract (GALLO and BIANCHI 1995; NAKANISHI et al. 1995), carcinogens possibly interacting with a genetically determined increased mutagen sensitivity in these patients (GALLO et al. 1995a).

Secondly, a biomarker should be useful in identifying dysplasias at risk of progressing to invasive SCC. For p53 protein, this would imply that p53 protein-positive dysplastic lesions should have an increased risk of further malignant degeneration in comparison with p53 protein-negative cases of dysplasia. This has not so far been found; in contrast, REGEZI et al. (1995) observed that both p53 protein-positive and p53 protein-negative dysplasias developed into SCC. Moreover, *p53* gene alterations occur early in oral carcinogenesis, but are not associated with disease progression (AHOMADEGBE et al. 1995). Therefore, it would be illogical to suppose that p53 protein was a biomarker able to identify dysplastic lesions with an increased risk of developing into SCC, as this implies cellular events connected with the later stages of oral carcinogenesis in which *p53* gene alterations are probably not involved. In summary, p53 protein may be useful in identifying SCC patients at risk of developing a second malignant primary tumour, but it appears not to be of any use in identifying tumour-free patients at risk of developing dysplasia or SCC or patients with dysplasia at risk of progressing to SCC.

5.4 Clinical Utility of p53 Analysis

5.4.1 Diagnostic Applications

Mutations in the *p53* gene may occur at different sites, a feature which may have diagnostic value in discerning between multiple primary tumours and recurrent or metastatic disease.

In the event of multiple primary tumours, different *p53* gene mutations can be found in the respective lesions, as has repeatedly been demonstrated (CHUNG et al. 1993; KOCH et al. 1994; ZARILAWA et al. 1994), whereas metastatic or recurrent tumours should retain the same mutation. As almost all head and neck cancers are of the squamous cell type, analysis of histological features is of no use in solving this diagnostic problem, and therefore availability of a non-morphological tool to identify tumours would be very useful, as treatment modalities for patients with a second primary oral SCC may be entirely different from those for patients with recurrent or metastatic disease.

The idea that *p53* gene mutations are maintained during tumour progression and metastasis has gained support from studies on primary SCC and their lymph node metastases. Results from these investigations can be summarised as follows. CHUNG et al. (1993) analysed three cases of primary SCC of the head, neck and lung and their respective regional lymph node metastases and noted identical mutations in primary tumour and metastasis exhibited by identical SSCP banding; no sequencing data were given. BURNS et al. (1994b) reported data using the technique of sequencing which demonstrated conservation of the *p53* gene mutation throughout progression to lymph node metastasis. KOCH et al. (1994) reported different mutations in two synchronous primary oral SCC; bilateral lymph node metastases contained the same mutated sequence as found in one of the primary SCC. AHOMADEGBE et al. (1995) observed identical mutations in primary tumour and lymph node metastasis in eight out of ten patients, whereas a mutation was only observed in the node metastasis in two patients. These studies suggest that mutant *p53* genes may indeed be useful in distinguishing between SCC and metastasis and/or recurrent disease.

Less clear-cut results were obtained by ZARILAWA et al. (1994), who reported a patient with a *p53* gene mutation in a lymph node metastasis not detected in the primary malignancy, a finding they explained by assuming that the mutation in the lymph node metastasis arose independently after metastatic spread or that mutation was present in the primary tumour in such a small fraction that it escaped detection.

As different *p53* gene mutations have been observed even within single biopsies of head and neck SCC (NEES et al. 1993), the presence of tumour clones in the primary lesion too small to be detected but with a higher propensity for metastasis may indeed explain differences in *p53* gene mutations between primary SCC and metastatic tumour deposits; therefore, the preliminary conclusion has to be that the same *p53* gene mutation present in tumours from several sites suggests one primary tumour that has metastasised, but that the presence of different mutations does not unequivocally rule out metastasis.

The value of *p53* gene mutation analysis as a reliable diagnostic tool to distinguish between multiple primary tumours and metastasising disease depends on the possibility of assessing whether an individual tumour harbours a single *p53* gene mutation or several clones with different *p53* gene mutations, even if some of these are only represented by a few tumour cells.

BRENNAN et al. (1995b) showed that application of such techniques yields clinically useful data; they demonstrated the presence of tumour cells not otherwise detected in surgical margins and excised lymph nodes from SCC patients by employing p53 mutant-specific probes.

5.4.2 Prognostic Significance

p53 protein is involved in control of genomic stability and cell cycle control in response to DNA damage. Loss of *p53* function (often seen as high p53 protein levels) would therefore be expected to correlate with aneuploidy and increased proliferation rates (GREENBLATT et al. 1994; HARTWELL and KASTAN 1994; BATSAKIS and EL-NAGGAR 1995). As these two features may be associated with poor prognosis, determination of p53 protein overexpression, although an indirect and admittedly imperfect means of estimating *p53* gene mutations, could be helpful in predicting tumour behaviour.

This assumption has been tested in various ways. LOWE et al. (1994) compared the therapeutic responsiveness of genetically defined tumours expression or devoid of the *p53* gene in mice. They found that tumours expressing the *p53* gene regressed after irradiation or chemotherapy, whereas *p53*-deficient tumours continued to enlarge; they therefore concluded that defects in *p53* function may be a significant impediment to successful cancer therapy. This study agrees very well with those of LIU et al. (1994, 1995) and CLAYMAN et al. (1995), who demonstrated that introduction of wild-type p53 into SCC cell lines via a recombinant adenoviral vector resulted in growth arrest and morphological changes consistent with apoptosis in vitro as well as significant tumour reduction in in vivo studies on nude mice. The influence of *p53* gene mutations on response to irradiation was analysed in SCC cell lines. JUNG et al. (1992) investigated whether *p53* mutations correlated with either a radiation-sensitive or radiation-resistant cellular phenotype, but did not find any difference. BRACHMAN et al. (1993), however, observed a trend toward increased radioresistance in SCC cell lines with abrogation of *p53* function.

It appears from these basic studies that normal *p53* functioning might have a beneficial effect on cancer treatment, probably by inducing apoptosis in the presence of oncogenic triggers (FISHER 1994). However, proof has to come from patient studies, which will be discussed in the following.

The value of p53 protein overexpression, as determined by immunohistochemistry, as a prognostic factor has been investigated by analysing correlations between this feature and clinico-pathological tumour parameters such as size, stage and histological grade by comparing p53 protein overexpression with cell-kinetic data and by evaluating the relationship between p53 protein overexpression and survival time.

The reports that correlate p53 protein immunohistochemistry with tumour cell kinetics will first be mentioned. BOURHIS et al. (1994) employed DNA flow cytometry after in vivo bromodeoxyuridine labelling and p53 protein immunohistochemistry. Their data suggest that overexpression of p53 protein is significantly more frequent in aneuploid tumours and significantly associated with a high proportion of cells in S phase. The authors conclude that overexpression of the *p53* gene is associated with rapid tumour cell proliferation. In contrast, HÖGMO et al. (1994) and TSUJI et al. (1995) failed to find a correlation between p53 immunostaining and DNA aberration, and MUKHOPADHYAY et al. (1994), who related p53 protein overexpression to in vitro bromodeoxyuridine labelling, observed no correlation between p53 positivity and cytokinetics in their series. WILSON et al. (1995) found no differences in DNA aneuploidy and proliferation rate measured by in vivo bromodeoxyuridine between p53 protein-positive and p53 protein-negative cases; however, when differentiating between strongly and weakly positive cases, the strongly positive tumours were more often aneuploid. NYLANDER et al. (1995a,b) found no correlation between *p53* gene mutations and p53 protein overexpression on the one hand and in vivo incorporation of iododeoxyuridine or number of cells expressing the immunohistochemically detectable proliferation marker PCNA on the other. A similar lack of correlation between p53 protein overexpression and expression of PCNA was observed by LAVIEILLE et al. (1995) and earlier by WARNAKULASURIYA and JOHNSON (1994), but with another proliferation marker, Ki-67, the latter authors observed an increased proportion of Ki-67-labelled cells in p53 protein-positive carcinomas. A positive correlation between p53 protein overexpression and the number of PCNA-positive cells was reported by NISHIOKA et al. (1993) and TSUJI et al. (1995).

Summarising the as yet rather limited data on the relationship between p53 protein overexpression in oral SCC, their proliferation rate and their ploidy status, it appears that this issue is far from clear. The cell-kinetic data obtained so far in various ways do not provide unequivocal support for the idea that p53 protein overexpression is associated with an increased proliferation rate or aneuploidy.

Another way to investigate whether p53 protein overexpression has prognostic significance is by analysing the association of this feature with other clinico-pathologic parameters influencing clinical outcome, such as histological grade, tumour size, clinical stage and presence of metastatic disease. Although some authors observed an association between p53 protein overexpression and tumour size as well as metastatic disease (GASPARINI et al. 1993) or between this feature and metastatic disease only (BOURHIS et al. 1994), most other authors do not confirm these findings, as no correlation between p53 protein overexpression and tumour stage, including metastatic disease, was found in their investigations (FIELD et al. 1991, 1993b, 1994; PAVELIC et al. 1992; GAPANY et al. 1993; NISHIOKA et al. 1993; HÖGMO et al. 1994; LEEDY et al. 1994; SCHIPPER and KELKER 1994; XU et al. 1994; AHOMADEGBE et al. 1995; BRENNAN et al. 1995a; LAVIEILLE et al. 1995; NAKANISHI et al. 1995; NYLANDER et al. 1995a,b). An inverse relationship between p53 protein overexpression and stage has even been reported (MUKHOPADHYAY et al. 1994).

As far as association of p53 protein overexpression and histological tumour features are concerned, data are as divergent as for clinical tumour parameters. No correlation between the presence of p53 protein and histological grade was observed by FIELD et al. (1991), PAVELIC et al. (1992), GAPANY et al. (1993), HÖGMO et al. (1994), SCHIPPER and KELKER (1994), XU et al. (1994a) BRENNAN et al. (1995a) or NAKANISHI et al. (1995). MUKHOPADHYAY et al. (1994) observed an inverse relationship between p53 protein overexpression and histological grade, p53 protein being most predominant in well-differentiated tumours. WATLING et al. (1992), however, found overexpression of p53 protein to be strongly associated with a histological malignancy grading scale, and LEE et al. (1993) found that p53 protein expression correlated with deeply invasive tumour growth.

Another way by which p53 gene mutations might influence prognosis has been proposed by HALD et al. (1994). These authors argued that mutated p53 proteins could be targets for cytotoxic T lymphocytes, thus inducing a possibly beneficial immune response of host to tumour. However, as peri-tumoural T cell infiltration did not correlate to p53 protein overexpression, T cell infiltration probably does not reflect an activation process induced by mutated p53 proteins, and it may be conluded that these mutated p53 proteins do not confer the immunogenic properties to tumour cells that are required to elicit a T cell-mediated cytotoxic attack.

The most conclusive evidence that p53 gene alterations are associated with prognosis needs to be provided by studies on patient survival. Such studies are few. FIELD et al. (1993b, 1994) noted no differences in survival time between patients with p53 protein-positive SCC and those with p53 protein-negative SCC, while AHOMADEGBE et al. (1995) failed to observe a different survival time between SCC patients with p53 gene mutations and those without. When comparing the outcome of radiotherapy in SCC patients with and without p53 protein overexpression, no differences were observed (WILSON et al. 1995).

BRACHMAN et al. (1992) observed that those patients with tumours in which p53 DNA sequence changes were detected had a shorter time to recurrence at the primary tumour site than those patients whose tumours had no p53 gene mutations. This trend towards earlier disease recurrence did not appear to be associated with tumour stage or type of treatment. A similar adverse influence of p53 gene alterations on survival was observed by LEE et al. (1993), who reported an increased risk of death from disease in patients with p53 gene mutations compared with patients without p53 gene mutations, and by GLUCKMAN et al. (1994) and TSUJI et al. (1995), who reported an association between p53 protein overexpression and decreased survival.

In contrast with these reports, SAUTER et al. (1992) observed that patients with p53 protein overexpression had a longer mean survival time than those without. They concluded that p53 protein overexpression may serve as a marker indicative of improved survival potential, whereas HÖGMO et al. (1994) failed to establish a significant impact of p53 positivity on prediction of survival.

Finally, it should be mentioned that there appears to be an association between p53 protein overexpression and response to chemotherapy – either negative, as observed by FIELD et al. (1993b), who reported an association between p53 protein overexpression and poor clinical outcome in a group of SCC patients with end-stage disease, or positive, as found by LAVIEILLE et al. (1995), who reported a significant correlation between complete response to induction chemotherapy and a high percentage of p53 staining in biopsies obtained before treatment.

From all these studies devoted to analysis of the influence of *p53* gene alterations on prognosis concerning oral SCC, irrespective of whether one considers cell kinetics, clinico-pathological parameters or disease-free survival time, no clear-cut picture emerges to indicate either a positive or a negative influence. It appears that so far detection of *p53* gene alterations has not fulfilled the characteristics of a useful prognostic factor as summarized by BATSAKIS and EL NAGGAR (1995): (a) significant and independent predictive value validated by clinical testing; (b) able to be determined by methods that are feasible, reproducible and widely available with appropriate quality control; (c) readily interpretable with clinical and therapeutic implications.

5.5 Alterations of *p53* in Oral Tumours Other Than Squamous Cell Carcinoma

Most data on *p53* gene alterations and p53 protein overexpression in oral tumours come from studies on SCC; much less attention has been paid to other oral tumours. In fact, the only studies performed have been devoted to p53 and salivary gland tumours; most of these concern pleomorphic adenomas and their malignant counterparts.

Overexpression of p53 protein was detected in benign pleomorphic adenomas and cell lines derived from this tumour (AZUMA et al. 1992; SOINI et al. 1992; DEGUCHI et al. 1993; RIGHI et al. 1994; GALLO et al. 1995b).

Some authors compared the expression of p53 protein in benign pleomorphic adenomas and carcinomas arising from pleomorphic adenoma. In general, the malignant tumours exhibited stronger positivity as well as more positive cells than the benign ones (GALLO et al. 1995b), and it has been proposed that involvement of p53 mutation may play an important role in the malignant transformation of salivary gland pleomorphic adenoma (DEGUCHI et al. 1993; RIGHI et al. 1994). As far as other salivary gland tumours are concerned, p53 protein overexpression has been reported to occur in muco-epidermoid carcinomas and undifferentiated carcinomas (SOINI et al. 1992), salivary duct carcinomas (HELLQUIST et al. 1994; ISHII and NAKAJIMA 1994; LI et al. 1995), adenoid cystic carcinomas, acinic cell carcinomas, polymorphous low-grade adenocarcinomas and epithelial myo-epithelial carcinomas (GALLO et al. 1995b).

Few data are available on correlations of p53 protein overexpression with other clinico-pathological features. SOINI et al. (1992) reported that in malignant salivary gland tumours the p53 protein positivity tended to be more evident in less-differentiated tumours. ISHII and NAKAJIMA (1994) reported a close correlation between p53 protein positivity and DNA aneuploidy in high-grade carcinomas of salivary gland tissue and, according to GALLO et al. (1995b), p53 protein positivity is an independent indication of clinical aggressiveness in patients with carcinoma of the parotid gland, as indicated by its correlation with regional and distant metastatic disease and a lower survival rate. It appears that p53 protein overexpression occurs in a variety of malignant salivary gland tumours. Its pur-ported predictive role as a marker of incipient malignancy in pleomorphic adenoma and its prognostic significance in patients with salivary gland carcino-mas both warrant further investigations.

5.6 Concluding Remarks

A vast amount of data on *p53* gene function, mutation and protein overexpression and its association with clinico-pathological parameters has appeared in the litera-ture during the past few years. As will have become apparent from the foregoing, *p53* gene alterations in oral SCC are frequently found and occur early in malignant transformation; it may be expected that further studies will augment our knowl-edge about the way in which *p53* is connected with regulation of cellular prolifera-tion and differentiation.

Whether determining *p53* gene status will provide useful knowledge applicable to clinical practice in the near future is debatable.

In a diagnostic sense, *p53*-mutant specific probes may represent a tool to detect tumour cells that are not visualised by conventional histological techniques, as outlined by BRENNAN et al. (1995b). Moreover, analysis of *p53* gene mutations by sequencing may be helpful in distinguishing multiple primary tumours from recurrent or metastatic disease, although more extensive application of this tech-nique requires evaluation of the prevalence of multiple *p53* gene mutations in one and the same lesion (NEES et al. 1993). Both DNA sequencing and preparation of mutant-specific probes, however, are not routinely employed in pathology, and they are very laborious. Therefore, it is not expected that they will be widely employed in the near future.

Overexpression of p53 protein as demonstrated by immunohistochemistry is more easily applicable in histopathological laboratories. However, its usefulness appears to be rather limited as far as diagnosis and prognosis are concerned, as has been discussed above. The confusing and contradictory data that have been published concerning impact of p53 protein overexpression on survival and the association of this feature with established clinico-pathological parameters is probably, at least in part, due to a lack of uniformity in immunohistochemical procedures.

Studies differ in the method of tissue preparation used (frozen versus paraffin-embedded material), in employing antibodies with different epitope specificities and in the use of antigen retrieval methods, all of which may not only influence the number of p53 protein-positive cases in a particular series, but also the number of p53 protein-labelled cells in an individual tumour (HALL and LANE 1994). Moreover, p53 protein positivity is scored in different ways. Methods vary from simply establishing whether there are any p53 protein-positive cells (GIROD et al. 1994a,b) to elaborate semi-quantitative methods in which both cell numbers and staining intensities are taken into account (PAVELIC et al. 1992).

This methodological diversity makes comparison of data from various series virtually impossible, and it will be apparent that it is necessary to formulate standard procedures for detection of p53 protein overexpression and positivity scoring in order to gain more insight into the significance of this feature in oral SCC.

References

Adamson R, Jones AS, Field JK (1994) Loss of heterozygosity studies on chromosome 17 in head and neck cancer using microsatellite markers. Oncogene 9: 2077–2082

Ahomadegbe JC, Barrois M, Fogel S, Le Bihan ML, Douc-Rasy S, Duvillard P, Armand JP, Riou G (1995) High incidence of p53 alterations (mutation, deletion, overexpression) in head and neck primary tumors and metastases; absence of correlation with clinical outcome. Frequent protein overexpression in normal epithelium and in early non-invasive lesions. Oncogene 10: 1217–1227

Azuma M, Kasai Y, Tamatani T, Sato M (1992) Involvement of p53 mutation in the development of human salivary gland pleomorphic adenomas. Cancer Lett 65: 61–67

Batsakis JG, El-Naggar AK (1995) p53: fifteen years after discovery. Adv Anat Pathol 2: 71–88

Battifora H (1994) p53 immunohistochemistry: a word of caution. Hum Pathol 25: 435–436

Berns A (1994) Is p53 the only real tumor suppressor gene. Curr Biol 4: 137–139

Birch JM (1992) Germline mutations in the p53 tumour suppressor gene; scientific, clinical and ethical challenges. Br J Cancer 66: 424–426

Birch JM (1994) Li-Fraumeni syndrome. Eur J Cancer 30: 1935–1941

Bourhis J, Bosq J, Wilson GD, Bressac B, Talbot M, Leridant AM, Dendale R, Janin N, Armand JP, Luboinski B, Malaise EP, Wibault P, Eschwege F (1994) Correlation between p53 gene expression and tumor-cell proliferation in oropharyngeal cancer. Int J Cancer 57: 458–462

Boyle JO, Hakim J, Koch W, Riet P van der, Hruban RH, Roa RA, Correo R, Eby YJ, Ruppert M, Sidransky D (1993) The incidence of p53 mutations increases with progression of head and neck cancer. Cancer Res 53: 4477–4480

Brachman DG, Graves D, Vokes E, Beckett M, Haraf D, Montay A, Dunphy E, Mick R, Yandell D, Weichselbaum RR (1992) Occurrence of p53 gene deletions and human papilloma virus infection in human head and neck cancer. Cancer Res 52: 4832–4836

Brachman DG, Beckett M, Graves D, Haraf D, Vokes E, Weichselbaum RR (1993) p53 mutation does not correlate with radiosensitivity in 24 head and neck cancer cell lines. Cancer Res 53: 3667–3669

Brennan JA, Boyle JO, Koch WM, Goodman SN, Hruban RH, Eby YJ, Cough MJ, Forastiere AA, Sidransky D (1995a) Association between cigarette smoking and mutation of the p53 gene in squamous cell carcinoma of the head and neck. N Engl J Med 332: 712–717

Brennan JA, Mao L, Hruban RH, Boyle JO, Eby YJ, Koch WM, Goodman SN, Sidransky D (1995b) Molecular assessment of histopathological staging in squamous cell carcinoma of the head and neck. N Engl J Med 332: 429–435

Burns JE, Baird MC, Clark LJ, Burns PA, Edington K, Chapman C, Mitchell R, Robertson G, Soutar D, Parkinson EK (1993) Gene mutations and increased levels of p53 protein in human squamous cell carcinomas and their cell lines. Br J Cancer 67: 1274-1284

Burns JE, Clark LJ, Yeudall WA, Mitchell R, Mackenzie K, Chang SE, Parkinson EK (1994a) The p53 status of cultured human premalignant oral keratinocytes. Br J Cancer 70: 591-595

Burns JE, McFarlane R, Clark LJ, Mitchell R, Robertson G, Soutar D, Parkinson EK (1994b) Maintenance of identical p53 mutations throughout progression of squamous cell carcinomas of the tongue. Oral Oncol Eur J Cancer 30B: 335-337

Caamano J, Zhang SY, Rosvold EA, Bauer B, Klein-Szanto AJP (1993) p53 alterations in human squamous cell carcinomas and carcinoma cell lines. Am J Pathol 142: 1131-1139

Chang F, Syrjänen S, Tervahauta A, Syrjänen K (1993) Tumourigenesis associated with the p53 tumour suppressor gene. Int J Cancer 68: 653-661

Chen YT, Xu L, Massey L, Zlotolow IM, Huvos AG, Garin-Chesa P, Old LJ (1994) Frameshift and nonsense p53 mutations in squamous carcinoma of head and neck: non-reactivity with three anti-p53 monoclonal antibodies. Int J Oncol 4: 609-614

Chung KY, Mukhopadhyay T, Kim, Casson A, Ro JY, Göpfert H, Hong WK, Roth JA (1993) Discordant p53 gene mutations in primary head and neck cancers and corresponding second primary cancers of the upper aerodigestive tract. Cancer Res 53: 1676-1683

Clayman GL, El Naggar AK, Roth JA, Zhang WW, Goepfert H, Taylor DL, Liu TJ (1995) In vivo molecular therapy with p53 adenovirus for microscopic residual head and neck squamous carcinoma. Cancer Res 55: 1-6

Coltrera MD, Zarbo RJ, Sakr WA, Gown AM (1992) Markers for dysplasia of the upper aerodigestive tract. Suprabasal expression of PCNA, p53 and CK19 in alcohol-fixed, embedded tissue. Am J Pathol 141: 817-825

Deguchi H, Hamano H, Hayashi Y (1993) c-myc, ras p21 and p53 expression in pleomorphic adenoma and its malignant form of the human salivary glands. Acta Pathol Jpn 43: 413-422

Demers GW, Halbert CL, Galloway DA (1994) Elevated wild type p53 protein in human epithelial cell lines immortalized by the human papillomavirus 16 E7 gene. Virology 198: 169-174

Eisenberg E, Krutchkoff DJ (1992) Lichenoid lesions of oral mucosa. Diagnostic criteria and their importance in the alleged relationship to oral cancer. Oral Surg Oral Med Oral Pathol 73: 699-704

El-Deiry WS, Tokino T, Velculescu VE, Levy DB, Parsons R, Trent JM, Lin D, Mercer E, Kinzler KW, Vogelstein B (1993) WAF1, a potential mediator of p53 tumor suppression. Cell 75: 817-825

Field JK, Spandidos DA, Malliri A, Gosney JR, Ylagnisis M, Stell PM (1991) Elevated p53 expression correlates with a history of heavy smoking in squamous cell carcinoma of the head and neck. Br J Cancer 64: 573-577

Field JK, Pavelic ZP, Spandidos DA, Stambrook PJ, Jones AS, Gluckman JL (1993a) The role of the p53 tumor suppressor gene in squamous cell carcinoma of the head and neck. Arch Otolaryngol Head Neck Surg 119: 1118-1122

Field JK, Malliri A, Butt SA, Gosney JR, Phillips D, Spandidos DA, Jones AS (1993b) p53 expression in end stage squamous cell carcinoma of the head and neck prior to chemotherapy treatment: expression correlates with a very poor clinical outcome. Int J Oncol 3: 431-435

Field JK, Zoumpourlis V, Spandidos DA, Jones AS (1994) p53 expression and mutations in squamous cell carcinoma of the head and neck: expression correlates with the patients use of tobacco and alcohol. Cancer Detect Prevent 18: 197-208

Fisher DE (1994) Apoptosis in cancer therapy: crossing the threshold. Cell 78: 539-542

Franceschi S, Gloghini A, Maestro R, Barzan L, Bidoli E, Talamini R, Vukosavljevic T, Carbone A, Boiocchi M (1995) Analysis of the p53 gene in relation to tobacco and alcohol in cancers of the upper aero-digestive tract. Int J Cancer 60: 872-876

Gallo O, Bianchi S (1995) p53 expression: a potential biomarker for risk of multiple primary malignancies in the upper aerodigestive tract. Oral Oncol Eur J Cancer 31B: 53-57

Gallo O, Bianchi S, Giovannucci-Uzzielli ML, Santoro R, Lenzi S, Salimbeni C, Abruzzese M, Alajmo E (1995a) p53 oncoprotein overexpression correlates with mutagen-induced chromosome fragility in head and neck cancer patients with multiple malignancies. Br J Cancer 71: 1008-1012

Gallo O, Franchi A, Bianchi S, Boddi V, Giannelli E, Alajmo E (1995b) p53 oncoprotein expression in parotid gland carcinoma is associated with clinical outcome. Cancer 75: 2037-2044

Gapany M, Pavelic ZP, Gapany SR, Pavelic L, Li YQ, Craven JM, Jones H, Biddinger P, Stambrook PJ, Gluckman JL (1993) Relationship between immunohistochemically detectable p53 protein and prognostic factors in head and neck tumors. Cancer Detect Prevent 17: 379-386

Gasparini G (1995) p53 and angiogenesis. J Clin Oncol 13: 1830

Gasparini G, Weidner N, Maluta S, Pozza F, Boracchi P, Mezzetti M, Testolin A, Bevilacqua P (1993) Intratumoral microvessel density and p53 protein: correlation with metastasis in head-and-neck squamous cells carcinoma. Int J Cancer 55: 739-744

Girod SC, Krueger GRF, Pape HD (1993) p53 and Ki67 expression in preneoplastic and neoplastic lesions of the oral mucosa. Int J Oral Maxillofac Surg 22: 285-288

Girod SC, Pape HD, Krueger GRF (1994a) p53 and PCNA expression in carcinogenesis of the oropharyngeal mucosa. Oral Oncol Eur J Cancer 30B: 419-423

Girod SC, Krämer C, Knüfermann R, Krueger GRF (1994b) p53 expression in the carcinogenesis in the oral mucosa. J Cell Biochem 56: 444-448

Gluckman JL, Stambrook PJ, Pavelic ZP (1994) Prognostic significance of p53 protein accumulation in early stage T1 oral cavity cancer. Oral Oncol Eur J Cancer 30B: 281

Greenblatt MS, Bennett WP, Hollstein M, Harris CC (1994) Mutations in the p53 tumor suppressor gene: clues to cancer etiology and molecular pathogenesis. Cancer Res 54: 4855-4878

Gusterson BA, Anbazhagan R, Warren W, Midgely C, Lane DP, O'Hare M, Stamps A, Carter R, Jayatilake H (1991) Expression of p53 in premalignant and malignant squamous epithelium. Oncogene 6: 1785-1789

Hald J, Rasmussen N, Claesson MH (1994) In vivo infiltration of mononuclear cells in squamous cell carcinoma of the head and neck correlates with the ability to expand tumour-infiltrating T-cells in vitro and with the expression of MHC class I antigens on tumour cells. Cancer Immunol Immunother 39: 383-390

Hall PA, Lane DP (1994) p53 in tumour pathology: can we trust immunohistochemistry? - revisited. J Pathol 172: 1-4

Hartwell LH, Kastan MB (1994) Cell cycle control and cancer. Science 266: 1821-1828

Hellquist HB, Karlsson MG, Nilsson C (1994) Salivary duct carcinoma - a highly aggressive salivary gland tumour with overexpression of c-erbB-2. J Pathol 172: 35-44

Hirano T, Franzen B, Kato H, Ebihara Y, Auer G (1994) Genesis of squamous cell lung carcinoma. Sequential changes of proliferation, DNA ploidy, and p53 expression. Am J Pathol 144: 296-302

Högmo A, Munck-Wikland E, Kuylenstierna R, Lindholm J, Auer G (1994) Nuclear DNA content and p53 immunostaining in oral squamous cell carcinoma - an analysis of a consecutive 10-year material. Int J Oncol 5: 915-920

Holmstrup P (1992) The controversy of a premalignant potential of oral lichen planus is over. Oral Surg Oral Med Oral Pathol 73: 704-706

Ishii K, Nakajima T (1994) Evaluation of malignant grade of salivary gland tumors: studies by cytofluorometric nuclear DNA analysis, histochemistry for nucleolar organizer regions and immunohistochemistry for p53. Pathol Int 44: 287-296

Jung M, Notario V, Dritschilo A (1992) Mutations in the p53 gene in radiation-sensitive and resistant human squamous carcinoma cells. Cancer Res 52: 6390-6393

Kaur J, Srivastava A, Ralhan R (1994) Overexpression of p53 protein in betel- and tobacco-related human oral dysplasia and squamous-cell carcinoma in India. Int J Cancer 58: 340-345

Koch WM, Boyle JO, Mao L, Hakim J, Hruban RH, Sidransky D (1994) p53 gene mutations as markers of tumor spread in synchromous oral cancers. Arch Otolaryngol Head Neck Surg 120: 943-947

Koch WM, Patel H, Brennan J, Boyle JO, Sidransky D (1995) Squamous cell carcinoma of the head and neck in the elderly. Arch Otolaryngol Head Neck Surg 121: 262-265

Kuttan NAA, Rosin MP, Ambika K, Priddy RW, Bhakthan NMG, Zhang L (1995) High prevalence of expression of p53 oncoprotein in oral carcinomas from India associated with betel and tobacco chewing. Oral Oncol Eur J Cancer 31B: 169-173

Lane DP (1994) The regulation of p53 function: Steiner Award Lecture. Int J Cancer 57: 623-627

Lane DP, Benchimol S (1990) p53: oncogene or anti-oncogene. Genes Dev 4: 1-8

Langdon JD, Partridge M (1992) Expression of the tumour suppressor gene p53 in oral cancer. Br J Oral Maxillofac Surg 30: 214-220

Lavieille JP, Brambilla E, Riva-Lavieille C, Reyt E, Charachon R, Brambilla C (1995) Immunohistochemical detection of p53 protein in preneoplastic lesions and squamous cell carcinoma of the head and neck. Acta Otolaryngol 115: 334-339

Lazarus P, Garewal HS, Sciubba J, Zwiebel N, Calcagnotto A, Fair A, Schaefer S, Richie JP Jr (1995) A low incidence of p53 mutations in pre-malignant lesions of the oral cavity from non-tobacco users. Int J Cancer 60: 458-463

Lee NK, Ye YW, Chen J, Li X, Waber PG, Nisen PD (1993) p53, retinoblastoma and human papillomavirus in squamous cell carcinoma and adjacent normal mucosa of the upper areodigestive tract. Arch Otolaryngol Head Neck Surg 119: 1125-1131

Leedy DA, Trune DR, Kronz JD, Weidner N, Cohen JI (1994) Tumor angiogenesis, the p53 antigen and cervical metastasis in squamous cell carcinoma of the tongue. Otolaryngol Head Neck Surg 111: 417-422

Levine AJ (1994) The road to the discovery of the p53 protein. The Steiner Cancer Prize Award Lecture. Int J Cancer 56: 775-776

Levine AJ, Momand J (1990) Tumor suppressor genes: the p53 and retinoblastoma sensitivity genes and gene products. Biochim Biophys Acta 1032: 119-136

Levine AJ, Momand J, Finlay CA (1991) The p53 tumour suppressor gene. Nature 351: 453-456

Levine AJ, Perry ME, Chang A, Silver A, Dittmer D, Wu M, Welsh D (1994) The 1993 Walter Hubert Lecture: the role of the p53 tumour-suppressor gene in tumorigenesis. Br J Cancer 69: 409-416

Lewensohn-Fuchs I, Munck-Wickland E, Berke Z, Magnusson KP, Pallesen G, Auer G, Lindholm J, Linde A, Aberg B, Rubio C, Kuylenstierna R, Wiman KG, Dalianis T (1994) Involvement of aberrant p53 expression and human papillomavirus in carcinoma of the head, neck and esophagus. Anticancer Res 14: 1281-1286

Li SH, Kim MS, Cherrick HM, Park NH (1992) Low p53 level in immortal, non-tumorigenic oral keratinocytes harboring HPV-16 DNA. Oral Oncol Eur J Cancer 28B: 129-134

Li X, Tsuji T, Wen S, Sobhan F, Wang Z, Shinozaki F (1995) Cytoplasmic expression of p53 protein and its morphological features in salivary gland lesions. J Oral Pathol Med 24: 201-220

Liu TJ, Zhang WW, Taylor DL, Roth JA, Goepfert H, Clayman GL (1994) Growth suppression of human head and neck cancer cells by the introduction of a wild type p53 gene via a recombinant adenovirus. Cancer Res 54: 3662-3667

Liu TJ, El-Naggar AK, McDonnell TJ, Steck KD, Wang M, Taylor DL, Clayman GL (1995) Apoptosis induction mediated by wild-type p53 adenoviral gene transfer in squamous cell carcinoma of the head and neck. Cancer Res 55: 3117-3122

Lowe SW, Bodis S, McClatchey A, Remington L, Ruley HE, Fisher DE, Housman DE, Jacks T (1994) p53 status and the efficacy of cancer therapy in vivo. Science 266: 807-810

Matthews JB, Scully C, Jovanovic A, van der Waal I, Yeudall WA, Prime SS (1993) Relationship of tobacco/alcohol use to p53 expression in patients with lingual squamous cell carcinomas. Oral Oncol Eur J Cancer 29B: 285-289

Melhem MF, Law JC, El-Ashmawy L, Johnson JT, Landreneau RJ, Srivastava S, Whiteside TL (1995) Assessment of sensitivity and specificity of immunohistochemical staining of p53 in lung and head and neck cancers. Am J Pathol 146: 1170-1177

Meltzer PS (1994) MDM2 and p53: a question of balance. J Natl Cancer Inst 86: 1265-1266

Min BM, Baek JH, Shin KH, Gujuluva CN, Cherrick HM, Park NH (1994) Inactivation of the p53 gene by either mutation or HPV infection is extremely frequent in human oral squamous cell carcinoma lines. Oral Oncol Eur J cancer 30B: 338-345

Momand J, Zambetti GP, Olson DC, George D, Levine AJ (1992) The mdm-2 oncogene product forms a complex with the p53 protein and inhibits p53-mediated transactivation. Cell 69: 1237-1245

Mukhopadhyay D, Chatterjee R, Chakraborty RN (1994) Association of p53 expression with cytokinetics and HPV capsid antigen prevalence in oral carcinomas. Cancer Lett 87: 99-105

Nakanishi Y, Noguchi M, Matsuno Y, Mukai K, Shimosato Y, Hirohashi S (1993) p53 expression in squamous cell carcinoma and dysplasia of the vocal cords and oral cavity. Appl Immunohistochem 1: 101-107

Nakanishi Y, Noguchi M, Matsuno Y, Saikawa M, Mukai K, Shimosato Y, Hirohashi S (1995) p53 expression in multicentric squamous cell carcinoma and surrounding squamous epithelium of the upper aerodigestive tract. Cancer 75: 1657-1662

Nees M, Homann N, Discher H, Andl T, Enders C, Herold-Mende C, Schuhmann A, Bosch FX (1993) Expression of mutated p53 occurs in tumor-distant epithelia of head and neck cancer patients: possible molecular basis for the development of multiple tumors. Cancer Res 53: 4189-4196

Nicol CJ, Harrison ML, Laposa RR, Gimelshtein IL, Wells PG (1995) A teratologic suppressor role for p53 in benzo (a) pyrene-treated transgenic p53 deficient mice. Nature Genet 10: 181-187

Nishioka H, Hiasa Y, Hayashi I, Kitahori Y, Konishi N, Sugimura M (1993) Immunohistochemical detection of p53 oncoprotein in human and squamous cell carcinomas and leukoplakias: comparison with proliferating cell nuclear antigen staining and correlation with clinicopathological findings. Oncology 50: 426-429

Nylander K, Stenling R, Gustafsson H, Zackrisson B, Roos G (1995a) p53 expression and cell proliferation in squamous cell carcinomas of the head and neck. Cancer 75: 87-93

Nylander K, Nilsson P, Mehle C, Roos G (1995b) p53 mutations, protein expression and cell proliferation in squamous cell carcinomas of the head and neck. Br J Cancer 71: 826-830

Ogden GR, Kiddie RA, Lunny DP, Lane DP (1992) Assessment of p53 protein expression in normal, benign and malignant oral mucosa. J Pathol 166: 389-394

Pavelic ZP, Gluckman JL, Gapany M, Reising J, Craven JM, Kelley DJ, Pavelic L, Gapany S, Biddinger P, Stambrook PJ (1992) Improved immunohistochemical detection of p53 protein in paraffin-embedded tissues reveals elevated levels in most head and neck and lung carcinomas: correlation with clinicopathological parameters. Anticancer Res 12: 1389-1394

Pavelic Z, Li YQ, Stambrook PJ, McDonald JS, Munck-Wikland E, Pavelic K, Dacic S, Danilovic Z, Pavelic L, Mugge RE, Wilson K, Nguyen C, Gluckman JL (1994) Overexpression of p53 protein is common in premalignant head and neck lesions. Anticancer Res 14: 2259-2266

Picksley SM, Lane DP (1994) p53 and Rb: their cellular roles. Curr Opin Cell Biol 6: 853-858

Ranasinghe A, MacGeoch C, Dyer S, Spurr N, Johnson NW (1993a) Some oral carcinomas from Sri Lankan betel tobacco chewers overexpress p53 oncoprotein but lack mutations in exons 5-9. Anticancer Res 13: 2065-2068

Ranasinghe AW, Warnakulasuriya KAAS, Johnson NW (1993b) Low prevalence of expression of p53 oncoprotein in oral carcinomas from Sri Lanka associated with betel and tobacco chewing. Oral Oncol Eur J Cancer 29B: 147-150

Regezi JA, Zarbo RJ, Regev E, Pisanty S, Silverman S, Ganit D (1995) p53 protein expression in sequential biopsies of oral dysplasias and in situ carcinomas. J Oral Pathol Med 24: 18-22

Righi PD, Li YQ, Deutsch M, McDonald JS, Wilson KM, Bejarano P, Stambrook PJ, Osterhage D, Nguyen C, Gluckman JL, Pavelic ZP (1994) The role of the p53 gene in the malignant transformation of pleomorphic adenomas of the parotid gland. Anticancer Res 14: 2253-2258

Sah VP, Attardi LD, Mulligan GJ, Williams BO, Bronson RT, Jacks T (1995) A subset of p53-deficient embryos exhibit exencephaly. Nature Genet 10: 175-180

Sakai E, Tsuchida N (1992) Most human squamous cell carcinomas in the oral cavity contain mutated p53 tumor-suppressor genes. Oncogene 7: 927-933

Sakai E, Rikimaru K, Ueda M, Matsumoto Y, Ishii N, Enomoto S, Yamamoto H, Tsuchida N (1992) The p53 tumor-suppressor gene and ras oncogene mutations in oral squamous cell carcinoma. Int J Cancer 52: 867-872

Sauter ER, Ridge JA, Gordon J, Eisenberg BL (1992) p53 overexpression correlates with increased survival in patients with squamous carcinoma of the tongue base. Am J Surg 164: 651-653

Sauter ER, Cleveland D, Trock B, Ridge JA, Klein-Szanto AJP (1994) p53 is overexpressed in fifty percent of pre-invasive lesions of head and neck epithelium. Carcinogenesis 15: 2269-2274

Scheffner M, Werness BA, Huibregtse JM, Levine AJ, Howley PM (1990) The E6 oncoprotein encoded by human papilloma virus types 16 and 18 promotes the degradation of p53. Cell 63: 1129-1136

Schipper JH, Kelker W (1994) Die Expression der Tumorsuppressor-gene p53 und Rb bei Patienten mit Plattenepithelkarzinomen im Kopf-/Halsbereich. HNO 42: 270-274

Shin DM, Kim J, Ro JY, Hittelman J, Roth JA, Hong WK, Hittelman WN (1994) Activation of p53 gene expression in premalignant lesions during head and neck tumorigenesis. Cancer Res 54: 321–326

Slootweg PJ, Koole R, Hordijk GJ (1994) The presence of p53 protein in relation to Ki-67 as cellular proliferation marker in head and neck squamous cell carcinoma and adjacent dysplastic mucosa. Oral Oncol, Eur J Cancer 30B: 138–141

Smith ML, Chen IT, Zhan Q, Chen CJ, Gilmer TM, Kastan MB, O'Connor PM, Fornace AJ (1994) Interaction of the p53-regulated protein Gadd 45 with proliferating cell nuclear antigen. Science 266: 1376–1380

Snijders PJF, Steenbergen RDM, Top B, Scott SD, Meijer CJLM, Walboomers JMM (1994) Analysis of p53 status in tonsillar carcinomas associated with human papillomavirus. J Gen Virol 75: 2769–2775

Soini Y, Kamel D, Nuorva K, Lane DP, Vähäkangas K, Pääkkö P (1992) Low p53 protein expression in salivary gland tumours compared with lung carcinomas. Virchows Arch [A] Pathol Anat 421: 415–420

Somers KD, Merrick MA, Lopez ME, Incognito LS, Schechter GL, Casey G (1992) Frequent p53 mutations in head and neck cancer. Cancer Res 52: 5997–6000

Soussi T, Legros Y, Lubin R, Ory K, Schlichtholz B (1994) Multifactorial analysis of p53 alteration in human cancer: a review. Int J Cancer 57: 1–9

Thomas S, Brennan J, Martel G, Frazer I, Montesano R, Sidransky D, Hollstein M (1994) Mutations in the conserved regions of p53 are infrequent in betel-associated oral cancers from Papua New Guinea. Cancer Res 54: 3588–3593

Tsuji T, Mimura Y, Wen S, Li X, Kanekawa A, Susaki K, Shinozaki F (1995) The significance of PCNA and p53 protein in some oral tumors. Int J Oral Maxillofac Surg 24: 221–225

Warnakulasuriya KAAS, Johnson NW (1992) Expression of p53 mutant nuclar phosphoprotein in oral carcinoma and potentially malignant oral lesions. J Oral Pathol Med 21: 404–408

Warnakulasuriya KAAS, Johnson NW (1994) Association of overexpression of p53 oncoprotein with the state of cell proliferation in oral carcinoma. J Oral Pathol Med 23: 246–250

Watling DL, Gown AM, Coltrera MD (1992) Overexpression of p53 in head and neck cancer. Head Neck 14: 437–444

Weidner N (1995) Intratumor microvessel density as a prognostic factor in cancer. Am J Pathol 147: 9–19

Werness BA, Levine AJ, Howley PM (1990) Association of human papillomavirus types 16 and 18 E6 proteins with p53. Science 248: 76–78

Wilson GD, Rickman PI, Dische S, Saunders MI, Robinson B, Daley FM, Ross DA (1995) p53 status of head and neck cancer: relation to biological characteristics and outcome of radiotherapy. Br J Cancer 71: 1248–1252

Wynford-Thomas D (1992) p53 in tumour pathology: can we trust immunocytochemistry? J Pathol 166: 329–330

Xu L, Chen YT, Huvos AG, Zlotolow IM, Rettig WJ, Old LJ, Garin-Chesa P (1994a) Over-expression of p53 protein in squamous cell carcinomas of head and neck without apparent gene mutations. Diagn Mol Pathol 3: 83–92

Xu L, Davidson BJ, Murty VVVS, Li RG, Sacks PG, Garin-Chesa P, Schantz SP, Chaganti RSK (1994b) TP53 gene mutations and CCND1 gene amplification in head and neck squamous cell carcinoma lines. Int J Cancer 59: 383–387

Yeudall WA (1992) Human papillomavirus and oral neoplasia. Oral Oncol Eur J Cancer 28B: 61–66

Yeudall WA, Paterson IC, Patel V, Prime SS (1995) Presence of human papillomavirus sequences in tumour-derived human oral keratinocytes expressing mutant p53. Oral Oncol Eur J Cancer 31B: 136–143

Zarilawa M, Schmid S, Pfaltz M, Ohgaki H, Kleihues P, Schäfer R (1994) p53 gene mutations in oropharyngeal carcinomas: a comparison of solitary and multiple primary tumors and lymph-node metastases. Int J Cancer 56: 807–811

Genomic Instability in Head and Neck Cancer

A.G.M. Scholes and J.K. Field

1 Introduction

Carcinogenesis is a multistage process, resulting from the accumulation of genetic alterations. Proliferation of normal cells is thought to be regulated by growth-promoting proto-oncogenes counterbalanced by growth-constraining tumour suppressor genes (TSG) (WEINBERG 1991). During tumour initiation and progression, proto-oncogenes may be activated by amplification, rearrangement or point mutation, whilst loss of function of TSG may be caused by deletion or mutation. Precisely how many genetic alterations are required for tumourigenesis is unclear; statistical analysis based on age-specific data suggests that five or six steps are generally necessary (RENAN 1993). In a molecular model specific for colorectal tumourigenesis, it has been proposed that mutations in at least four to five genes are required for the formation of a malignant tumour (FEARON and VOGELSTEIN 1990). In the case of head and neck cancer, however, it has been suggested that a greater number of genetic lesions are required (RENAN 1993), and it is evident from allelotype analysis that the process is complex (FIELD et al. 1995b).

Current Topics in Pathology
Volume 90, G. Seifert (Ed.)
© Springer-Verlag Berlin Heidelberg 1996

Determination of the critical genetic events in head and neck carcinogenesis will conceivably allow early detection and direct future treatment of these cancers. In this chapter, potentially important chromosome regions identified by cytogenetic and loss of heterozygosity (LOH) analysis in squamous cell carcinomas of the head and neck (SCCHN) will be reviewed. Recent evidence regarding the role of DNA repair genes in genomic instability and problems associated with the development of a molecular progression model for SCCHN will be discussed.

2 Cytogenetic Analysis in Squamous Cell Carcinoma of the head and Neck

Characterisation of particular chromosome aberrations in tumour cells by cytogenetic analysis has been the first step in identifying genes which may be involved in cancer development. These aberrations include whole chromosomal loss or gain, chromosomal rearrangements, such as inversions and translocations, deletions

Table 1. Summary of chromosome aberrations detected in head and neck squamous cell carcinomas by cytogenetic analysis

Chromosome	Regions with aberrations
1	1p, 1q, 1p11–p12, 1p13, 1p22, 1p36, 1q21, 1q25, 1q32
2	2q, 2q33–q36
	3p, 3q, 3pter–p23, 3p11, 3p13, 3p13–p23, 3p14–p25, 3p21, 3p21–qter, 3p26–qter, 3cent–qter
4	4p, 4q, 4q11–q21, 4q21, 4q21–qter
5	5p, 5p11, 5q, 5q12–q23
6	6q15–q26, 6q21–q25
7	7p, 7q, 7cent–p15, 7p11, 7p21–p22, 7q22–q34, 7q33–qter
8	8p, 8q, 8p11.2, 8p22–p23, 8 cent, 8cent–q21.2, 8q10
9	9p, 9p21–p24, 9 cent, 9q32
10	10p, 10q, 10pter–q21.2, 10q11.2, 10q22–q26
11	11p, 11q, 11p15, 11q13, 11q13–q21, 11q13–q23, 11q23
12	12p, 12p11.2
13	13p, 13q, 13p11–p13, 13q32–qter
14	14p, 14q, 14p11–q11
15	15p, 15p11–q11, 15q10
16	16p
17	17p, 17q
18	18q, 18q21, 18q21–qter, 18q22, 18q22–q23
19	19p, 19q, 19pter–cen, 19p13, 19p13.1
20	20p, 20p13
21	21p, 21q
22	22p, 22q

Compilation of aberrations detected by Hauser-Urfer and Stauffer 1985; Jin et al. 1990; Allegra et al. 1992; Cowan 1992; Mitelman 1991; Osella et al. 1992; Owens et al. 1992; Jin and Mertens 1993; Jin et al. 1993; Rao et al. 1994; Van Dyke et al. 1994; Jin et al. 1995 and Speicher et al. 1995.

and amplifications. Identification of chromosomal regions frequently deleted or duplicated may indicate possible sites of TSG or oncogenes, respectively; chromosomal bands frequently rearranged may represent sites of oncogene activation (COWAN 1992). Review of cytogenetic studies using cultures derived from SCCHN shows that the majority of autosomal chromosome arms may be affected (Table 1). A problem with the use of cell lines, however, is that the rearrangements observed may not be represented in the primary tumour. Indeed, a comparison of karyotypic changes in cell lines with those of the corresponding primary carcinoma identified clonal evolution in all cell lines (SREEKANTAIAH et al. 1994). This has been largely overcome by the use of short-term cultures, although different culture conditions may favour the proliferative growth of different cell populations (JIN et al. 1993). A consistent abnormality common to all SCCHN has not been identified, but it is clear that there is a recurrent clustering of aberrations on several chromosomal regions. In a study of short-term cultures from SCCHN, JIN et al. (1995) found the chromosomal bands most frequently involved were, in order of decreasing frequency, 8p11–q11, 1p11–q11, 3p11–q11, 11q13, 13p11–q11, 1p13, 5p11–q11, 7p11–q11, 15p11–q11 and 14p11–q11. It is notable that COWAN (1992) reported deletions of the following specific regions at high frequency: 3pter–p23, 4q11–q21, 4q11–q221, 4q21–qter, 8pter–p23, 8p23–p21 and 10pter–p11.2. In addition, chromosome region 7cent–p15 was duplicated at high frequency (COWAN 1992).

3 Allelic Imbalance

Analysis of allelic imbalance (i.e. LOH analysis) has a major advantage over cytogenetic techniques as it has a greatly enhanced resolution, especially if closely spaced microsatellite markers are used. This technique allows the determination of specific chromosome regions containing deletions (allelic loss), which has led to the identification of a number of TSG, including the retinoblastoma gene (RB) and adenomatous polyposis coli gene (APC) (MARSHALL 1991; WEINBERG 1991).

Whilst early studies mainly used restriction fragment-length polymorphisms to detect allelic loss, recent studies have used microsatellite markers. Microsatellites are short, simple repeat sequences (typically di-, tri- or tetranucleotides) usually found in intergenic DNA or within the introns of genes. Dinucleotide repeats are very common, are relatively uniformly distributed throughout the genome and are often highly polymorphic as a result of variation in the number of repeated units from one allele to another. Polymerase chain reaction (PCR)-based amplification of specific microsatellite repeats can be carried out using primers which flank the area of interest (WEBER and MAY 1989). Radioactively labelled products may be detected by autoradiography, following electrophoresis. Alternatively, the products may be visualised and sized on silver-stained acrylamide gels. Determination of allelic loss for informative markers is made by comparison of the relative intensity of normal and tumour alleles from the same patient. LOH may be determined by the absence of, or reduced, allelic amplification in the tumour

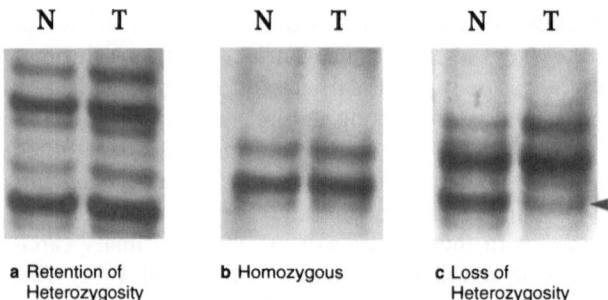

a Retention of   **b** Homozygous   **c** Loss of
Heterozygosity   Heterozygosity

Fig. 1a–c. Representative allelic imbalance (loss of heterozygosity). a Retention of heterozygosity. b Homozygosity. c Allelic imbalance (*arrowhead*). "Stutter" or "shadow bands" may be seen in both the normal (*N*) and tumour (*T*) lanes. (From Field et al. 1995b, with permission)

sample. Complete loss is not always seen, due to contamination of the tumour with non-neoplastic cells (Fig. 1).

3.1 Possible Target Regions in Squamous Cell Carcinoma of the Head and Neck

Certain regions frequently show allelic imbalance in SCCHN, particularly on chromosome arms 3p, 5q, 9p, 9q, 11p, 11q, 13q, 17p and 18q (Maestro et al. 1993; Adamson et al. 1994; Ah-See et al. 1994; Lydiatt et al. 1994; Nawroz et al. 1994; Scholnick et al. 1994; Field et al. 1995b; Rowley et al. 1995); these are detailed below. Other chromosomal regions which show LOH at lower frequency include 1p, 1q, 2p, 6p, 6q, 8p, 8q, 17q and 19q (Field et al. 1995b); although all of these are not discussed in detail, it is possible that genetic alterations at these sites may play an important role in the pathogenesis of certain tumours.

The findings reported in cytogenetic and allelic imbalance studies do not always agree; this may be due to the interpretation of LOH data. In general, papers reporting allelic imbalance define reduced intensity of one allele as indicative of LOH, although these studies cannot readily distinguish between allele deletion and low-level amplification or duplication. Thus apparent LOH may not necessarily be indicative of the presence of a TSG, and this should be taken into consideration when interpreting allelic imbalance studies (Field et al. 1995b; Jin et al. 1995).

3.1.1 Chromosome 1

Chromosome 1p frequently demonstrates cytogenetic abnormalities in SCCHN, particularly at 1p22 and 1p11–p12 (Jin et al. 1990, 1993; Owens et al. 1992), whereas LOH analysis has demonstrated allelic loss of this chromosome arm in only 14%–30% of tumours (Ah-See et al. 1994; Nawroz et al. 1994; Field et al. 1995b). The study by Field et al. (1995b), however, used the greatest number of microsatellite markers and identified a minimal area of loss at 1p31.2–p21.3. Thus, although loss of this region may not be as frequent as that at other chromosomal sites in SCCHN, retention of heterozygosity of markers outside this region in the majority of tumours suggests this chromosomal locus may be important in the pathogenesis of a number of head and neck tumours.

3.1.2 Chromosome 3

Allele loss on the short arm of chromosome 3 is common in SCCHN. Initial studies in early-passage cell lines defined the commonly deleted region as 3p14–26 (LATIF et al. 1992). Later studies of paired tumour and normal mucosa have suggested the presence of at least three TSG on 3p. MAESTRO et al. (1993) demonstrated LOH at 3p in 74% of SCCHN and defined three regions of loss, 3p24–pter, 3p21.3 and 3p14–cen. In a study of oral carcinomas, WU et al. (1994) identified LOH at 3p in 52% of tumours and mapped three distinct regions of loss, which appear to overlap with those described by MAESTRO et al. (1993), 3p13–p21.1, 3p21.3–p23 and 3p25. Other studies of SCCHN have found more than 60% loss using markers mapping within these regions, for example to 3p13–p14 and 3p21 (EL-NAGGAR et al. 1993; AH-SEE et al. 1994; SCHOLNICK et al. 1994). Frequent deletion of these regions is not unique to SCCHN and has been demonstrated in many tumour types, including lung cancer (HIBI et al. 1992; KILLARY et al. 1992). A TSG locus at 3p21–p22, for example, has previously been defined, and a number of putative TSG have been isolated from this region (KILLARY et al. 1992). Recently, a human mismatch repair gene, *h*MLH1 (see Sect. 4) has been located on chromosome 3p21.3–p23 (BRONNER et al. 1994). Studies of inactivation of these genes in SCCHN have not been reported.

The similar finding of three discrete regions of loss on chromosome 3p in lung cancer (HIBI et al. 1992) raises the possibility that aetiological factors common to both lung and head and neck cancer, such as smoking, may be associated with LOH on 3p. Our studies have found LOH on 3p to correlate with nodal metastases and TNM stage IV tumours (FIELD et al. 1994a), suggesting these alterations may occur as later events in the progression of SCCHN. WU et al. (1994) showed that, in contrast to TNM stage I tumours, the majority of stage II–III oral carcinomas showed 3p LOH, although the sample size was small. Notable, however, was the finding that three out of the five stage IV tumours examined did not show loss, but two of these were from young subjects and were not associated with known aetiological factors; the third was associated with chewing of betel nut leaf quid (WU et al. 1994).

3.1.3 Chromosome 5

The long arm of chromosome 5 contains the APC gene at 5q21, which has been linked with familial adenomatous polyposis (FAP) (KINZLER et al. 1991). FAP is characterised clinically by the presence of multiple polyps throughout the colon and rectum, at least one of which may become malignant. Allele loss on chromosome 5q has been demonstrated in 25%–43% of SCCHN, often involving the 5q21–q22 region (AH-SEE et al. 1994; FIELD et al. 1995b). A study of oral SCC in Japan has demonstrated LOH at the APC locus in 73%, but APC gene mutations in only 12.5% of tumours (UZAWA et al. 1994).

3.1.4 Chromosome 8

Cytogenetic studies of short-term cultures from head and neck carcinomas have reported frequent aberrations on chromosome 8, specifically at 8p11–q11, 8pter–p23 and 8p23–p21 (COWAN 1992; JIN et al. 1995). Frequent LOH (40%) has also been demonstrated on the p arm of this chromosome in SCCHN (KIARIS et al. 1994); an area of minimal loss was identified between markers D8S87 (8p12) and ANK1 (8p21.2–p11) (Fig. 2), suggesting the presence in this region of one or more putative TSG which may play a role in the development of these tumours. Chromosome 8p has not been examined in detail in SCCHN by other workers; only one microsatellite marker was used in the allelotype studies by AH-SEE et al. (1994) and NAWROZ et al. (1994). Studies of other tumour types, however, including colorectal, prostate, bladder, breast, lung and hepatocellular carcinomas, have also indicated the localisation of candidate TSG in the 8p22–p11 region (EMI et al. 1992; FUJIWARA et al. 1993; KNOWLES et al. 1993; TRAPMAN et al. 1994; KERANGUEVEN et al. 1995).

3.1.5 Chromosome 9

A common region of loss in SCCHN, seen in up to 72% of tumours and also in pre-invasive (severely dysplastic and carcinoma in situ) lesions, is at 9p21–p22 (LYDIATT et al. 1994; VAN DER RIET et al. 1994; EL-NAGGAR et al. 1995a). A high frequency of loss on chromosome 9p21–p23 has been demonstrated in a number of other tumour types, including non-small cell lung carcinoma (NSCLC) (MEAD et al. 1994; NOBORI et al. 1994; NEVILLE et al. 1995). The cyclin-dependent kinase-4 inhibitor genes, p15 and p16, which inhibit progression through the G_1 phase of the cell cycle, both map to 9p21. Deletions and mutations of these putative TSG have recently been reported in NSCLC (WASHIMI et al. 1995; XIAO et al. 1995). Sequence analysis of p16 in primary SCCHN with chromosome 9p loss has demonstrated that point mutations are infrequent (CAIRNS et al. 1994; ZHANG et al. 1994). The rarity of p16 point mutations does not necessarily indicate that p16 is not the target gene in tumours with 9p21 LOH. Using newly cloned markers around the p16 locus, CAIRNS et al. (1995) have convincingly demonstrated that small homozygous deletions represent an important mechanism of inactivation of 9p21 in many tumour types, including SCCHN. Fine mapping of these deletions implicates a 170-kb minimal region that includes p16 and excludes p15 (CAIRNS et al. 1995).

It has been suggested that an alternative mechanism for inactivation of p16 may be methylation of the 5' CpG-rich region, which results in a complete block of gene transcription (MERLO et al. 1995). More than 70% LOH in SCCHN has also been reported at 9p22–q23.3, suggesting that this may be an additional TSG locus on chromosome 9p (NAWROZ et al. 1994).

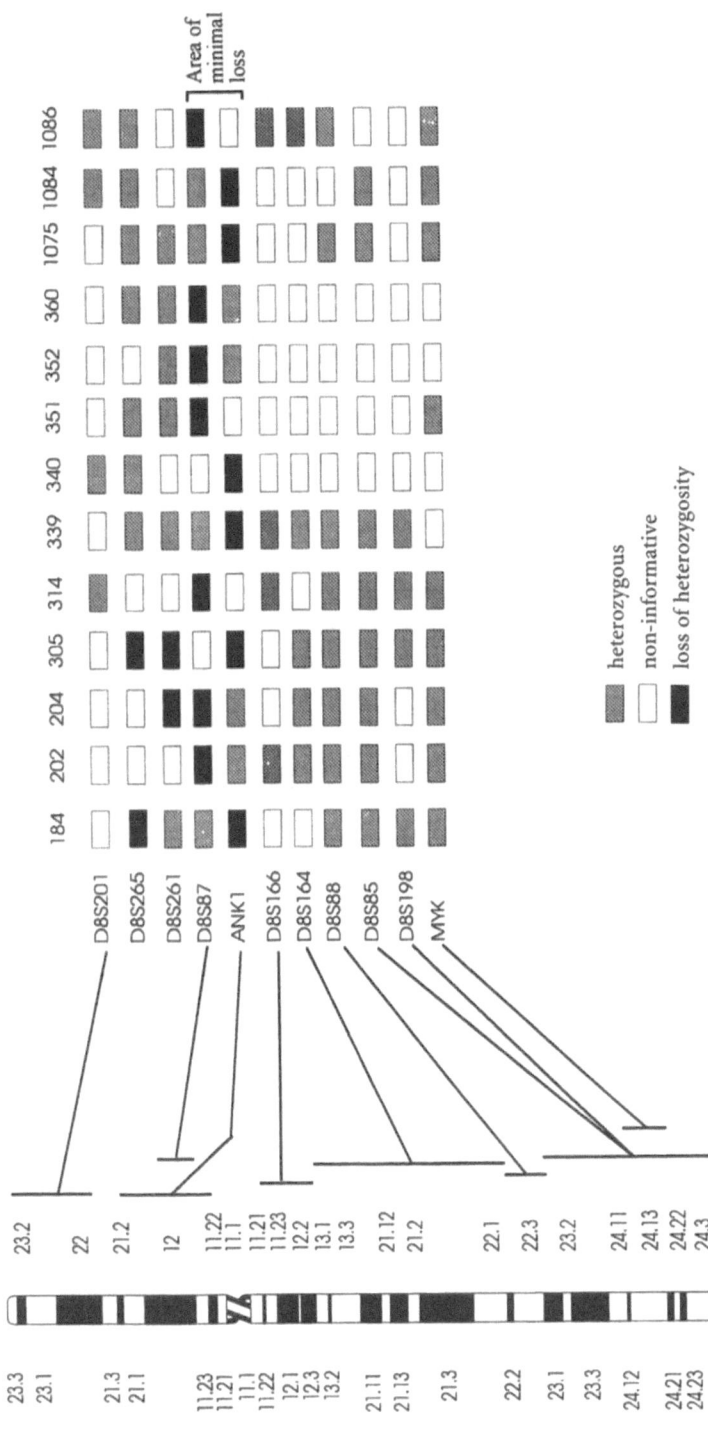

Fig. 2. Representative results of loss of heterozygosity on chromosome 8 in 13 patients exhibiting allele deletions with microsatellite markers D8S87 or ANK1. (From KIARIS et al. 1994, with permission)

Putative TSG located on the long arm of chromosome 9 include those related to Gorlin's syndrome (basal cell naevus syndrome) and the Ferguson-Smith syndrome (multiple self-healing squamous epitheliomata), mapped to 9q31 and 9q22–q31, respectively (Gailani et al. 1992; Goudie et al. 1993). LOH on chromosome 9q has been found in 35% of SCCHN, at 9q31–q34 and 9q22.1–q32; thus it is possible that the gene or genes associated with these familial cancers may also be involved in some sporadic head and neck carcinomas (Ah-See et al. 1994).

3.1.6 Chromosome 11

The short arm of chromosome 11 contains genes associated with Wilms' tumour, a childhood renal tumour with both a hereditary and a non-hereditary form. A candidate gene has been isolated at 11p13, although other genes in the region may play an important role in tumour development (Gessler et al. 1990). LOH at 11p15.5 has been found in 50% of SCCHN, suggesting the presence of a TSG in this region (Lydiatt et al. 1994). Indeed, fine mapping of chromosome 11p in breast cancer suggests the presence of three potential TSG at 11p15 (Negrini et al. 1995). Furthermore, multiple regions of LOH on chromosome 11p have been identified in NSCLC (Bepler and Garcia-Blanco 1994). The H-*ras* proto-oncogene is located at 11p15.5, and this region has been studied in detail by Kiaris et al. (1994, 1995) for H-*ras* mutations, overexpression by competitive reverse transcription (RT)-PCR and instability. Mutations in H-*ras* were not detected in any of the 120 SCCHN samples analysed, but 54% overexpressed this gene and five out of 14 samples exhibited 3'-VTR (variable tandem repeat) instability.

The long arm of chromosome 11 contains the MEN1 locus, associated with anterior pituitary insulinomas, at 11q12–q13. The 11q13 region also contains a number of proto-oncogenes, including *int-1*, *hst-1* and *bcl-1*/PRAD-1/cyclin D1. It is now recognised that the most likely candidate *bcl-1* gene is the PRAD-1/cyclin D1 proto-oncogene (Hunter and Pines 1994). Allelic imbalance on chromosome 11q, at 11q13 or 11q23, has been demonstrated in 45% of SCCHN (Ah-See et al. 1994). In cases of allelic imbalance, it can be difficult to distinguish between amplification and deletion of an allele. Ah-See et al. (1994) concluded, following Southern blot analysis, that the imbalance found at 11q13 was largely due to deletion rather than amplification, suggesting the possible loss of a TSG at this site.

Amplification of 11q13, however, has been demonstrated in 30%–50% of SCCHN (Berenson et al. 1989; Somers et al. 1990; Leonard et al. 1991). The target gene of greatest prognostic significance at this locus appears to be PRAD-1/cyclin D1. There is compelling evidence that D-type cyclins are fundamental to cell cycle regulation (for a review, see Hunter and Pines 1994). Two- to 12-fold amplification of the cyclin D1 gene has been demonstrated in 34%–37% of SCCHN (Callender et al. 1994; Jares et al. 1994) and has been found to correlate with mRNA overexpression, aggressive or late-stage tumours, advanced local invasion and presence of lymph node metastases (Callender et al. 1994; Jares et al. 1994). Overexpression of cyclin D1 has also been detected immunohistochemically in 63% of SCCHN and was found to correlate with a poor prognosis, being associated with a more rapid and frequent recurrence of disease and shortened survival (MICHALIDES et al. 1995).

The 11q22–q24 region is commonly lost in breast cancer, and recently refined mapping has defined two independent areas of loss at 11q23 (NEGRINI et al. 1995). The finding of frequent loss at 11q23 in SCCHN (AH-SEE et al. 1994) raises the possibility of involvement of putative TSG in this region in the pathogenesis of head and neck tumours.

3.1.7 Chromosome 13

The RB TSG is located on the long arm of chromosome 13 at 13q14.2. Inactivation of the RB gene has been reported in a number of tumour types (other than retinoblastoma), including carcinomas of the oesophagus and lung (HUANG et al. 1993; REISSMANN et al. 1993). Detailed analysis of the long arm of chromosome 13 in 60 SCCHN using ten microsatellite markers has demonstrated LOH in at least one 13q marker in 52% of tumours (YOO et al. 1994). A high frequency of LOH was found at a marker mapping to 13q14.3, just telomeric to the RB gene. Function of the RB gene appeared to be largely unaffected, as the majority of SCCHN showed normal nuclear immunostaining for RB protein. Similar findings of allelic loss at 13q14 in the presence of RB protein expression have been reported in ovarian and breast cancer (BORG et al. 1992; DODSON et al. 1994); thus it is possible that another TSG is contained at 13q14. This is supported by the study carried out by SCHOLNICK et al. (1994), which found LOH at 13q14.3 in 59% of squamous cell carcinomas of the supraglottic larynx. Other regions of chromosome 13q showing LOH less frequently in SCCHN include 13q32 (LYDIATT et al. 1994).

3.1.8 Chromosome 17

The p53 TSG, contained on chromosome 17p, is commonly involved in the pathogenesis of human tumours, including SCCHN. Frequent LOH involving TP53, the p53 locus at 17p13.1, has been found in a number of studies of SCCHN (ADAMSON et al. 1994; NAWROZ et al. 1994; SCHOLNICK et al. 1994). Detailed study of chromosome 17 has shown LOH on 17p in 50% of SCCHN, often involving the TP53 locus (42%), but more frequently involving the CHRNB1 locus at 17p11.1–p12 (56%) (ADAMSON et al. 1994). Consideration of tumours from the hypopharynx alone increased LOH at CHRNB1 to 77%, strongly suggesting the presence of a TSG at this locus which is involved in the development of these carcinomas. Fine mapping with additional microsatellite markers is required to further define this region. In addition, 34% of SCCHN showed LOH on 17q (ADAMSON et al. 1994).

Mutations of p53 are frequent in many tumour types (HOLLSTEIN et al. 1991; GREENBLATT et al. 1994). Initial investigations of p53 expression in SCCHN demonstrated that approximately 60% of these tumours had immunohistochemically detectable p53, thus suggesting, but not necessarily indicating, the presence of p53 gene mutations (for a review, see FIELD et al. 1993). Immunostaining for p53 correlated with the patients' history of smoking (FIELD et al. 1991, 1994b).

Tumours from eight out of 12 non-smokers were p53 negative, whereas 36 out of 45 from heavy smokers were p53 positive. In addition, tumours from all but two of the 12 patients who had stopped smoking for more than 5 years prior to presentation immunostained for p53, suggesting that p53 gene alterations were an early event in the development of these cancers (Field et al. 1991, 1994b). Sequence analysis has recently confirmed the correlation between p53 mutations and heavy smoking (Brennan et al. 1995; Liloglou et al., unpublished). In addition to smoking, Field et al. (1994b) also correlated p53 data with the patients' history of alcohol consumption. A possible synergistic effect of these two "carcinogens" was demonstrated by logistic regression analysis ($p < 0.05$), thereby indicating that both smoking and alcohol consumption are probably linked to aberrant p53 expression in head and neck cancer. These findings have recently been corroborated by Brennan et al. (1995). The majority of molecular studies have now demonstrated that 40% or more of SCCHN contain p53 mutations (Somers et al. 1992; Boyle et al. 1993; Brennan et al. 1995; for a review, see Greenblatt et al. 1994). As the p53 TSG plays an important role in arresting the cell cycle to permit repair of damaged DNA and inducing apoptosis if damage is irreparable, loss of p53 function presumably results in genomic instability and the accumulation of genetic lesions. Other genes involved in maintaining genomic stability are discussed in Sect. 4.

Inactivation of p53 may also occur by non-genetic mechanisms, through interation with human papillomavirus (HPV) proteins. The E6 protein from high-risk HPV types, such as HPV-16, can complex with and facilitate the rapid degradation of p53 (Werness et al. 1990; Scheffner et al. 1990; Hubbert et al. 1992). Cells expressing HPV-16 E6 do not manifest a p53-mediated response to DNA damage (Kessis et al. 1993). Presumably E6-mediated degradation of p53 abrogates its negative growth-regulatory effect and can result in genomic instability. In addition, HPV-16 E7 protein binds to the hypophosphorylated form of the RB TSG product (pRB) and may therefore prevent pRB-mediated suppression of cell growth (Münger et al. 1989). High-risk HPV types have been detected in SCCHN, but prevalence figures vary greatly between studies; this variation may be due in part to different sensitivities of detection systems used (for a review, see Snijders et al. 1994). A particular association between HPV-16/33 and tonsillar carcinomas, however, has been demonstrated (Snijders et al. 1992). We have recently detected HPV-16 in 21% of SCCHN (excluding tonsillar carcinomas) by PCR, using HPV general and type-specific primers (Snijders et al., 1996).

3.1.9 Chromosome 18

LOH on chromosome 18q has been reported in a range of cancers, many studies concentrating on the DCC (deleted in colorectal cancer) locus at 18q21.1. In a detailed study, Rowley et al. (1995) found LOH on 18q in 49% of SCCHN. The most frequent region of loss was 18q21.1–q21.3 using the marker D18S35 (33%), whereas loss at the DCC locus was found in only 12% of samples. Only one sample showed loss at both D18S35 and DCC, raising the possibility that another putative TSG may be located in this region (Rowley et al. 1995).

3.2 Allelotype Analysis of Squamous Cell Carcinoma of the Head and Neck - Fractional Allele Loss

Genetic changes at particular chromosome loci may occur as independent genetic events; they are, however, part of a complex tumour progression process. Allele losses are irreversible and will remain, and accumulate, as the cell proliferates. It may be that evaluation of the degree of genetic alteration or fractional allele loss (FAL), as determined by allelotype analysis, will provide useful molecular correlates of tumour behaviour.

FAL for a particular tumour is defined as the number of chromosomal arms on which allele loss is observed divided by the number of chromosomal arms for which allelic markers are informative (VOGELSTEIN et al. 1989). In an allelotype of colorectal carcinomas, a positive correlation between high FAL and development of recurrent disease has been found. In addition, patients with a tumour containing high FAL were significantly more likely to die with or from their cancer (VOGELSTEIN et al. 1989).

In the most comprehensive allelotype of SCCHN (FIELD et al. 1995b), 80 carcinoma samples were analysed using a total of 145 microsatellite markers on 39 chromosome arms (Fig. 3). FAL values were calculated for 52 of these carcinomas which had LOH information on nine to 39 chromosome arms (Fig. 4). This group of 52 tumours was composed of 36 previously untreated tumours and 16 previously treated tumours. The median FAL value for these tumours was 0.22 (mean, 0.25; range, 0.0–0.8), demonstrating that on average alleles were lost from 25% of

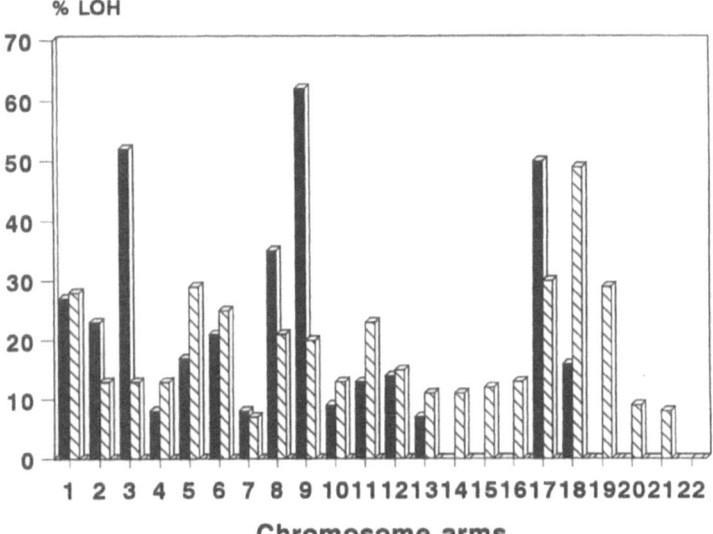

Fig. 3. Allelotype of squamous cell carcinoma of the head and neck. Frequency of allele loss on each chromosome arm in 80 carcinomas using 145 microsatellite markers. *Black bars*, p arm; *shaded bars*, q arm. *LOH*, loss of heterozygosity. (From FIELD et al. 1995b, with permission)

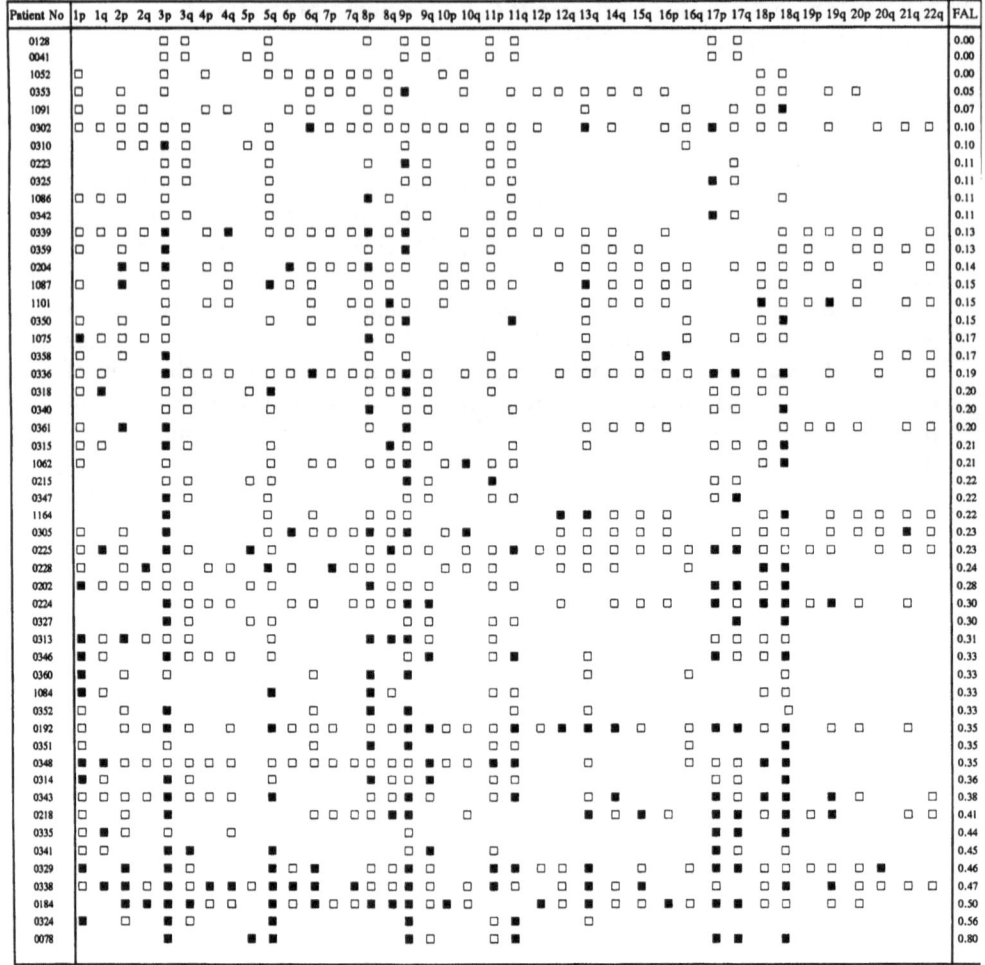

Fig. 4. Individual allelotypes for 52 squamous cell carcinomas of the head and neck examined on nine or more informative chromosome arms (range, nine to 36). Fractional allele loss (*FAL*) data is shown for each tumour sample. *Black boxes*, loss of heterozygosity (LOH); *white boxes*, retention of heterozygosity. Chromosome arms which were not informative or not examined are not shown. Each *square* represents the summation of LOH results on a single chromosome arm using all of the informative markers. (From Field et al. 1995b, with permission)

the chromosome arms examined. Tumours were divided into two subgroups – those with FAL greater than the median value and those with FAL less than the median value – and were correlated with clinico-pathological data (tumour site, tumour grade, TNM staging, nodes at pathology and patient history of smoking and drinking). A positive correlation was found between FAL and tumour grade ($p = 0.06$) and nodes at pathology ($p = 0.01$). The FAL data was also related to clinical outcome by log-rank analysis; FAL greater than the median value correlated with poor survival ($p < 0.032$), even when previously untreated tumours were analysed separately ($p < 0.019$). Analysis of 40 advanced tumours (TNM III and IV) also demonstrated a correlation between FAL and prognosis. Thus accumulated genetic damage, as provided by allelotype analysis, provides a useful molecular indicator of the behaviour of head and neck carcinomas.

4 DNA Repair

The importance of DNA repair mechanisms in tumour avoidance has recently received much attention. Although the molecular processes involved in DNA repair have been studied in bacteria (*Escherichia coli*) and yeast (*Saccharomyces cerevisiae*) for many years, it is only recently that research has been focused on these processes in human cells. Fortunately, human cells use DNA repair mechanisms analogous to those in micro-organisms, and it is now recognised that a predisposition to certain cancers is caused by defects in these pathways.

4.1 Mismatch Repair and Familial Cancer

Insertion of an incorrect base or the addition of an extra nucleotide is a relatively common DNA biosynthetic error. Microsatellite repeat sequences are particularly susceptible to errors due to slipped-strand mispairing during replication (KUNKEL 1993; RICHARDS and SUTHERLAND 1994). The role of the mismatch repair system is to recognise these mispairs and eliminate them from newly synthesised DNA strands.

Repair of mismatched DNA in *E. coli* requires a number of genes, including *mutS*, *mutL* and *mutH*. Similarly, studies with *S. cerevisiae* have identified three mismatch repair genes, a *mutS* homologue (MSH2) and two *mutL* homologues PMS1 and MLH1. Mutations in these genes result in a general elevation of spontaneous mutation rates and a dramatic destabilisation of microsatellite repeats (MODRICH 1991; STRAND et al. 1993).

The finding of widespread alterations in microsatellite repeats in familial colorectal cancer was a clue that defects in the human mismatch repair system might be involved. Hereditary non-polyposis colorectal cancer (HNPCC) is one of the most common familial cancer syndromes, characterised by early-onset carcinomas of the colon. In addition to colorectal cancer, a subset of affected individuals are also predisposed to endometrial, haematological, gastric, pancreatic, ovarian, skin and urinary tract cancers (LYNCH et al. 1993). Tumours from HNPCC patients have been found to harbour frequent mutations within simple microsatellite repeat sequences, suggesting the occurrence of numerous replication errors during tumour development (AALTONEN et al. 1993; IONOV et al. 1993). Cell lines derived from these tumours display a mutator phenotype and can acquire mutations at rates more than 100-fold greater than that of normal cells (PARSONS et al. 1993; BHATTACHARYYA et al. 1994; ESHLEMAN et al. 1995). Four human mismatch repair genes have now been identified; the *h*MSH2 gene encodes a protein homologue of bacterial *mutS*, while *h*MLSH1, *h*PMS1 and *h*PMS2 encode distinct *mutL* homologues (Fishel et al. 1993; Leach et al. 1993; Bronner et al. 1994; Nicolaides et al. 1994; Papadopoulos et al. 1994). The majority of HNPCC cases are attributable to a defect in any one of these four genes. Normal cells from the affected individual contain one functional and one defective copy of the involved repair gene, whereas in tumour cells the wild-type allele is inactivated by somatic mutation, resulting in defects in both copies of the affected gene (Leach et al. 1993; Nicolaides et al. 1994). Thus it appears that genetic destabilisation in HNPCC tumours is due to the functional loss of critical mismatch repair activity.

4.2 Microsatellite Instability in Sporadic Cancers

If instability of microsatellite sequences is used as a marker of deficiency in human mismatch repair, it would appear that this mechanism is associated with the development of some non-familial cancers. Microsatellite instability (MI) has been demonstrated in sporadic cancers, including colon, breast, gastric, pancreatic, lung and endometrial carcinomas (Han et al. 1993; Risinger et al. 1993; Thibodeau et al. 1993; Rhyu et al. 1994; Merlo et al. 1994; Shridhar et al. 1994; Yee et al. 1994). The stage at which MI occurs, however, appears to vary with the tumour type. Genomic instability is apparently an early event in colorectal cancer, as MI has been detected in adenomas (Shibata et al. 1994) and at similar frequency in ulcerative colitis-associated colorectal dysplasias and cancers (Suzuki et al. 1994). MI has also been detected in early-stage breast cancer (Yee et al. 1994). In contrast, genomic instability appears to be a late event in gastric carcinomas, as MI has been detected significantly more frequently in poorly differentiated advanced-stage tumours than in well-differentiated early-stage tumours and has been infrequently detected in dysplastic tissue (Han et al. 1993; Chong et al. 1994; Rhyu et al. 1994).

4.2.1 Squamous Cell Carcinoma of the Head and Neck

The presence of MI in SCCHN has recently been examined (Field et al. 1995a; Fig. 5). Fifty-six tumours were assessed using a total of 34 microsatellite markers on ten chromosomes; 25 of these tumours were examined with a minimum of ten (range, 10–34) microsatellite markers. Alteration observed in two or more markers was regarded as indicative of MI. Of the 25 SCCHN examined in detail, seven tumours (28%) were found to have MI in two or more microsatellite markers; three of these tumours contained alterations in at least 20 markers. The level of MI was assessed with clinico-pathological parameters and survival data in these 25 SCCHN patients. No correlations were found between MI and tumour site, previous treatment, degree of histological differentiation, nodal metastases, TNM stage or history of alcohol consumption. MI was detected in TNM stage I carcinomas, however, indicating that genomic instability may occur in the early stages of

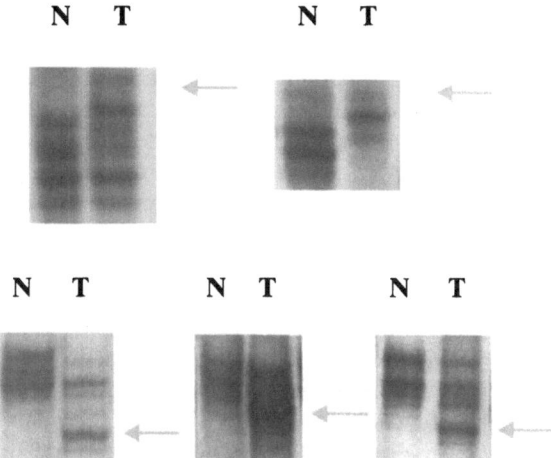

Fig. 5. Representative microsatellite instability detected in squamous cell carcinoma of the head and neck in patient no. 184 (*top*) and patient no. 224 (*bottom*). *Arrows* represent novel alleles. *N*, normal; *T*, tumour

tumour progression. There was a significant association between MI and smoking history, with instability being more frequent in tumours from non-smokers compared to smokers ($p = 0.02$). In a study of MI in SCCHN by Mao et al. (1994), a similar percentage (29%) of tumours to that found by Field et al. (1995a) exhibited microsatellite alterations with at least one marker.

Whether MI in SCCHN results from mutations in known mismatch repair genes is unknown. It is possible that alterations in other genes may be responsible, as many sporadic colorectal cancers which exhibit MI do not contain mutations in any of the four known human mismatch repair genes (Liu et al. 1995). We have previously reported that a history of heavy smoking correlates with overexpression of the p53 TSG (Field et al. 1991, 1992, 1994b), and these results are now supported by the demonstration of a significantly higher rate of p53 mutations in SCCHN from smokers compared with non-smokers (Liloglou et al., unpublished). The contrasting association of smoking history with MI and p53 mutations suggests that MI is a distinctive mechanism from that mediated by TSG in head and neck carcinogenesis. MI may occur relatively early in the progression of some SCCHN, particularly in non-smokers.

5 Conclusion

The characterisation of genetic aberrations in SCCHN by cytogenetic and allelic imbalance investigations has greatly increased our knowledge of the molecular mechanisms involved in the development of this disease. The cytogenetic studies of Jin et al. (1993, 1995) and Cowan (1992) and the three allelotype analyses (Ah-See et al. 1994; Nawroz et al. 1994; Field et al. 1995b) demonstrate the complexity of the genetic mechanisms involved in the pathogenesis of SCCHN. Apart from the involvement of *ras* and *myc* oncogenes (Field et al. 1989; Kiaris et al. 1995) and the p53 TSG (Field et al. 1991), it is now apparent that alterations at many additional chromosome loci may also play a role in head and neck carcinogenesis (1p31.2-p21.3, 3p25, 3p21.3-p23, 3p13-p14, 5q21-q22, 8p21.2-p11, 9p21-23, 11p15.5, 11q13, 13q14, 17p11.1-p12, 18q21.1-q21.3; see Sect. 3). Fractional allele loss analysis has demonstrated that increased accumulation of this genetic damage correlates with a poor clinical outcome (Field et al. 1995b). The recent finding in SCCHN of MI, which has been associated with DNA repair defects in HNPCC, provides a completely new approach to investigating molecular mechanisms in cancer of the head and neck (Mao et al. 1994; Field et al. 1995a).

The correlation of specific genetic alterations with histopathological progression in colorectal cancer has permitted the development of a molecular model in which the accumulation of specific genetic changes is responsible for successive phases of clonal expansion (Fearon and Vogelstein 1990; Boland et al. 1995). The development of such a model for head and neck cancer would have advantages in terms of early diagnosis, prognosis and management. From the data available to date, it would appear that mutation of the p53 TSG and LOH at 9p21-22 may be early events in the pathogenesis of SCCHN. p53 mutations have been demonstrated in pre-malignant lesions of the head and neck and increase in frequency with increasing severity of dysplasia and tumour progression (Boyle et al. 1993; El-Naggar et al. 1995b; Scholes et al., unpublished). LOH at 9p21-22 has been found at similar frequency in severely dysplastic lesions and carcinomas (van der Riet et al. 1994). LOH on 9p has also been found in severe dysplasia by El-Naggar et al. (1995a), but at a substantially lower frequency compared with carcinomas (28% and 72%, respectively). Amplification of the cyclin D1 gene appears to be a late event, correlating with advanced-stage tumours and metastases (Callender et al. 1994; Jares et al. 1994). Overexpression of the c-*myc* oncogene has been associated with a poor prognosis (Field et al. 1989), whereas *ras* overexpression has been correlated with a favourable prognosis (Kiaris et al. 1995).

It is important to recognise that the genetic alterations which occur during tumour progression in smokers may differ from those in non-smokers. Our studies have shown that immunohistochemical detection of p53 in SCCHN correlates with a history of heavy smoking (Field et al. 1991, 1992, 1994b). In addition, we have found a significantly higher prevalence of p53 mutations by sequence analysis in SCCHN from smokers compared with non-smokers (Liloglou et al., unpublished). In contrast, MI is more common in SCCHN from non-smokers than smokers (Field et al. 1995a), as are multiple allelic deletions (Lydiatt et al. 1994). It is of interest that *ras* mutations are uncommon in head and neck carcinomas from Europeans (Kiaris et al. 1995), but are frequently found in oral tumours in India (Saranath et al. 1991); the differing results in Indian subjects may be related to their habit of chewing tobacco.

Further characterisation of the genetic changes involved in head and neck carcinogenesis is imperative for improvements in the diagnosis, prognosis and therapy of these tumours. Of particular importance is the investigation of pre-malignant lesions, the malignant potential of which cannot be determined by conventional histopathological methods. Elucidation of the specific genetic alterations that are important in the initial stages of carcinogenesis will be critical in predicting which of these lesions progress to malignancy, thereby allowing early intervention.

References

Aaltonen LA, Peltomäki P, Leach FS, Sistonen P, Pylkkänen L, Mecklin J-P, Järvinen H, Powell SM, Jen J, Hamilton SR, Petersen GM, Kinzler KW, Vogelstein B, de la Chapelle A (1993) Clues to the pathogenesis of familial colorectal cancer. Science 260: 812–816

Adamson R, Jones AS, Field JK (1994) Loss of heterozygosity studies on chromosome 17 in head and neck cancer using microsatellite markers. Oncogene 9: 2077–2082

Ah-See KW, Cooke TG, Pickford IR, Soutar D, Balmain A (1994) An allelotype of squamous carcinoma of the head and neck using microsatellite markers. Cancer Res 54: 1617–1621

Allegra E, Garozzo A, Grillo A, Catalano GB (1992) Cytogenetic alterations in laryngeal carcinomas. Arch Otolaryngol Head Neck Surg 118: 1320–1322

Bepler G, Garcia-Blanco MA (1994) Three tumor-suppressor regions on chromosome 11p identified by high-resolution deletion mapping in human non-small-cell lung cancer. Proc Natl Acad Sci USA 91: 5513–5517

Berenson JR, Yang J, Mickel R (1989) Frequent amplification of the bcl-1 locus in head and neck squamous cell carcinomas. Oncogene 4: 1111–1116

Bhattacharyya NP, Skandalis A, Ganesh A, Groden J, Meuth M (1994) Mutator phenotypes in human colorectal carcinoma cell lines. Proc Natl Acad Sci USA 91: 6319–6323

Boland CR, Sato J, Appleman HD, Bresalier RS, Feinberg AP (1995) Microallelotyping defines the sequence and tempo of allelic losses at tumour suppressor gene loci during colorectal cancer progression. Nature Med 1: 902–909

Borg Å, Zhang Q-X, Alm P, Olsson H, Sellberg G (1992) The retinoblastoma gene in breast cancer: allele loss is not correlated with loss of gene protein expression. Cancer Res 52: 2991–2994

Boyle JO, Hakim J, Koch W, van der Riet P, Hruban RH, Roa RA, Correo R, Eby YJ, Ruppert JM, Sidransky D (1993) The incidence of p53 mutations increases with progression of head and neck cancer. Cancer Res 53: 4477–4480

Brennan JA, Boyle JO, Koch WM, Goodman SN, Hruban RH, Eby YJ, Couch MJ, Forastiere AA, Sidransky D (1995) Association between cigarette smoking and mutation of the p53 gene in squamous cell carcinoma of the head and neck. N Engl J Med 332: 712–717

Bronner CE, Baker SM, Morrison PT, Warren G, Smith LG, Lescoe MK, Kane M, Earabino C, Lipford J, Lindblom A, Tannergård P, Bollag RJ, Godwin AR, Ward DC, Nordenskjold M, Fishel R, Kolodner R, Liskay RM (1994) Mutation in the DNA mismatch repair gene homologue hMLH1 is associated with hereditary non-polyposis colon cancer. Nature 368: 258–261

Cairns P, Mao L, Merlo A, Lee DJ, Schwab D, Eby Y, Tokino K, van der Riet P, Blaugrund JE, Sidransky D (1994) Rates of p16 (MTS1) mutations in primary tumors with 9p loss. Science 265: 415–416

Cairns P, Polascik TJ, Eby Y, Tokino K, Califano J, Merlo A, Mao L, Herath J, Jenkins R, Westra W, Rutter JL, Buckler A, Gabrielson E, Tockman M, Cho KR, Hedrick L, Bova GS, Isaacs W, Koch W, Schwab D, Sidransky D (1995) Frequency of homozygous deletion at p16/CDKN2 in primary human tumours. Nature Genet 11: 210–212

Callender T, El-Naggar AK, Lee MS, Frankenthaler R, Luna MA, Batsakis JG (1994) PRAD-1 (CCND1)/cyclin D1 oncogene amplification in primary head and neck squamous cell carcinoma. Cancer 74: 152–158

Chong JM, Fukayama M, Hayashi Y, Takizawa T, Koike M, Konishi M, Kikuchi-Yanoshita R, Miyaki M (1994) Microsatellite instability in the progression of gastric carcinoma. Cancer Res 54: 4595–4597

Cowan JM (1992) Cytogenetics in head and neck cancer. Otolaryngol Clin North Am 25: 1073–1087

Dodson MK, Cliby WA, Xu H-J, DeLacey KA, Hu S-X, Keeney GL, Li J, Podratz KC, Jenkins RB, Benedict WF (1994) Evidence of functional RB protein in epithelial ovarian carcinomas despite loss of heterozygosity at the RB locus. Cancer Res 54: 610–613

El-Naggar AK, Lee MS, Wang G, Luna MA, Goepfert H, Batsakis JG (1993) Polymerase chain reaction-based restriction fragment length polymorphism analysis of the short arm of chromosome 3 in primary head and neck squamous carcinoma. Cancer 72: 881–886

El-Naggar AK, Hurr K, Batsakis JG, Luna MA, Goepfert H, Huff V (1995a) Sequential loss of heterozygosity at microsatellite motifs in preinvasive and invasive head and neck squamous carcinoma. Cancer Res 55: 2656–2659

El-Naggar AK, Lai S, Luna MA, Zhou X-D, Weber RS, Goepfert H, Batsakis JG (1995b) Sequential p53 mutation analysis of pre-invasive and invasive head and neck squamous carcinoma. Int J Cancer 64: 196–201

Emi M, Fujiwara Y, Nakajima T, Tsuchiya E, Tsuda H, Hirohashi S, Maeda Y, Tsuruta K, Miyaki M, Nakamura Y (1992) Frequent loss of heterozygosity on chromosome 8p in hepatocellular carcinoma, colorectal cancer and lung cancer. Cancer Res 52: 5368–5372

Eshleman JR, Lang EZ, Bowerfind GK, Parsons R, Vogelstein B, Willson JKV, Veigl ML, Sedwick WD, Markowitz SD (1995) Increased mutation rate at the *hprt* locus accompanies microsatellite instability in colon cancer. Oncogene 10: 33–37

Fearon ER, Vogelstein B (1990) A genetic model for colorectal tumorigenesis. Cell 61: 757–767

Field JK, Spandidos DA, Stell PM, Vaughan ED, Evan GI, Moore JP (1989) Elevated expression of the c-*myc* oncoprotein correlates with poor prognosis in head and neck squamous cell carcinoma. Oncogene 4: 1463–1468

Field JK, Spandidos DA, Malliri A, Yiagnisis M, Gosney JR, Stell PM (1991) Elevated p53 expression correlates with a history of heavy smoking in squamous cell carcinoma of the head and neck. Br J Cancer 64: 573–577

Field JK, Spandidos DA, Stell PM (1992) Overexpression of the p53 gene in head and neck cancer, linked with heavy smoking and drinking. Lancet 339: 520–503

Field JK, Pavelic ZP, Spandidos DA, Stambrook PJ, Jones AS, Gluckman JL (1993) The role of the p53 tumour suppressor gene in squamous cell carcinoma of the head and neck. Arch Otolaryngol Head Neck Surg 119: 1118–1122

Field JK, Tsiriyotis C, Howard P, Jones AS (1994a) Allele loss on chromosome 3 in squamous cell carcinoma of the head and neck correlates with poor clinical prognostic indicators. Int J Oncol 4: 543–549

Field JK, Zoumpourlis V, Spandidos DA, Jones AS (1994b) p53 expression and mutations in squamous cell carcinoma of the head and neck: expression correlates with the patients' use of tobacco and alcohol. Cancer Detect Prevent 18: 197–208

Field JK, Kiaris H, Howard P, Vaughan ED, Spandidos DA, Jones AS (1995a) Microsatellite instability in squamous cell carcinoma of the head and neck. Br J Cancer 71: 1065–1069

Field JK, Kiaris H, Risk JM, Tsiriyotis C, Adamson R, Zoumpourlis V, Rowley H, Taylor K, Whittaker J, Howard P, Beirnie JC, Gosney JR, Woolgar J, Vaughan ED, Spandidsos DA, Jones AS (1995b) Allelotype of squamous cell carcinoma of the head and neck: fractional allele loss correlates with survival. Br J Cancer 72: 1180–1188

Fishel R, Lescoe MK, Rao MRS, Copeland NG, Jenkins NA, Garber J, Kane M, Kolodner R (1993) The human mutator gene homolog *MSH2* and its association with hereditary nonpolyposis colon cancer. Cell 75: 1027–1038

Fujiwara Y, Emi M, Ohata H, Kato Y, Nakajima T, Mori T, Nakamura Y (1993) Evidence for the presence of two tumor suppressor genes on chromosome 8p for colorectal carcinoma. Cancer Res 53: 1172–1174

Gailani MR, Bale SJ, Leffell DJ, DiGiovanna JJ, Peck GL, Poliak S, Drum MA, Pastakia B, McBride OW, Kase R, Greene M, Mulvihill JJ, Bale AE (1992) Developmental defects in Gorlin syndrome related to a putative tumor suppressor gene on chromosome 9. Cell 69: 111–117

Gessler M, Poustka A, Cavenee W, Neve RL, Orkin SH, Bruns GAP (1990) Homozygous deletion in Wilms tumours of a zinc-finger gene identified by chromosome jumping. Nature 343: 774–778

Goudie DR, Yuille MAR, Leversha MA, Furlong RA, Carter NP, Lush MJ, Affara NA, Ferguson-Smith MA (1993) Multiple self-healing squamous epitheliomata (ESS1) mapped to chromosome 9p22–q31 in families with common ancestry. Nature Genet 3: 165–169

Greenblatt MS, Bennett WP, Hollstein M, Harris CC (1994) Mutations in the p53 tumor suppressor gene: clues to cancer etiology and molecular pathogenesis. Cancer Res 54: 4855–4878

Han H-J, Yanagisawa A, Kato Y, Park J-G, Nakamura Y (1993) Genetic instability in pancreatic cancer and poorly differentiated type of gastric cancer. Cancer Res 53: 5087–5089

Hauser-Urfer IH, Stauffer J (1985) Comparative chromosome analysis of nine squamous cell carcinoma lines from tumors of the head and neck. Cytogenet Cell Genet 39: 35–39

Hibi K, Takahashi T, Yamakawa K, Ueda R, Sekido Y, Ariyoshi Y, Suyama M, Tagaki H, Nakamuran Y, Takahashi T (1992) Three distinct regions involved in 3p deletion in human lung cancer. Oncogene 7: 445–449

Hollstein M, Sidransky D, Vogelstein B, Harris CC (1991) p53 mutations in human cancers. Science 253: 49–53

Huang Y, Meltzer SJ, Yin J, Tong Y, Chang EH, Srivastava S, McDaniel T, Boynton RF, Zou Z-Q (1993) Altered messenger RNA and unique mutational profiles of p53 and Rb in human esophageal carcinomas. Cancer Res 53: 1889–1894

Hubbert NL, Sedman SA, Schiller JT (1992) Human papillomavirus type 16 E6 increases the degradation rate of p53 in human keratinocytes. J Virol 66: 6237–6241

Hunter T, Pines J (1994) Cyclins and cancer II: cyclin D and CDK inhibitors come of age. Cell 79: 573–582

Ionov Y, Peinado MA, Malkhosyan S, Shibata D, Perucho M (1993) Ubiquitous somatic mutations in simple repeated sequences reveal a new mechanism for colonic carcinogenesis. Nature 363: 558–561

Jares P, Fernández PL, Campo E, Nadal A, Bosch F, Aiza G, Nayach I, Traserra J, Cardesa A (1994) PRAD-1/cyclin D1 gene amplification correlates with messenger RNA overexpression and tumor progression in human laryngeal carcinomas. Cancer Res 54: 4813–4817

Jin Y, Mertens F (1993) Chromosome abnormalities in oral squamous cell carcinomas. Oral Oncol Eur J Cancer 29B: 257–263

Jin Y, Higashi K, Mandahl N, Heim S, Wennerberg J, Biörkland A, Dictor M, Mitelman F (1990) Frequent rearrangement of chromosomal bands 1p22 and 11q13 in squamous cell carcinomas of the head and neck. Genes Chromosomes Cancer 2: 198–204

Jin Y, Mertens F, Mandahl N, Heim S, Olegard C, Wennerberg J, Biorklund A, Mitelman F (1993) Chromosome abnormalities in eighty-three head and neck squamous cell carcinomas: influence of culture conditions on karyotypic pattern. Cancer Res 53: 2140–2146

Jin Y, Mertens F, Jin C, Åkervall J, Wennerberg J, Gorunova L, Mandahl N, Heim S, Mitelman F (1995) Nonrandom chromosome abnormalities in short-term cultured primary squamous cell carcinomas of the head and neck. Cancer Res 55: 3204–3210

Kessis TD, Slebos RJ, Nelson WG, Kastan MB, Plunkett BS, Han SM, Lorincz AT, Hedrick L, Cho KR (1993) Human papillomavirus 16 E6 expression disrupts the p53-mediated cellular response to DNA damage. Proc Natl Acad Sci USA 90: 3988–3992

Kerangueven R, Essioux L, Dib A, Noguchi T, Allione F, Geneix J, Longy M, Lidereau R, Eisinger F, Pébusque M-J, Jacquemier J, Bonaïti-Pellié C, Sobol H, Birnbaum D (1995) Loss of heterozygosity and linkage analysis in breast carcinoma: indications for a putative third susceptibility gene on the short arm of chromosome 8. Oncogene 10: 1023–1026

Kiaris H, Jones AS, Spandidos DA, Vaughan ED, Field JK (1994) Loss of heterozygosity on chromosome 8 in squamous cell carcinoma of the head and neck. Int J Oncol 5: 579–582

Kiaris H, Spandidos DA, Jones AS, Vaughan ED, Field JK (1995) Mutations, expression and genomic instability of the H-ras proto-oncogene in squamous cell carcinomas of the head and neck. Br J Cancer 72: 123–128

Killary AM, Wolf ME, Giambernardi TA, Naylor SL (1992) Definition of a tumor suppressor locus within human chromosome 3p21–p22. Proc Natl Acad Sci USA 89: 10877–10881

Kinzler KW, Nilbert MC, Su L-K, Vogelstein B, Bryan TM, Levy DB, Smith KJ, Preisinger AC, Hedge P, McKechnie D, Finniear R, Markham A, Groffen J, Boguski MS, Altschul SF, Horii A, Ando H, Miyoshi Y, Miki Y, Nishisho I, Nakamura Y (1991) Identification of FAP locus genes from chromosome 5q21. Science 253: 661–665

Knowles MA, Shaw ME, Proctor AJ (1993) Deletion mapping of chromosome 8 in cancers of the urinary bladder using restriction fragment length polymorphisms and microsatellite polymorphisms. Oncogene 8: 1357–1364

Kunkel TA (1993) Slippery DNA and diseases. Nature 365: 207–208
Latif F, Fivash M, Glenn G, Tory K, Orcutt ML, Hampsch K, Delisio J, Lerman M, Cowan J, Beckett M, Weichselbaum R (1992) Chromosome 3p deletions in head and neck carcinomas: statistical ascertainment of allelic loss. Cancer Res 52: 1451–1456
Leach FS, Nicolaides NC, Papadopoulos N, Liu B, Jen J, Parsons R, Peltomaki P, Sistonen P, Aaltonen LA, Nystrom-Lahti M et al (1993) Mutations of a mutS homolog in hereditary nonpolyposis colorectal cancer. Cell 75: 1215–1225
Leonard JH, Kearsley JH, Chenevix-Trench G, Hayward NK (1991) Analysis of gene amplification in head-and-neck squamous cell carcinomas. Int J Cancer 48: 511–515
Liu B, Nicolaides NC, Markowitz S, Willson JKV, Parsons RE, Jen J, Papadopolous N, Peltomäki P, de la Chapelle A, Hamilton SR, Kinzler KW, Vogelstein B (1995) Mismatch repair gene defects in sporadic colorectal cancers with microsatellite instability. Nature Genet 9: 48–55
Lydiatt WM, Davidson BJ, Shah J, Schantz SP, Chaganti RSK (1994) The relationship of loss of heterozygosity to tobacco exposure and early recurrence in head and neck squamous-cell carcinoma. Am J Surg 168: 437–440
Lynch HT, Smyrk TC, Watson P, Lanspa SJ, Lynch JF, Lynch PM, Cavalieri RJ, Boland CR (1993) Genetics, natural history, tumor spectrum, and pathology of hereditary nonpolyposis colorectal cancer: an updated review. Gastroenterology 104: 1535–1549
Maestro R, Gasparotto D, Vukosavljevic T, Barzan L, Sulfaro S, Boiocchi M (1993) Three discreet regions of deletion at 3p in head and neck cancers. Cancer Res 53: 5775–5779
Mao L, Lee DJ, Tockman MS, Erozan YS, Askin F, Sidransky D (1994) Microsatellite alterations as clonal markers for the detection of human cancer. Proc Natl Acad Sci USA 91: 9871–9875
Marshall CJ (1991) Tumor suppressor genes. Cell 64: 313–326
Mead LJ, Gillespie MT, Irving LB, Campbell LJ (1994) Homozygous and hemizygous deletions of 9p centromeric to the interferon genes in lung cancer. Cancer Res 54: 2307–2309
Merlo A, Mabry M, Gabrielson E, Vollmer R, Baylin SB, Sidransky D (1994) Frequent microsatellite instability in primary small cell lung cancer. Cancer Res 54: 2098–2101
Merlo A, Herman JG, Mao L, Lee DJ, Gabrielson E, Burger PC, Baylin SB, Sidransky D (1995) 5' CpG island methylation is associated with transcriptional silencing of the tumour suppressor p16/CDKN2/MTS1 in human cancers. Nature Med 1: 686–692
Michalides R, van Veelen N, Hart A, Loftus B, Wientjens E, Balm A (1995) Overexpression of cyclin D1 correlates with recurrence in a group of forty-seven operable squamous cell carcinomas of the head and neck. Cancer Res 55: 975–978
Mitelman F (1991) Catalog of chromosome aberrations in cancer. Wiley-Liss, New York
Modrich P (1991) Mechanisms and biological effects of mismatch repair. Annu Rev Genet 25: 229–253
Münger K, Werness BA, Dyson N, Phelps WC, Harlow E, Howley PM (1989) Complex formation of human papillomavirus E7 proteins with the retinoblastoma tumor suppressor gene product. EMBO J 8: 4099–4105
Nawroz H, Vanderriet P, Hruban RH, Koch W, Ruppert JM, Sidransky D (1994) Allelotype of head and neck squamous cell carcinoma. Cancer Res 54. 1152–1155
Negrini M, Rasio D, Hampton GM, Sabbioni S, Rattan S, Carter SL, Rosenberg AL, Schwartz GF, Shiloh Y, Cavenee WK, Croce CM (1995) Definition and refinement of chromosome 11 regions of loss of heterozygosity in breast cancer: identification of a new region at 11q23.3. Cancer Res 55: 3003–3007
Neville EM, Stewart M, Myskow M, Donnelly RJ, Field JK (1995) Loss of heterozygosity at 9p23 defines a novel locus in non-small cell lung cancer. Oncogene 11: 581–585
Nicolaides NC, Papadopoulos N, Liu B, Wei Y, Carter KC, Ruben SM, Rosen CA, Haseltine WA, Fleischmann RD, Fraser CM, Adams MD, Venter JC, Dunlop MG, Hamilton SR, Peterson GM, de la Chappelle A, Vogelstein B, Kinzler KW (1994) Mutations of two PMS homologues in hereditary nonpolyposis colon cancer. Nature 371: 75–80
Nobori T, Miura K, Wu DJ, Lois A, Takabayashi K, Carson DA (1994) Deletions of the cyclin-dependent kinase-4 inhibitor gene in multiple human cancers. Nature 368: 753–756
Osella P, Carlson A, Wyandt H, Milunsky A (1992) Cytogenetic studies of eight squamous cell carcinomas of the head and neck: deletion of 7q, a possible primary chromosomal event. Cancer Genet Cytogenet 59: 73–78

Owens W, Field JK, Howard T, Stell PM (1992) Multiple cytogenetic aberrations in squamous cell carcinoma of the head and neck. Oral Oncol Eur J Cancer 28B: 17–22

Papadopoulos N, Nicolaides NC, Wei YF, Ruben SM, Carter KC, Rosen CA, Haseltine WA, Fleischmann RD, Fraser CM, Adams MD, Venter JC, Hamilton SR, Petersen GM, Watson P, Lynch HT, Peltomaki P, Mecklin JP, de la Chapelle A, Kinzler KW, Vogelstein B (1994) Mutation of a *mutL* homolog in hereditary colon cancer. Science 263: 1625–1629

Parsons R, Li G-M, Longley MJ, Fang W-h, Papadopoulos N, Jen J, de la Chapelle A, Kinzler KW, Vogelstein B, Modrich P (1993) Hypermutability and mismatch repair deficiency in RER + tumor cells. Cell 75: 1227–1236

Rao PH, Sreekantaiah C, Schantz SP, Chaganti RS (1994) Cytogenetic analysis of 11 squamous cell carcinomas of the head and neck. Cancer Genet Cytogenet 77: 60–64

Reissmann PT, Koga H, Takahashi R, Figlin RA, Holmes EC, Piantadosi S, Cordon-Cardo C, Slamon DJ (1993) Inactivation of the retinoblastoma susceptibility gene in non-small-cell lung cancer. The Lung Cancer Study Group. Oncogene 8: 1913–1919

Renan MJ (1993) How many mutations are required for tumorigenesis? Implications from human cancer data. Mol Carcinog 7: 139–146

Rhyu MG, Park WS, Meltzer SJ (1994) Microsatellite instability occurs frequently in human gastric carcinoma. Oncogene 9: 29–32

Richards RI, Sutherland GR (1994) Simple repeat DNA is not replicated simply. Nature Genet 6: 114–116

Risinger JI, Berchuck A, Kohler MF, Watson P, Lynch HT, Boyd J (1993) Genetic instability of microsatellites in endometrial carcinoma. Cancer Res 53: 5100–5103

Rowley H, Jones AS, Field JK (1995) Chromosome 18: a possible site for a tumour suppressor gene deletion in squamous cell carcinoma of the head and neck. Clin Otol 20: 266–271

Saranath D, Chang SE, Bhoite LT, Panchal RG, Kerr IB, Mehta AR, Johnson NW, Deo MG (1991) High frequency mutation in codons 12 and 61 of H-ras oncogene in chewing tobacco-related human oral carcinoma in India. Br J Cancer 63: 573–578

Scheffner M, Werness BA, Huibregtse JM, Levine AJ, Howley PM (1990) The E6 oncoprotein encoded by human papillomavirus types 16 and 18 promotes the degradation of p53. Cell 63: 1129–1136

Scholnick SB, Sun PC, Shaw ME, Haughey BH, El-Mofty SK (1994) Frequent loss of heterozygosity for Rb, TP53 and chromosome arm 3p, but not NME1 in squamous cell carcinomas of the supraglottic larynx. Cancer 73: 2472–2479

Shibata D, Peinado MA, Ionov Y, Malkhosyan S, Perucho M (1994) Genomic instability in repeated sequences is an early somatic event in colorectal tumorigenesis that persists after transformation. Nature Genet 6: 273–281

Shridhar V, Siegfried J, Hunt J, Alonso MM, Smith DI (1994) Genetic instability of microsatellite sequences in many non-small cell lung carcinomas. Cancer Res 54: 2084–2087

Snijders PJF, Cromme FV, van den Brule AJC, Schrijnemakers HFJ, Snow GB, Meijer CJLM, Walboomers JMM (1992) Prevalence and expression of human papillomavirus in tonsillar carcinomas, indicating a possible viral etiology. Int J Cancer 51: 845–850

Snijders PJF, van den Brule AJC, Meijer CJLM, Walboomers JMM (1994) Papillomaviruses and cancer of the upper digestive and respiratory tracts. In: Zur Hausen H (ed) Human pathogenic papillomaviruses. Springer, Berlin Heidelberg New York, pp 177–198 (Current topics in microbiology and immunology, vol 186)

Snijders PJF, Scholes AGM, Hare CA, Jones AS, Vaughan ED, Woolgar JA, Meijer CJLM, Walboomers JMM, Field JK (1996) Prevalence of mucosotropic human papillomaviruses in squamous cell carcinomas of the head and neck. Int J Cancer 66: 1–6

Somers KD, Cartwright SL, Schechter GL (1990) Amplification of the int-2 gene in human head and neck squamous cell carcinomas. Oncogene 5: 915–920

Somers KD, Merrick MA, Lopez ME, Incognito LS, Schechter GL, Casey G (1992) Frequent p53 mutations in head and neck cancer. Cancer Res 52: 5997–6000

Speicher MR, Howe C, Crotty P, du Manoir S, Costa J, Ward DC (1995) Comparative genomic hybridization detects novel deletions and amplifications in head and neck squamous cell carcinomas. Cancer Res 55: 1010–1013

Sreekantaiah C, Rao PH, Xu L, Sacks PG, Schantz SP, Chaganti RSK (1994) Consistent chromosomal losses in head and neck squamous cell carcinoma cell lines. Genes Chromosomes Cancer 11: 29–39

Strand M, Prolla TA, Liskay PM, Petes TD (1993) Destabilization of tracts of simple repetitive DNA in yeast by mutations affecting DNA mismatch repair. Nature 365: 274–276

Suzuki H, Harpaz N, Tarmin L, Yin J, Jiang HY, Bell JD, Hontanosas M, Groisman GM, Abraham JM, Meltzer SJ (1994) Microsatellite instability in ulcerative colitis-associated colorectal dysplasias and cancers. Cancer Res 54: 4841–4844

Thibodeau SN, Bren G, Schaid D (1993) Microsatellite instability in cancer of the proximal colon. Science 260: 816–819

Trapman J, Sleddens HFBM, van der Weiden MM, Dinjens WNM, Konig JJ, Schroder FH, Faber PW, Bosman FT (1994) Loss of heterozygosity of chromosome 8 microsatellite loci implicates a candidate tumor suppressor gene between the loci D8S87 and D8S133 in human prostate cancer. Cancer Res 54: 6061–6064

Uzawa K, Yoshida H, Susuki H, Tanzawa H, Shimazaki J, Seino S, Sato K (1994) Abnormalities of the adenomatous polyposis coli gene in human oral squamous cell carcinoma. Int J Cancer 58: 814–817

Van der Riet P, Nawroz H, Hruban RH, Corio R, Tokino K, Koch W, Sidransky D (1994) Frequent loss of chromosome 9p21-22 early in head and neck cancer progression. Cancer Res 54: 1156–1158

Van Dyke DL, Worsham MJ, Benninger MS, Krause CJ, Baker SR, Wolf GT, Drumheller T, Tilley BC, Carey TE (1994) Recurrent cytogenetic abnormalities in squamous cell carcinomas of the head and neck region. Genes Chromosomes Cancer 9: 192–206

Vogelstein B, Fearon ER, Kern SE, Hamilton SR, Preisinger AC, Nakamura Y, White R (1989) Allelotype of colorectal carcinomas. Science 244: 207–211

Washimi O, Nagatake M, Osada H, Ueda R, Koshikawa T, Seki T, Takahashi T, Takahashi T (1995) In vivo occurrence of p16 (MTS1) and p15 (MTS2) alterations preferentially in non-small cell lung cancers. Cancer Res 55: 514–517

Weber JL, May PE (1989) Abundant class of human DNA polymorphisms which can be typed using the polymerase chain reaction. Am J Hum Genet 44: 388–396

Weinberg R (1991) Tumor suppressor genes. Science 254: 1138–1146

Werness BA, Arnold JL, Howley PM (1990) Association of human papillomavirus types 16 and 18 E6 proteins with p53. Science 248: 76–79

Wu CL, Sloan P, Read AP, Harris R, Thakker N (1994) Deletion mapping on the short arm of chromosome 3 in squamous cell carcinoma of the oral cavity. Cancer Res 54: 6484–6488

Xiao S, Li D, Corson JM, Vijg J, Fletcher JA (1995) Codeletion of p15 and p16 genes in primary non-small cell lung carcinoma. Cancer Res 55: 2968–2971

Yee CJ, Roodi N, Verrier CS, Parl FF (1994) Microsatellite instability and loss of heterozygosity in breast cancer. Cancer Res 54: 1641–1644

Yoo GH, Xu HJ, Brennan JA, Westra W, Hruban RH, Koch W, Benedict WF, Sidransky D (1994) Infrequent inactivation of the retinoblastoma gene despite frequent loss of chromosome 13q in head and neck squamous cell carcinoma. Cancer Res 54: 4603–4606

Zhang SY, Klein-Szanto AJ, Sauter ER, Shafarenko M, Mitsunaga S, Nobori T, Carson DA, Ridge JA, Goodrow TL (1994) Higher frequency of alterations in the p16/CDKN2 gene in squamous cell carcinoma cell lines than in primary tumors of the head and neck. Cancer Res 54: 5050–5053

Oncogenes and Growth Factor Receptors As Diagnostic and Prognostic Markers in Precancers and Cancers of the Oral Mucosa*

A. BURKHARDT

1 Introduction

Cancer, if not in essence a genetic disease, is at least to a large extent determined in its behaviour by the interaction of a number of genetically coded products, which may enhance its growth (oncogenes) or suppress it (tumour suppressor genes or anti-oncogenes). However, the genetic changes of various cancers show considerable individual variations some of which maybe determined by geographic or aetiological factors. Overall, 50%–96% of oral carcinomas have abnormal karyotypes (OWEN et al. 1992; HITTELMAN et al. 1993), and there is a high frequency of breakpoints and deletions (OWEN et al. 1992; PATEL et al. 1993; PARTRIDGE et al. 1994; FÜZESI et al. 1994). All chromosomes may be involved, and it is noteworthy that those chromosomes encoding some of the well-known oncogenes (or tumour suppressor genes) are frequently altered, such as chromosome 1, 3, 7 (epidermal growth factor receptor, EGFR), 8 (*myc*), 9 (MTS), 11 (*ras*, *bcl1*, *int1*), 13 (*erb*), 17 (*neu*, p53) and 18 (PATEL et al. 1993; VORAVUD 1993; TSUJI et al. 1994). Details are outlined in the chapter by Scholes and Field in this volume.

Proto-oncogenes are present in all cells, and in humans some 40 different types are known. They code for proteins which normally have important functions in growth regulations and differentiation of cells and tissues such as growth factors, growth factor receptors, and gene expression regulators. Especially in embryogenesis, many of these genes are temporarily expressed. Also in normal and altered tissue with deregulated growth, these genes may under certain circum-

---

* Dedicated to Professor Dr. Gerhard Seifert, ordinarius emeritus of Pathology, University of Hamburg, on the occasions of his 75th birthday who so decisively influenced the endeavours of Oral Pathology in Germany and the scientific work of the author.

stances (for example, by transduction by retroviruses or physical/chemical factors) be rearranged, activated, overexpressed or mutated and become oncogenes. Activation of oncogenes leads to an enhanced cellular growth potential, and some growth receptors may be activated by false signals; mutation of antioncogenes may result in loss of function and thus has the same effect as oncogene overexpression. Oncogenes may induce abnormal growth factors or growth factor receptors. Oncogene tumour suppressor gene alterations maybe instrumental in tumour initiation, but most such changes are acquired during the promotion phase of carcinogenesis or even later during tumour progression. Thus precancerous lesions or early carcinomas as a rule exhibit fewer changes of oncogene/tumour suppressor gene expression than do progressed tumours. On the other hand, the extent of oncogene activation or tumour suppressor mutation without question influences tumour behaviour and may thus be of prognostic value for established carcinomas. In lesions considered potentially premalignant, determination of these changes maybe instrumental in differentiating true premalignant precancerous lesions from harmless aberrations like hyperplasia.

2 Methodological Problems

The demonstration of oncogene/tumour suppressor gene alterations in normal tissues and in tumours may be achieved by molecular biochemical methods on tissue homogenates or by specific staining of tissue sections (in situ demonstration). Both methods may show either the specific DNA/RNA sequences of the oncogene/tumour suppressor gene or the gene products, i.e. the proteins. Single-stranded nucleic acids have a tendency to form double-stranded helices (hybrids) with nucleotides in complementary sequence. Using labelled (radioactive isotopes, biotinylated sequences) nucleic acids makes it possible to demonstrate specific DNA/RNA sequences by hybridisation in tissue homogenates. The sensitivity maybe greatly enhanced by polymerase chain reaction (PCR). In situ localization maybe achieved by in situ hybridisation or immunohistochemical staining of the gene product proteins. Certainly the biochemical method of determination is more sensible, may be suitable for exact quantification, is generally more specific, and is able to identify even minor mutations. However, the specificity makes it very sensitive to contamination (e.g. traces of DNA) and other methodological faults; thus single publications without confirmation by other groups should be regarded sceptically. Also it must be kept in mind that mere oncogene expression is a widerspread phenomenon in tissues of different histogenesis, and quantitative analysis is necessary prior to propagating it as being of diagnostic or prognostic relevance (Rivière et al. 1990). Furthermore, examining a tissue homogenate never provides conclusive evidence of the cell fraction the substance identified is derived from, and of how high the concentrations in the tumour cells actually were. Tissue samples may contain less than 10% vital tumour cells.

In situ hybridisation and immunohistochemistry have the advantage of localising the positive signal, even to a specific cellular compartment (nucleus, cytoplasm, cell membrane). However sensitivity is low compared with that of biochemical methods as a rule, not allowing, for example, distinction of mutant and non-mutant protein, and hybridisation may give false-positive results due to the occurrence of intervening repetitive sequences of nucleic acids. Also quantification is only roughly possible. For practical reasons, positive histochemical staining either by hybridisation or immunotechnique is considered to mark amplification or overexpression of the gene under consideration.

Most biochemical examinations of oncogenes/tumour suppressor genes have been applied to larger solid tumours, especially breast carcinomas and colonic carcinomas. A larger tumour mass makes it possible to select an area with a high percentage of vital tumour cells and little tumour stroma. This limits our knowledge of oncogene expression to progressed tumours with many secondary genetic changes. However, the more interesting early alterations seem to be of greater interest, as they may give insight into aetiological and prognostic factors. Precise correlation to histomorphology is impossible in tissues composed of heterogeneous cell populations, so that the assessment of precancerous lesions by this method is limited. In extensive multifocal lesions (e.g. in the mammary ductal system), a higher percentage of atypical cells may be harvested in tissue blocs; in lesions of superficial covering epithelium with only focal atypias no meaningful results can be expected.

A new method combining the histomorphological localisation with molecular genetic analysis by microdissection of paraffin-embedded tissue is promising to bridge this gap. By this method, YOUNGSON et al. (1995) were able to demonstrate that a single copy of HER 2/neu identified by molecular gene analysis in breast carcinomas or normal tissue resulted in a negative immunostaining, while fourfold to eightfold amplification was detected by positive immunostaining, thus confirming conventional wisdom.

Unfortunately, there are very little reliable data on gene expression in oral carcinomas and even less for oral precancerous lesions (reviewed in BURKHARDT 1985; TALACKO et al. 1991; FIELD 1991, 1992; SCULLY and BURKHARDT 1993; SCULLY 1993; BRACHMAN 1994). The meaning of these factors for diagnostic and prognostic assessment of cancerous and precancerous oral lesions is thus still very limited. In any case it seems of the utmost importance to distinguish results obtained by molecular genetic studies from in-situ demonstration on the one hand and results on progressed and early or precancerous lesions on the other.

3 Oncogenes

3.1 Growth Factor and Growth Factor Receptor-Related Genes

Epidermal growth factor (EGF) a polypeptide of 6000 daltons, stimulates the replication and also differentiation of a number of different cell types (CASTELLANI et al. 1994). EGF is counteracted by inhibitory growth regulators – so-called chalones, probably also polypeptides – which have not yet been defined in the oral mucosa (IVERSEN 1985). EGF, probably of fibroblastic origin

(SHIRASUNA et al. 1991) is normally found in small amounts in the subepithelial region of the oral mucosa, but is not expressed by epithelial cells. It is increased in dysplastic and malignant epithelial proliferations (SHIRASUNA et al. 1991). The fact that also in these circumstances the epithelium does not express EGF seems to indicate that the autocrine hypothesis (SPORN and TODARO 1980), i.e. permanent stimulation of tumour cells by self-secreted growth factor, does not apply to oral carcinomas. In squamous cell carcinoma cell lines, EGF even has a growth inhibitory function (KAMATA and ENOMOTO 1994).

Fibroblast growth factors (FGF 1 and FGF 2) on the other hand have been shown to be expressed by cells of oral squamous cell carcinomas in high frequency and enhanced intensity as compared to normal oral epithelium, and it has been speculated that these growth factors may contribute to cancer cell growth (MYOKEN et al. 1994). Also transforming growth factor-alpha (TGF-α) is produced by squamous cells and squamous cell carcinoma cells, and there may be EGFR/TGF-α autocrine stimulation in these carcinomas (REISS et al. 1991; WONG 1993). Eosinophils may be a further source of TGF-α (WONG 1993). TGF-α is increased in oral leukoplakias compared with normal mucosa and decreases during treatment with retinoids, suggesting that it maybe an intermediate endpoint in cancer chemoprevention (BEENKEN et al. 1994). Human oral carcinoma cell lines produce more TGF-α than normal keratinozytes, but presence of a neutralising antibody in conditioned medium failed to produce a decrease in cell replication (PRIME et al. 1994a), casting doubt on the importance of this mechanism. Transforming growth factor-beta (TGF-β) is produced by normal and malignant keratinocytes and inhibits epithelial replication. Malignant cells may become refractory to this inhibition (PRIME et al. 1994b).

EGF and TGF-α act by binding to a specific receptor (EGFR). The EGFR is found on many cell lines, but especially on proliferating epithelial cells. Normally it is found in high concentration on basal cells of stratified squamous epithelium of skin and mucous membranes (CHRISTENSEN et al. 1992a). It is a 170kDa transmembranous (COHAN et al. 1982) glycoprotein with tyrosine kinase activity (DOWNWARD et al. 1984a). It consists of an outer portion, which binds EGF and TGF-α, a transmembranous portion, and a cytoplasmic portion which contains the tyrosine kinase. DOWNWARD et al. (1984b) in a study on the Avian erythroblastose virus (AV) found a significant homology of the cytoplasmic portion of the EGFR and the v-*erb* B oncoprotein sequence. The EGFR has been shown to be a product of the c-*erb*B-1 protooncogene. The observation that the ligand enhances cellular replication and that during carcinogenesis changes in the receptor are found have led to the proposition that overexpression of the receptor in a number of neoplasms is paramount to their growth potential and thus its aggressiveness.

The prognostic implication of the expression of EGFR in tumours, especially mammary, gastric, cervical, and urinary bladder carcinomas has been intensively investigated. A number of studies in patients with breast carcinomas showed that patients with EGFR-positive tumours had a reduced recurrence-free survival and a shorter overall survival time than patients with EGFR-negative tumours (SAINSBURY et al. 1985a,b, 1987; COSTA et al. 1988; LEWIS et al. 1990), although other studies could not show significant differences (FOEKENS et al. 1990; SPYRATOS et al. 1990).

In the oral mucosa, EGFR expression has been reported in potentially premalignant lesions such as leukoplakias and preferentially in well-differentiated squamous cell carcinomas and cell lines derived from them (YAMAMOTO et al. 1986; EISBRUCH et al. 1987; WONG 1987; WONG and BISWAS 1988; PARTRIDGE et al. 1988; WEICHSELBAUM et al. 1989; ISHITOYA et al. 1989; OH et al. 1989; TODD et al. 1989; EL-ZAYAT et al. 1991; KIM et al. 1991; SHIRASUNA et al. 1991; YAMADA et al. 1992). In leukoplakia, EGFR expression has been found to be increased compared with normal mucosa (BEENKEN et al. 1994). In dysplasias of the oral mucosa, CHRISTENSEN et al. 1992a noted an extension of the EGFR-positive cells from the normally positive basal cell layer to all cells and cell layers.

SAKAI et al. (1990) could demonstrate EGFR by immunohistochemistry in four of 28 cases of oral carcinomas with a location mainly in the cytoplasm, but seldom on the cell surface; a strong expression was observed in mitotic cells. PARTRIDGE et al. (1988) studied 20 oral carcinomas and found variations of receptor expression, but no correlation to prognosis. ISHITOYA et al. (1989) reported overexpression in 53% of 15 carcinomas, SAKAI et al. (1990) reported the same in four of 28 cases. TALACKO et al. (1991), in a study of 35 oral squamous cell carcinomas, noted an extremely heterogeneous expression of EGFR, but noted that poorly differentiated carcinomas had a tendency to express high levels especially in the proliferating "basal" portion of the tumour. Also CHRISTENSEN et al. (1992a,b) found a varied distribution and staining pattern and stronger expression in poorly differentiated carcinomas with staining of all tumour cells in 40 oral and 15 laryngeal squamous cell carcinomas. A study on laryngeal carcinomas confirms the association of EGFR expression and poor tumour differentiation (SCAMBIA et al. 1991), while other studies on head and neck squamous cell carcinomas could not confirm this relationship (SANTINI et al. 1991). SARANATH et al. (1992) observed amplification and overexpression of the EGFR gene in 25% of 84 primary oropharyngeal cancers, while RIKIMARU et al. (1992), in a study of four cases, noted that EGF binding capacity of the tumour cells does not always parallel amplification of the EGFR gene.

YAMADA et al. (1992) report that, of 47 oral carcinomas, 51% contained EGFR-positive cells as determined by immunohistochemistry, and one of 25 cases exhibited fourfold gene amplification on molecular genetic analysis. In contrast to most authors, they report an association of EGFR expression with well-differentiated carcinomas. Some clinical studies indicate that, in oral lesions too, high expression of EGFR is associated with a poor prognosis (OZANNE et al. 1986; HENDLER et al. 1989). OHI et al. (1993) in a study of 68 patients with squamous cell carcinomas found positive reactions in all tumours and noted that 28 of 36 patients in whom staining was stronger than that in the normal cells, but only 12 of 32 patients in whom the staining intensity was equal to or weaker than that in basal cells had lymph node metastasis. In vitro studies showed that overexpression of EGFR is not an invariable characteristic of human oral squamous carcinoma-derived cell lines (PRIME et al. 1994a). In experimental carcinogenesis in the hamster cheek pouch using inoculation of dimethyl-benzanthracene (DMBA) or DMBA plus herpes simplex virus (HSV)-1, amplification and overexpression of c-erb B 1 has been observed (OH et al. 1989).

The avian erythroblastosis virus encodes a v-erb B protein which is a crippled EGFR lacking the EGF binding site. It is similar to the *neu* oncogene initially identified in rat neuroblastomas. In humans, the equivalent is c-*erb* B 2 or HER 2 (human *erb*-B related) gene on chromosome 17. The product of the c-*erb* B 2 is a membrane-bound 185kDa receptor protein with tyrosine kinase activity also termed p185. It exhibits amino acid sequence homology to the EGFR encoded by the c-*erb* B 1 gene. C-*erb* B 2 has been found to be frequently amplified or overexpressed in adenocarcinomas, e.g. of the breast, stomach, kidneys, ovaries and pancreas.

SLAMON et al. (1987) investigated the prognostic relevance of the c-*erb* B 2 oncogene in breast carcinomas and found that overexpression was correlated with shorter recurrence-free survival and shorter overall survival of the patients. These results have been confirmed by a number of authors (TANDON et al. 1989; WALKER et al. 1989; WRIGHT et al. 1989; BORG et al. 1990; BORRESEN et al. 1990; PAIK et al. 1990; TOIKKANEN et al. 1992; for review, see ANDERSON 1992).

Overexpression of c-*erb* B 2 was not observed in hyperplastic or dysplastic intraductal lesions of the mammary gland, but in 56%–77% of preinvasive intraductal carcinomata in situ and most often in those lesions associated with invasive carcinoma (ALLRED et al. 1992).

C-*erb* B 2 has been demonstrated in basal cells of oral mucosa (GULLICK et al. 1987). A number of molecular genetic studies could not demonstrate amplification of c-*erb* B 2 in oral or oropharyngeal cancers (EASTY et al. 1986; RIVIÈRE et al. 1990; MERRITT et al. 1990; SOMERS et al. 1990; TALACKO et al. 1991; LEONARD et al. 1991; FIELD 1992). Amplification, overexpression and rearrangements of the gene in human oral squamous carcinomas were observed by LI et al. (1992) by DNA und RNA dot blot hybridisation. Transcription of c-*erb* B 2 could be detected in normal squamous epithelium and in oral carcinomas by RIVIÈRE et al. (1990). In contrast to molecular studies, immunohistochemically positive staining for the protein may be obtained in premalignant and malignant oral mucosal lesions.

BEEKEN et al. (1994) observed increased staining of oral leukoplakias as compared with normal mucosa. In a spectrum of 86 specimens from normal, hyperplastic, dysplastic and malignant human oral mucosa, HOU et al. (1992) noted a progressive increase in c-*erb* B 2 expression. In oral squamous cell carcinomas, FIELD et al. (1992) demonstrated a positive cytoplasmatic staining in 60% of 75 specimens, CRAVEN et al. (1992) in contrast found cell surface staining in 41% of 93 specimens. Both found no correlation to tumour differentiation, stage or survival. In our own experience, expression of EGFR and c-*erb* B 2 in precancerous oral lesions and carcinomas may be very inconsistent and in contrast to breast carcinomas may not yet be considered as a standard diagnostic procedure. Correlations with prognosis have to be considered with caution.

3.2 Guanosine Triphosphate Binding Oncogenes

The group of guanosine triphosphate (GTP) binding oncogenes is represented by the so-called *ras* gene family on chromosome 11 (Harvey-*ras*, Kirsten-*ras*, N-*ras*) of three closely related genes, which encode a 21 kDa protein (ras p21) localized on the inner side of the plasma membrane with exhibition of GTPase activity. The mutant p21 probably binds to GTP or guanosine diphosphate (GDP), resulting in reduced enzymatic degradation thus creating a prolonged signal for cell proliferation. Such mutations have been demonstrated to be instrumental in the initiation and promotion of chemical carcinogenesis and are found in a number of neoplasias notably in bladder carcinomas and also in carcinomas of the breast, pancreas, stomach, lung, uterus, thyroid and liver (GULBIS and GALAND 1993). The importance of the *ras* oncogenes in oral precancerous and malignant lesions has not been fully elucidated.

In experimental DMBA-induced cancers amplification of H-*ras* or N-*ras* was found (WONG and BISWAS 1988; SHIN et al. 1993); in carcinomas induced in mice by 4-nitroquinoline 1-oxide, H-*ras* mutations were detected in ten of 14 invasive carcinomas, two of four carcinomata in situ, one of five dysplastic lesions and in none of two normal tissues (YUAN et al. 1994). In oral squamous papillomas, *ras* mutations were found in ten of 24 specimens in the spinous layer (SATOH et al. 1990.) ANDERSON et al. (1994) discuss a strong association between human papilloma virus (HPV) infection and activation of the H-*ras* gene in oral verrucous carcinoma. In their material, 6% of 27 oral squamous cell carcinomas demonstrated point mutations in the H-*ras* gene, and three of these contained both HPV-DNA and H-*ras* gene point mutations.

The study by FIELD and SPANDIDOS in 1987 gave first hints of an involvement of the *ras* mutations in oral squamous cell carcinomas, as all 14 oral squamous cell carcinomas of their series exhibited significantly higher expression of H-*ras* and K-*ras*. In the study by HOWELL et al. (1989), four of five patients with oral squamaous cell carcinomas were constitutionally heterozygous at the c-H-*ras* 1 locus, and the tumour had lost heterozygosity in one case.

A number of publications have reported various involvement of the ras mutations in oral precancerous lesions and carcinomas (AZUMA et al. 1987; SHENG et al. 1990; MERRITT et al. 1990; RUMSBY et al. 1990; FREER et al. 1990).

KANNAN et al. (1994) studied the expression of *ras* p21 by immunohistochemistry in normal, premalignant and malignant lesions of the oral mucosa. In normal keratinizing mucosa, expression was found in the basal and lower spinal cells, while non-keratinizing epithelium was negative. All other lesions showed more or less similar expression patterns, mostly confined to the basal or basaloid cells of leukoplakia or carcinoma and an increase with malignancy. The occurrence of *ras* p21 was often parallelled by positive EGFR expression, suggesting a relationship of both to cell proliferation.

HOWELL et al. (1990) found K-*ras* overexpression in only one of 11 oral carcinomas, and YEUDALL et al. (1993) demonstrated mutant H-*ras* gene in only one of 12 oral carcinomas. Some studies revealed that there are apparently important geographic differences concerning *ras* gene changes in oral carcinomas which again may reflect differences in etiology. RUMSBY et al. (1990), CHANG et al. (1991), and WARNAKULASURIYA et al. (1992) reported H-*ras* mutations to be infrequent in oral squamous cell carcinomas among British white caucassian populations, while SARANATH et al. (1989) found N-*ras* amplification in seven and K-*ras* amplification in 23 of 23 oral cancers associated with tobacco chewing in India and in a subsequent study H-*ras* mutations in 20 of 57 tumours also in India (SARANATH et al. 1991). Studies on H-*ras* 1 restriction fragment length polymorphism (RFLP) by BHOITE et al. (1993) revealed that the heterozygous genotype occurred more frequently in normal individuals in India (53%) than in cancer patients (36%), thus limiting the utility of H-*ras* RFLP as a genetic marker for cancer risk.

In a study from Taiwan, six of 33 (18%) tumour specimens from betel quid chewers contained K-*ras* codon 12 mutations and four contained more than one mutation (KUO et al. 1994). In Japan, expression of *ras* p21 product was detected in 44 of 67 specimens (65.7%) of oral cancer, with the highest incidence in patients in the fifth decade and in tumours of the buccal mucosa (SATOH et al. 1992). HOELLERING and SHULER (1989) detected H-*ras* mRNA and p21 in all five oral squamous cell carcinomas examined and noted a non-uniform distribution with high expression in areas of high proliferation and also in dysplastic epithelium. In a study in Belgrade by MILASIN et al. (1994) five of nine specimens (55%) of carcinomas of the lip vermilion harboured mutations, four in codon 12 and one in codon 13.

In the United States, an immunohistological study by McDONALD et al. (1994) revealed that 15 of 22 primary carcinomas (68%) stained positive for H-*ras*, ten for K-*ras* (45%), and seven for N-*ras* (32%). This was associated with increased tumour size and later stages of disease, but there was no correlation to lymph node involvement, site, differentiation, sex, age or race. The authors conclude that overexpression of the *ras* gene family occurs as a relatively late, but important event in oral squamous cell carcinoma. Two Japanese studies also associate *ras* expression to poor prognosis (AZUMA et al. 1987; TSUJI et al. 1989). In contrast, FIELD (1992) reports that overexpression of the p21 *ras* in squamous cell carcinomas correlates with favourable prognosis in the disease-free group of cancer patients and conclude that it may be an important event in early stages of cancer. The relationship of *ras* mutation to etiology (tobacco, chewing habits), stage of disease and geographical distribution certainly awaits further clarification.

3.3 Nuclear Protein-Related Oncogenes

The members of the so-called *myc* oncogene family (c-*myc*, l-*myc* and n-*myc*) code for a nuclear protein of 62 kDa and are involved in DNA binding and regulation of transcription, activating cell replication and influencing differentiation and apoptosis. Especially amplification and elevated expression of c-*myc* (on chromosome 8) are found in a number of malignant lymphomas and solid tumours, e.g. small-cell carcinomas of lung, breast and ovarian carcinomas, and are as a rule associated with poor prognosis.

C-*myc* overexpression could be demonstrated in all of 14 squamous cell carcinomas of the head and neck (FIELD and SPANDIDOS 1987; FIELD 1991). Most subsequent studies confirmed overexpression with or without amplification of the c-*myc* gene in oral carcinomas (YOKOTA et al. 1986; VOLLING et al. 1988; BERENSON et al. 1989; SARANATH et al. 1989; LEONARD et al. 1991).

SAKAI et al. (1990) in an immunohistological study found positive staining of all of 27 oral carcinomas for the c-*myc* oncogene product and noticed three staining patterns: nuclear staining, perinuclear staining, and diffuse cytoplasmic staining. A pronounced staining was seen in mitotic cells.

Ten of 14 oral squamous cell carcinomas associated with tobacco chewing showed molecular lesions in *myc* genes (SARANATH et al. 1994b). Two of eight carcinomas in the series examined by HAUGHEY et al. (1992) exhibited increased c-*myc* copy numbers, and amplification may also be found in metastatic tumour tissue. This is considered to indicate an increased metastatic potential of tumour cells with c-*myc* amplification (HAUGHEY et al. 1992).

Oral cancer cell lines may also show overexpression of c-*myc* mRNA (INAGAKI et al. 1994). RIVIÈRE et al. (1990) could demonstrate transcription of c-*myc* in normal tongue mucosa and primary and metastatic oral squamous cell carcinomas. In oral papillomas, the c-*myc* oncogene product was demonstrated by immunohistochemistry in 17 of 25 specimens (70.8%) and was located mainly in basal cells (SATOH et al. 1992). In a study of oral precancerous and early invasive oral lesions, c-*myc* nuclear labelling correlated with progressive histological atypia (EVERSOLE and SAPP 1993), but some hyperkeratotic lesions without dysplasia were positive for the c-*myc* oncoproteins, possibly labelling those few cases of non-dysplastic leukoplakias transforming into carcinoma that are not detected by conventional assessment of dysplasia. Most studies link c-*myc* amplification or overexpression to advanced stages of oral carcinomas and correlate it with tumour progression and poor prognosis (YOKOTA et al. 1986; FIELD et al. 1986, 1989; BUTT et al. 1990; FIELD 1991). FIELD et al. (1989) in a study of 44 squamous cell carcinomas of the head and neck found c-*myc* expression in 21 cases (48%), and decreased survival was documented for these patients. No correlation could be established to age, sex, tumour stage, lymph node metastasis of differentiation in this study.

An immunohistochemical study of 30 tumours with 11 strongly positive for c-*myc* (37%), five moderately positive, and 14 (47%) negative (GAPANY et al. 1992), revealed a correlation between negative c-*myc* reaction and number of metastatic nodes. The authors speculate that loss of c-*myc* oncoprotein might be associated with aggressive behaviour of squamous cell carcinomas.

For c-*myc* oncogene too, further studies are necessary for establishing a clear link to prognostic assessment. L-*myc* may be increased in squamous carcinoma cell lines (YIN et al. 1991). N-*myc* alterations may be frequently present in normal healthy individuals and in oral cancer patients in India (SARANATH et al. 1994a).

3.4 Protein Kinases and Other Oncogenes

A number of membrane-associated protein kinases may function as proto-oncogenes and oncogenes. Of these the oncogenes *abl*, *fes*, *mos* and *raf* have been investigated in oral carcinomas. None was significantly amplified or overexpressed (SPANDIDOS et al. 1985; FIELD and SPANDIDOS 1987; SARANATH et al. 1989; MERRITT et al. 1990; LEONARD et al. 1991; FIELD 1992). Of the various oncogenes without a defined mechanism of action, int-1, int-2 (SOMERS et al. 1990), hst-1 (MULLER et al. 1994) and bcl-1 (BERENSON et al. 1989) and bcl-2 have been demonstrated to be increased in head and neck carcinomas. The bcl-1 and -2 oncogenes inhibit apoptosis (programmed cell death) and may delay terminal differentiation in epithelial cells with subsequent hyperkeratosis (DAWSON et al. 1995). Bcl-1 amplification was found in eight of 23 head and neck carcinomas, and this was seen more often in poorly differentiated squamous carcinomas and may be associated with poor prognosis (BERENSON et al. 1989).

Chromosome 11q13 (which contains bcl-1) amplification is common in oral squamous cell carcinomas (JIN et al. 1990; MULLER et al. 1994; GAFFEY et al. 1995). The same region contains several other putative oncogenes such as cyclin D 1 (PRAD 1, CCND 1), hst-1, int-2, EMSI, and the gene for the drug detoxifying enzyme glutathione-S-transferase-pi (GST-pi) (GAFFEY et al. 1995). GAFFEY et al. 1995 examined squamous cell carcinomas of the head and neck, both by Southern blot hybridisation and immunohistochemistry. Anticyclin D 1 labelled 44% of the tumours (with a prevalence of hypopharyngeal cancer), while cytoplasmatic immunoreactivity for GST-pi was found in 85%. Twenty-four tumours showed twofold to tenfold amplification of 11q13 loci, two of these were coamplified for GST-pi. No correlations to grade of malignancy, invasive pattern, stage, or survival was noticed.

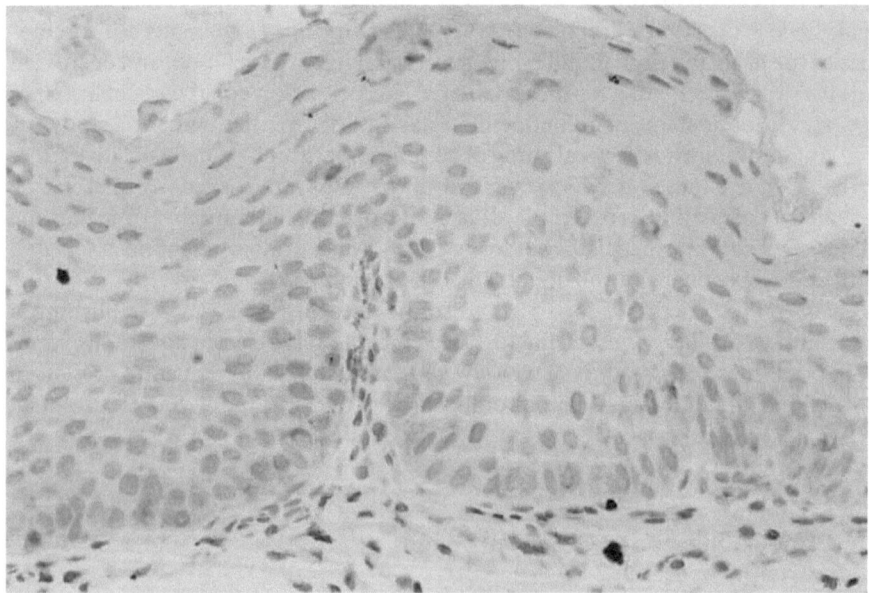

Fig. 1. Bcl-2 expression confined to single cells of the basal cell layer of a hyperplastic oral mucosal lesion (clinical manifestation: leukoplakia of the floor of the mouth in a 55-year-old male patient). There is weak positive staining of the cytoplasm of the basal cells indicating the presence of the 25 kDa protein within the mitochondria. This pattern of expression is found for the products of a number of oncogenes and suppressor genes

The *bcl-2* encodes a *bcl-2* protein (BCLP) which is located in mitochondria and is regularly found in centrocytic malignant lymphomas. In oral mucosa, normal basal cells are negative for BCLP, but in hyperplastic lesions like leukoplakia it maybe expressed (Fig. 1).

4 Tumour Suppressor Genes

Of the various known tumour suppressor genes, p53 has been most intensively investigated in tumours of various organs and in oral lesions. In view of its importance it is separately treated in the chapter by Slootweg (this volume). Further tumour suppressor genes, Rb and DCC, have been described in oral cancer cell lines (KIM et al. 1993). The MTS 1/CDK 41 gene on chromosome 9p21 is supposed to encode a 16 kDa cyclin kinase inhibitor that is instrumental in tumour suppression. It was found to be mutated in cell lines derived from primary and metastatic oral squamous cell carcinomas (YEUDALL et al. 1994). A correlation of expression of a putative metastasis suppressor gene, the nm 23-2/NDP kinase alpha gene, with the metastatic potential of metastatic clones from a spontaneous rat oral squamous cell carcinoma could not be established (HENDERSON 1993).

References

Allred DC, Clark GM, Molina R, Tandon AK, Schnitt SJ, Gilchrist KW, Osborne CK, Tormey DC, McGuire WL (1992) Overexpression of HER-2/neu and its relationship with other prognostic factors change during the progression of in situ to invasive breast cancer. Hum Pathol 23: 974–979

Anderson TJ (1992) C-erbB-2 oncogene in breast cancer. Hum Pathol 23: 971–972

Anderson JA, Irish JC, McLachlin CM, Ngan BY (1994) H-ras oncogene mutation and human papillomavirus infection in oral carcinomas. Arch Otolaryngol Head Neck Surg 120: 755–760

Azuma M, Furumoto N, Kawamata H, et al (1987) The relation of ras oncogene product p21 expression to clinico pathological status and clinical outcome in squamous cell head and neck cancer. Cancer J 1: 375–380

Beenken SW, Huang P, Sellers M, Peters G, Listinsky C, Stockard C, Hubbard W, Wheeler R, Grizzle W (1994) Retinoid modulation of biomarkers in oral leukoplakia/dysplasia. J Cell Biochem Suppl 19: 270–277

Berenson JR, Yang J, Mickel RA (1989) Frequent amplification of the bcl-1 locus in head and neck squamous cell carcinomas. Oncogene 4: 1111–1116

Bhoite LT, Saranath D, Nair R, Deo MG, Sanghavi V, Mehta A (1993) H-ras-1 restriction fragment length polymorphism in normal individuals and oral cancer patients in India. J Oral Pathol Med 22: 298–302

Borg A, Tandon AK, Sigurdsson H, Clark GM, Fernö M, Fuqua S, Killander D, Mc Guire W (1990) Her-2/neu amplification predicts poor survival in node-positive breast cancer. Cancer Res 50: 4332–4337

Borresen AL, Ottestad L, Gaustad A, Andersen TI, Heikkilä R, Jahnsen T, Tveit K, Nesland J (1990) Amplification and protein over-expression of the neu/HER-2/c-erb B-2 protooncogene in human breast carcinomas: relationship to loss of gene sequences on chromosome 17, family history and prognosis. Br J Cancer 62: 585–590

Brachman DG (1994) Molecular biology of head and neck cancer. Semin Oncol 21: 320–329

Burkhardt A (1985) Advanced methods in the evaluation of premalignant lesions and carcinomas of the oral mucosa. J Oral Pathol 14: 751–778

Butt SA, Field JK, Gosney JR, Reed T, Stell PM (1990) Immunohistochemical study of c-myc expression in head and neck cancer: a prognostic indicator. In Vivo 4: 88

Castellani R, Visscher DW, Wykes S, Sarkar FH, Crissman JD (1994) Interaction of transforming growth factor-alpha and epidermal growth factor receptor in breast carcinoma. Cancer 73: 344–349

Chang SE, Bhatia P, Johnson NW (1991) Ras mutations in United Kingdom examples of oral malignancies are infrequent. Int J Cancer 48: 409–412

Christensen ME, Therkildsen MH, Hansen BL, Hansen GN, Brelau P (1992a) Epidermal growth factor receptor expression on oral mucosa dysplastic epithelia and squamous cell carcinomas. Eur Arch Otorhinolaryngol 249: 243–247

Christensen ME, Therkildsen MH, Hansen BL, Hansen GN, Bretlau P (1992b) Immunohistochemical detection of epidermal growth factor receptor in laryngeal squamous cell carcinomas. Acta Otolaryngol Stockh 112: 734–738

Cohan S, Ushiro H, Stoscheck C, Chinkers M (1982) A native 170000 epidermal growth factor receptor-kinase complex from shed plasma membrane vesicles. J Biol Chem 257: 1523–1531

Costa S, Stamm H, Almendral A, Ludwig H, Wyss R, Fabbro D, Ernst A, Takahaschi A, Eppenberger U (1988) Predictive value of EGF receptor in breast cancer. Lancet 2: 1258

Craven JM, Pavelic Z, Stambrook PJ (1992) Expression of c-erbB-2 gene in human head and neck carcinoma. Anticancer Res 12: 2273–2276

Dawson CW, Eliopoulos AG, Dawson J, Young LS (1995) BHRF1, a viral homoloque of the Bcl-2 oncogene, disturbs epithelial cell differentiation. Oncogene 10: 69–77

Downward J, Parker P, Waterfield MD (1984a) Autophosphorylation sites on the epidermal growth factor receptor. Nature 311: 483–485

Downward J, Yarden Y, Mayes E, Scrace G, Totty N, Stockwell P, Ullrich A, Schlessinger J, Waterfield MD (1984b) Close similarity of epidermal growth factor receptor and v-erb-B oncogene protein sequences. Nature 307: 520–527

Easty DM, Easty GC, Bacici A (1986) Biological studies on ten human squamous cell lines: an overview. Eur J Cancer Clin Oncol 22: 617–634

Eisbruch A, Blick M, Lee JS, Sacks PG, Gutterman J (1987) Analysis of the epidermal growth factor receptor gene in fresh human head and neck tumours. Cancer Res 47: 3603–3605

El-Zayat AAE, Pingree TE, Mock PM, Clark GM, Otto RA, von Hoff DD (1991) Epidermal growth factor receptor amplification in head and neck cancer. Cancer J 4: 373–381

Eversole LR (1992) Immunohistochemical detection of ras 21 in oral squamous cell carcinomas. Oral Surg Oral Med Oral Pathol 74: 469–472

Eversole LR, Sapp JP (1993) C-myc oncoprotein expression in *oral* precancerous and early cancerous lesions. Eur J Cancer B Oral Oncol 29B: 131–135

Field JK (1991) The biology of oncogenes and their role in malignant transformation. In: Johnson NW (ed) Risk markers for oral diseases, vol 2, Oral Cancer. Cambridge University Press, Cambridge, pp 257–293

Field JK (1992) Oncogenes and tumor-suppressor genes in squamous cell carcinoma of the head and neck. Oral Oncol Eur J Cancer Vol 28b: 67–76

Field JK, Spandidos DA (1987) Expression of oncogenes in human tumours with special reference to the head and neck region. Oral Pathol 16: 97–107

Field JK, Lamothe A, Spandidos DA (1986) Clinical relevance of oncogene expression in head and neck tumours. Anticancer Res 6: 595–600

Field JK, Spandidos DA, Stell PM, Vaughan ED, Evan KI, Moore JP (1989) Elevated expression of the c-myc oncoprotein correlates with poor prognosis in head and neck squamous cell carcinoma. Oncogene 4: 1463–1468

Field JK, Spandidos DA, Yiagnisis M (1992) C-erb-B-2 expression in squamous cell carcinoma of the head and neck. Anticancer Res 12: 613–620

Foekens JA, van Putten WL, Portengen H, Rodenburg CJ, Reubi JC, Berns PMJJ, Henzen-Logmans SC, van der Burg MEL, Alexieva-Figusch J, Klijn JGM (1990) Prognostic value of pS2 protein and receptors for epidermal growth factor (EGR-R), insulin-like growth factor-

1 (IGF-1-R) and somatostatin (SS-R) in patients with breast and ovarian cancer. J Steroid Biochem Mol Biol 37: 815–821

Freer E, Savage NW, Seymour CJ, Dunn TL, Lavin MF, Gardiner RA (1990) Ras oncogene product expression in normal and malignant oral mucosa. Aust Dent J 35: 141–146

Füzesi L, Braun S, Gunawan B, Schmitz HJ, Mittermayer C (1994) Cytogenetic findings in squamous cell carcinoma of the oral cavity. Int J Oral Maxillofac Surg 23: 153–155

Gaffey MJ, Iezzoni JC, Meredith SD, Boyd JC, Stoler MH, Weiss LM, Zukerberg LR, Levine PA, Arnold A, Williams ME (1995) Cyclin D 1 (PRAD1, CCND1) and gluathione-S-transferase gene expression in head and neck squamous cell carcinoma. Hum Pathol 26: 1221–1226

Gapany M, Pavelic ZP, Kelley DJ (1992) Prognostic relevance of c-myc oncoprotein detection in head and neck tumors. Proceedings of the Third International Conference on Head and Neck Cancer, July 26–30, San Francisco, CA, p 123 (abstr)

Gulbis B, Galand P (1993) Immunodetection of the p21-ras products in human normal and preneoplastic tissues and solid tumors: a review. Hum Pathol 24: 1271–1285

Gullick WJ, Berger MS, Bennett PLP, Rothbard JB, Waterfield MD (1987) Expression of the c-erbB-2 protein in normal and transformed cells. Int J Cancer 40: 246–254

Haughey BH, von Hoff DD, Windle BE, Wahl GM, Mock PM (1992) C-myc oncogene copy number in squamous carcinoma of the head and neck. Am J Otolaryngol 13: 168–171

Henderson BR (1993) Expression of the nm23-2/NDP kinase alpha gene in rat mammary and oral carcinoma cells of varying metastatic potential. Br J Cancer 68: 874–878

Hendler FJ, Shum-Siu A, Oeschsli M, Nanu L, Richards C, Ozanne BW (1989) Increased EGF-R1 binding predicts a poor survival in squamous tumours. Cancer Cells 7: 347–351

Hittelman WN, Voravud N, Shin DM, Lee JS, Ro JY, Hong WK (1993) Early genetic changes during upper aerodigestive tract tumorigenesis. J Cell Biochem Suppl 17(F): 233–236

Hoellering J, Shuler CF (1989) Localization of H-RAS mRNA in oral squamous cell carcinomas. J Oral Pathol Med 18: 74–78

Hou L, Shi D, Tu SM, Zhang HZ, Hung MC, Ling D (1992) Oral cancer progression and c-erb B 2/neu proto-oncogene expression. Cancer-Lett 65: 215–220

Howell RE, Wong FSH, Fenwick RG (1989) Loss of Harvey ras heterozygosity in oral squamous carcinoma. J Oral Pathol 18: 79–83

Howell RE, Wong FSH, Fenwick RG (1990) A transforming Kirsten ras oncogene in an oral squamous carcinoma. J Oral Pathol Med 19: 301– 305

Inagaki T, Matsuwari S, Takahashi R, Shimada K, Fujie K, Maeda S (1994) Establishment of human oral-cancer cell lines (KOSC-2 and -3) carrying p53 and c-myc abnormalities by geneticin treatment. Int J Cancer 56: 301–308

Ishitoya J, Toriyama M, Oguchi N (1989) Gene amplification and overexpression of EGF receptor in squamous cell carcinomas of the head and neck. Br J Cancer 59: 559–562

Iversen OH (1985) What is New in endogenous growth stimulators and inhibitors (chalones). Path Res Pract 180: 77–80

Jin Y, Higashi K, Mandahl N (1990) Frequent rearrangement of chromosomal bands 1p22 and 11q13 in squamous cell carcinomas of the head and neck. Genes Chrom Cancer 2: 198–204

Kamata N, Enomoto S (1994) Cell cycle arrest induced by epidermal growth factor on human squamous cell carcinoma cell lines. Kokubyo Gakkai Zasshi 61: 446–453

Kannan S, Balaram P, Chandran GJ, Pillai MR, Mathew B, Nair MK (1994) Co-expression of ras p21 and epidermal growth factor receptor during various stages of tumour progression in oral mucosa. Tumour Biol 15: 73–81

Kim K, Akoto-Amanfu E, Cherrick HM, Park NH (1991) Anchorage independent growth and the expression of cellular proto-oncogenes in normal human epidermal keratinocytes and in human squamous cell carcinoma cell lines. Oral Surg Oral Med Oral Pathol 71: 303–311

Kim Ms, Li SL, Bertolami CN, Cherrick HM, Park NH (1993) State of p53, Rb and DCC tumor suppressor genes in human oral cancer cell lines. Anticancer Res 13: 1405–1413

Kuo MYP, Jeng JH, Chiang CP, Hahn LJ (1994) Mutations of Ki-ras oncogene codon 12 in betel quid chewing-related human oral squamous cell carcinoma in Taiwan. J Oral Pathol Med 23: 70–74

Leonard JH, Kearsley JH, Chenevix-Trench G, Hayward NK (1991) Analysis of gene amplification in head and neck squamous cell carcinomas. Int J Cancer 48: 511–515

Lewis S, Locker A, Todd JH, Bell JA, Nicholson R, Elston CW, Blamey RW, Ellis IO (1990) Expression of epidermal growth factor receptor in breast carcinoma. J Clin Pathol 43: 385–389

Li B, Wang M, Wen Y, Chen J (1992) Erb-B oncogene in human oral squamous cell carcinomas. Hua-Hsi-I-Ko-Ta-Hsueh-Hsueh-Pao 23: 284–287

McDonald JS, Jones H, Pavelic ZP, Pavelic LJ, Stambrook PJ, Gluckman JL (1994) Immunohistochemical detection of the H-ras, K-ras and N-ras oncogenes in squamous cell carcinoma of the head and neck. J Oral Pathol Med 23: 342–346

Merritt WD, Weissler MC, Turk BF, Gilmer TM (1990) Oncogene amplification in squamous cell carcinoma of the head and neck. Arch Otolaryngol Head Neck Surg 116: 1394–1398

Milasin J, Pujié N, Dedovic, Nikolic Z, Petrovic V, Dimitrijevic B (1994) High incidence of H-ras oncogene mutations in squamous cell carcinoma of lip vermilion. J Oral Pathol Med 23: 298–301

Muller D, Million R, Lidereau R, Engelmann A, Bronner G, Flesch H, Eber M, Methlin G, Abecassis J (1994) Frequent amplification of 11q13 DNA markers is associated with lymph node involvement in human head and neck squamous cell carcinomas. Oral Oncol Eur J Cancer 30: 113–120

Myoken Y, Myoken Y, Okamoto T, Sato JD, Takada K (1994) Immunocytochemical localization of fibroblast growth factor-1 (FGF-1) and EGF-2 in oral squamous cell carcinoma. J Oral Pathol Med 23: 451–456

Oh JS, Paik D, Christensen R, Akoto-Amanfu E, Kim K, Park NH (1989) Herpes simplex virus enhances the 7,12-dimetylbenzanthracene (DMBA)-induced carcinogenesis and amplification and overexpression of c-erb-B-1 protooncogene in hamster buccal pouch epithelium. Oral Surg Oral Med Oral Pathol 68: 428–435

Ohi K, Suzuki M, Koike S, Satake J, Matsu-Ura K, Takasaka T (1993) Expression of epidermal growth factor receptor in squamous cell carcinoma of the head and neck. Nippon Jibiinkoka Gakkai Kaiho 96: 2039–2043

Owen W, Field JK, Howard PJ, Stell PM (1992) Multiple cytogenetic aberrations in squamous cell carcinomas of the head and neck. Oral Oncology, Eur J Cancer 28B: 17–21

Ozanne B, Richards CS, Hendler F, Burns D, Gusterson B (1986) Overexpression of the EGF receptor is a hallmark of squamous cell carcinomas. J Pathol 149: 9–14

Paik S, Hazan R, Fisher ER, Sass RE, Fisher B, Redmond C, Schlessinger J, Lippman ME, King C (1990) Pathologic findings from the national surgical adjuvant breast and bowel project; prognostic significance of erbB-2 protein overexpression in primary breast cancer. J Clin Oncol 8: 103–112

Partridge M, Gullick WJ, Langdon JD, Sherriff M (1988) Expression of epidermal growth factor receptor on oral squamous cell carcinoma. Br J Oral Maxillofac Surg 26: 381–389

Partridge M, Kiguwa S, Langdon JD (1994) Frequent deletion of chromosome 3p in oral squamous cell carcinoma. Eur J Cancer B Oral Oncol 30B: 248–251

Patel V, Yeudall WA, Gardner A, Mutlu S, Scully C, Prime SS (1993) Consistent chromosomal anomalies in keratinocyte cell lines derived from untreated malignant lesions of the oral cavity. Genes Chromosom Cancer 7: 109–115

Prime SS, Game SM, Matthews JB, Stone A, Donnelly MJ, Yeudall WA, Patel V, Sposto R, Silverthorne A, Scully C (1994a) Epidermal growth factor and transforming growth factor alpha characteristics of human oral carcinoma cell lines. Br J Cancer 69: 8–15

Prime SS, Matthews JB, Patel V, Game SM, Donnelly M, Stone A, Paterson IC, Sandy JR, Yeudall WA (1994b) TGF-beta receptor regulation mediates the response to exogenous ligand but is independent of the degree of cellular differentiation in human oral keratinocytes. Int J Cancer 56: 406–412

Reiss M, Stash EB, Vellucci VF (1991) Activation of the autocrine transforming growth factor α pathway in human squamous carcinoma cells. Cancer Res 51: 6254–6262

Rikimaru K, Tadokoro K, Yamamoto T, Enomoto S, Tsuchida N (1992) Gene amplification and overexpression of epidermal growth factor receptor in squamous cell carcinoma of the head and neck. Head Neck 14: 8–13

Rivière A, Wilckens C, Löning T (1990) Expression of c-erb B2 and c-myc in squamous epithelia and squamous cell carcinomas of the head and neck and the lower female genital tract. J Oral Pathol Med 19: 408–413

Rumsby G, Carter RL, Gusterson BA (1990) Low incidence of ras oncogene activation in human squamous cell carcinomas. Br J Cancer 61: 365–368

Sainsbury JRC, Fandon JR, Harris AL, Sherbet GV (1985a) Epidermal growth factor receptors on human breast cancers. Brit J Surg 72: 186–188

Sainsbury JRC, Malcolm AJ, Appleton DR, Farndon JR, Harris AL (1985b) Presence of epidermal growth factor receptors as an indicator of poor prognosis in patients with breast cancer. J Clin Pathol 38: 1225–1228

Sainsbury JRC, Farndon JR, Needham GK, Malcolm AJ, Harris AL (1987) Epidermal-growth-factor receptor status as predictor of early recurrence and of death from breast cancer. Lancet 20: 1398–1402

Sakai H, Kawano K, Okamura K, Hashimoto N (1990) Immunohistochemical localization of c-myc oncogene product and EGF receptor in oral squamous cell carcinoma. J Oral Pathol Med 19: 1–4

Santini J, Formento JL, Francoual M (1991) Characterization, quantification, and potential clinical value of the epidermal growth factor receptor in head and neck squamous cell carcinomas. Head Neck 13: 132–139

Saranath D, Panchal RG, Nair R, Mehta AR, Sanghavi V, Sumegi J, Klein G, Deo MG (1989) Oncogene amplification in squamous cell carcinoma of the oral cavity. Jpn J Cancer Res 80: 430–437

Saranath D, Chang SE, Bhoite LT, Panchal RG, Kerr IB, Mehta Ar, Johnson NW, Deo MG (1991) High frequency mutation in codons 12 and 61 of H-ras oncogene in chewing tobacco-related human oral carcinoma in India. Br J Cancer 63: 573–578

Saranath D, Panchal RG, Nair R, Mehta AR, Sanghavi VD, Deo MG (1992) Amplification and overexpression of epidermal growth factor receptor gene in human oropharyngeal cancer. Eur J Cancer B Oral Oncol 28B(2): 139–143

Saranath D, Panchal RG, Deo MG, Sanghavi V, Mehta AR (1994a) Restriction fragment length polymorphisms of the human N-myc gene in normal healthy individuals and oral cancer patients in India. Indian J Biochem Biophys 31: 177–193

Saranath D, Bhoite LT, Deo MG, Tandle AT, D'Costa J, Kolhapure RN, Govardhan MK, Banerjee K (1994b) Detection and cloning of potent transforming gene(s) from chewing tobacco-related human oral carcinomas. Eur J Cancer B Oral Oncol 30B: 268–277

Satoh M, Hatakeyama S, Sashima M, Suzuki A (1990) Immunohistochemical detection of ras p21 in oral papilloma. J Oral Pathol Med 19: 490–491

Satoh M, Sashima M, Hatakeyama S, Yoshimura N, Otsu T, Suzuki A (1992) Immunohistochemical localization of c-myc oncogene product in oral papilloma. J Oral Pathol Med 21: 97–99

Scambia G, Panici PB, Battaglia F (1991) Receptors for epidermal growth factor and steroid hormones in primary laryngeal tumors. Cancer 67: 1347–1351

Scully C (1993) Oncogenes, tumour suppressors and viruses in oral squamous carcinoma. J Oral Pathol Med 22: 337–347

Scully C, Burkhardt A (1993) Tissue markers of potentially malignant human oral epithelial lesions. J Oral Pathol Med 22: 246–256

Sheng ZM, Barrois M, Klijanienko J, Micheau C, Richard JM, Riou G (1990) Analysis of the c-Ha-ras-1 gene for deletion mutation amplification and expression in lymph node metastases of human head and neck carcinomas. Br J Cancer 62: 398–404

Shin DM, Chiao PJ, Sacks PG, Shin HJ, Hong WK, Hittelman WN, Tainsky MA (1993) Activation of ribosomal protein S2 gene expression in a hamster model of chemically induced oral carcinogenesis. Carcinogenesis 14: 163–166

Shirasuna K, Hayashido Y, Sugiyama M, Yoshioka H, Matsuya T (1991) Immunohistochemical localization of epidermal growth factor (EGF) and EGF receptor in human oral mucosa and its malignancy. Virchows Archiv A Pathol Anat 418: 349–353

Slamon DJ, Clark GM, Wong SG, Levin WJ, Ullrich A, McGuire W (1987) Human breast cancer: correlation of relapse and survival with amplification of the HER-2/neu oncogene. Science 235: 177–182

Somers KD, Cartwright SL, Schechter GL (1990) Amplification of the int-2 gene in human head and neck squamous cell carcinomas. Oncogene 5: 915–920

Spandidos DA, Kerr IB, Field JK (1985) Multiple transcriptional activation of cellular oncogenes in head and neck solid tumours. Anticancer Res 5: 221–224

Sporn MB, Todaro SJ (1980) Autocrine secretion and malignant transformation of cells. N Engl J M 303: 878–880

Spyratos F, Delarue JC, Andrieu C, Lidereau R, Champeme MH, Hacene K, Brunet M (1990) Epidermal growth factor receptors and prognosis in primary breast cancer. Breast Cancer Res Treat 17: 83–89

Talacko AA, Shirlaw PJ, Johnson NW (1991) Growth factors and their receptors as markers of the high risk lesion, with special reference to epidermal growth factors. In: Johnson NW (ed) Risk markers for oral Diseases, vol 2, Oral cancer. Cambridge University Press, Cambridge, pp 294–316

Tandon AK, Clark GM, Chamness GC, Ullrich A, McGuire WL (1989) HER-2/neu oncogene protein and prognosis in breast cancer. J Clin Oncol 7: 1120–1128

Todd R, Donoff BR, Gertz R (1989) TGF-α and EGF receptor mRNAs in human oral cancers. Carcinogenesis 10: 1553–1556

Toikkanen S, Helin H, Isola J, Joensuu H (1992) Prognostic significance of HER-2 oncoprotein expression in breast cancer: a 30-year follow-up. J Clin Oncol 10: 1044–1048

Tsuji T, Sasaki K, Hiraoka F, Shinozaki F (1989) The immunohistochemical detection of ras p21 and its correlation with differentiation in oral cancer. J Tumour Marker Oncol 4: 415–419

Tsuji T, Mimura Y, Maeda K, Ida M, Sasaki K, Shinozaki F (1994) Numerical aberrations of chromosome 17 detected by FISH with DNA-specific probe in oral tumors. Anticancer Res 14: 1689–1693

Volling P, Jungelhuelsing M, Tesch H, Stennert E (1988) Onkogene bei Plattenepithelkarzinomen im Kopf-Hals-Bereich. Laryngol Rhinol Otol 67: 160–164

Voravud N, Shin DM, Ro JY, Hong WK, Hittelman WN (1993) Increased polysomies of chromosomes 7 and 17 during head and neck multistage tumorigenesis. Cancer Res 53: 2874–2883

Walker RA, Gullick WJ, Varley JM (1989) An evaluation of immunoreactivity for c-erbB-2 protein as a marker of poor short-term prognosis in breast cancer. Br J Cancer 60: 426–429

Warnakulasuriya KAAS, Chang SE, Johnson NW (1992) Point mutations in the Ha-ras oncogene are detectable in formalin-fixed tissues of oral squamous cell carcinomas, but are infrequent in British cases. J Oral Pathol Med 21: 225–229

Weichselbaum R, Dunphy E, Beckett M (1989) Epidermal growth factor receptor gene amplification and expression in head and neck cancer cell lines. Head Neck Surg 11: 437–442

Wong DTW (1987) Amplification of the c-erb B 1 oncogene in chemically induced oral carcinomas. Carcinogenesis 8: 1963–1967

Wong DTW (1993) TGF-alpha and oral carcinogenesis. Eur J Cancer B Oral Oncol 29B: 3–7

Wong DTW, Biswas DK (1988) Expression of c-erb oncogene during dimethylbenanthracene-induced tumorigenesis in hamster cheek pouch. Oncogene 2: 67–72

Wright C, Angus B, Nicholson S, Sainsbury J, Cairns J, Gullick WJ, Kelly P, Harris AL, Horne CH (1989) Expression of c-erbB-2 oncoprotein: a prognostic indicator in human breast cancer. Cancer Res 49: 2087–2090

Yamada T, Takagi M, Shioda S (1992) Evaluation of epidermal growth factor receptor in squamous cell carcinoma of the oral cavity. Oral Surg Oral Med Oral Pathol 73: 67–70

Yamamoto T, Kamata N, Kawano H (1986) High incidence of amplification of the epidermal growth factor receptor gene in human squamous carcinoma cell lines. Cancer Res 46: 414–416

Yeudall WA, Torrance LK, Elsegood KA, Speight P, Scully C, Prime SS (1993) Ras gene point mutations is a rare event in premalignant tissues and malignant cells and tissues from oral mucosal lesions. Eur J Cancer B Oral Oncol 29B: 63–67

Yeudall WA, Crawford RY, Ensley JF, Robbins KC (1994) MTS1/CDK41 is altered in cell lines derived from primary and metastatic oral squamous cell carcinoma. Carcinogenesis 15: 2683–2686

Yin XY, Donovan-Peluso M, Whiteside TL (1991) Gene amplification and gene dosage in cell lines derived from squamous cell carcinoma of the head and neck. Genes Chromosom Cancer 3: 443–454

Yokota J, Tsunetsugu-Yokota Y, Battifora H, Le Fevre C, Cline MJ (1986) Alterations of myc myb ras Ha protooncogenes in cancers are frequent and show clinical correlation. Science 231: 261–265

Youngson BJ, Anelli A, Van Zee KJ, Borgen PI, Norton L, Rosen PP (1995) Microdissection and molecular genetic analysis of HER2/neu in breast carcinoma. Am J Surg Pathol 19: 1354–1358

Yuan B, Heniford BW, Ackermann DM, Hawkins BL, Hendler FJ (1994) Harvey ras point mutations are induced by 4-nitroquinoline 1 oxide in murine oral squamous epithelia, while squamous cell carcinomas and loss of heterozygosity occur without additional exposure. Cancer Res 54: 5310–5317

Subject Index

Index of Volumes 87–89 Current Topics in Pathology